ADVANCED LAPAROSCOPY

Edited by **Ali Shamsa**

Advanced Laparoscopy
Edited by Ali Shamsa

Published by InTech
Janeza Trdine 9, 51000 Rijeka, Croatia

Publishing Process Manager Niksa Mandic

Technical Editor Teodora Smiljanic

Cover Designer InTech Design Team

Additional hard copies can be obtained from orders@intechopen.com

Advanced Laparoscopy, Edited by Ali Shamsa
p. cm.
ISBN 978-953-307-674-4

For EU product safety concerns:
IN TECH d.o.o., Prolaz Marije Krucifikse Kozulić 3, 51000 Rijeka, Croatia,
info@intechopen.com or visit our website at intechopen.com.

Meet the editor

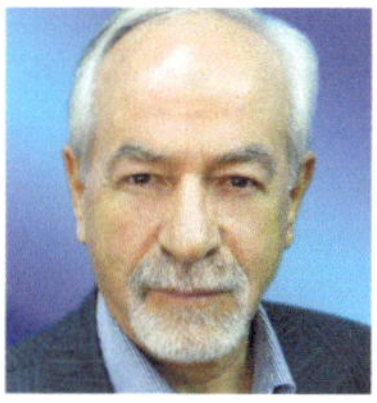

As an eminent member of the medical profession, Dr. Ali Shamsa has proven successful in the capacity of administrator-Chancellor of Mashhad University of Medical Sciences, full Professor of Urology, researcher and educator. He has excelled in kidney transplantation and is widely renown for his advancement in the field of infertility. He routinely performs surgery and carries out transplantation procedures in the many medical centers and hospitals located in the municipality of Mashhad. He has been a member of the National Board of Urology for over twenty years. He attends as many of the national and international medical conferences and congresses pertaining to his specialty as possible. He is also an accomplished author of medical literature in both English and Persian language, and his many articles have been published in both national and international scientific journals. His love of writing has produced numerous memoirs and travelogues as well.

Contents

Preface

The twentieth century was one of medical wonders. In the beginning of the century, the greatest surgeon was the one who placed the greatest concentration on the meaning of medical operations—he who inflicted the great surgery—the great incision.

But by the end of the century the greatest surgeon was the person who used the smallest incision for his surgical operations (the smaller the incision the greater the surgeon). Especially since this method could have the same results as the former methods of surgery, with a shorter duration of recovery and patient's hospitalization needed.

The greatest surgeons, such as my mentor, Professor J.P. Blandy from the United Kingdom, with his generalization of TURP, and his compatriot Prof. John Wickham in developing PNL and laparoscopy, and even robotic laparoscopy, have progressed in great strides. We witnessed the big bang of laparoscopy in 1991 with the laparoscopic nephrectomy done by Ralph Clayman and his Iranian compatriot Louis Kavousi. Clayman himself, in his lecture at the World congress for endourology in 2008, addressed and explained the struggles and hardships that existed in the newly discovered scientific course for carrying out laparoscopic nephrectomy.

The media had difficulties in promoting laparascopy. Prof. D.D. Gour from Bombay was the first person who innovated retroperitoneoscopy and showed us that even if a little more difficult, it was a less dangerous option for kidney and adrenal laparascopy.

Today, as we have reached the end of first decade of the 21st Century, we are confronted with new progress in laparoscopic methods like performing laparoscopy through the orifices of the human body such as the mouth or vagina, and da Vinci robotic laparoscopy.

Have all the problems of human limb surgery been solved by laparoscopy? Is it possible to apply laparascopy to every surgical operation? The answers are negative! In urology there is a total use of laparoscopy of the upper urogenital tract, kidneys and adrenal glands (adrenalectomy, nephrectomy, and pyeloplasty, partial nephrectomy), but there is no common agreement on prostate and/or vesico ureteral reflux, for example. The present book, published by InTech, has been written by a number of highly outstanding authors from al over the world. Every author provides information concerning treatment of different diseases. based on his or her knowledge, experience and skills. Most of the chapters are very useful and innovative to me as to a reader. This book is not merely devoted to urology sciences. There are also clear results and conclusions on the treatment of many diseases, for example well-differentiated papillary mesothelioma. The chapter "The Impact of Visceral Fat Accumulation on Laparoscopy-Assisted Distal Gastrectomy" and other chapters vastly contribute to the practice of laparoscopy in urology and other areas. We should not forget nor neglect that laparoscopy is in use more extensively than before, and it is hoped that in the future new subjects such as use of laparascopy in treatment of kidney cysts, simple nephrectomy, pyeloplasty, donor nephrectomy and even robotic laparoscopy will be researched further.

In the end I have to thank the InTech staff, specially Mrs. Natalia Reinic and Mr. Niksa Mandic, two kind friends who have always helped me and granted me the honor of editing this book.

31/7/2011

Ali Shamsa, M.D.
Professor of Urology and Kidney Tx
Mashhad University of Sciences, Iran

1

Risks Associated with Laparoscopic Surgery

Tülün Öztürk
Celal Bayar University
Turkey

1. Introduction

Laparoscopic surgical (LS) procedures aim to achieve a satisfactory therapeutic result while minimizing the traumatic and metabolic stress of the intervention. Tissue trauma is significantly less than that with conventional open procedures, thus results in the additional benefit of reduced post-operative pain. Other advantages of LS procedures include smaller incisional sites, lower risks of wound complications, reduced postoperative pain and complications, shorter hospital stay, more rapid return to normal activities, and cost savings (Carther, 2011; Nicholsen, 2011; Leonard & Cunningham, 2002).

Despite these advantages, laparoscopic surgery may result in serious complications due to the important physiologic changes which occur during the procedure. In complicated surgical cases of extended duration, the prolonged steep head-down position and carbon dioxide insufflation results in a pneumoperitoneum which often has adverse haemodynamic and respiratory consequences (Russoa et al., 2009). Negative aspects of laparoscopic surgery in terms of the surgical procedure itself include poor visualization and traumatic injuries to viscera and blood vessels associated with blind trocar insertion.

The physiologic changes associated with laparoscopy include those associated with tilting the patient to facilitate instrumentation and surgical exposure, the pressure effects of instilled gas into a closed cavity, and the systemic effects of the gas, almost universally CO_2, that is instilled (and absorbed or embolized).

Initially performed in healthy patients, laparoscopy is now used for complicated gastrointestinal (eg. distal gastrectomy for gastric cancer patients with comorbid diseases, laparoscopic hepatic resection for colorectal cancer liver metastases, and laparoscopic resection or debulking of presacral and retrorectal space tumors) and genitourinary procedures. (Russoa et al., 2009).

2. Physiologic changes and complications related to patient positioning

During laparoscopy, the patient is placed in a variety of positions in order to maximise the surgical visual field and facilitate instrumentation. The head-down (Trendelenburg) positioning is commonly used in gynecological operations, prostatectomy, and colorectal procedures, and usually is combined with lithotomy. The steep head-down tilt is frequently used for laparoscopic gynecologic and urologic procedures. The head-up position (reverse Trendelenburg) is used for cholecystectomy, invasive urological surgery, and gastric bypass surgery, whereas the lateral decubitus position is used for nephrectomy. The tilting of a patient during laparoscopy results in important physiologic responses and potential serious complications. During laparoscopy, it is difficult to clearly separate the effects of anesthesia, position, and pneumoperitoneum. Because abdominal insufflation adds to the deleterious physiologic effects of the head-down tilt position, special attention by the anesthesiologist must be given to patients undergoing laparoscopic surgery in this position.

2.1 Hemodynamic effects of positioning during laparoscopy

In a study of hemodynamic changes using transthoracic echocardiography in patients undergoing gynaecological laparoscopic operations, the Trendelenburg position increased central venous pressure (CVP), pulmonary capillary wedge pressure (PCWP) and pulmonary arterial pressures (PAP) and decreased cardiac output (CO) (Russo et al, 2009). Pneumoperitoneum increased these pressures further, mostly at the beginning of the laparoscopy, and cardiac output decreased towards the end of the laparoscopy. In recent years, gynaecological laparoscopic operations of longer duration with an even steeper head-down position are being performed.

In the study by Meininger et al, ASA I-III patients undergoing total endoscopic radical prostatectomy with 4 hours of pneumoperitoneum in the Trendelenburg position experienced no significant hemodynamic compromise. Placing the patient in the Trendelenburg position caused a significant increase in CVP (from 9.9 ± 3.4 to 15.1 ± 2.3 mm Hg), whereas all other hemodynamic parameters [cardiac index (CI), heart rate (HR), mean arterial pressure (MAP), systemic vascular resistance index (SVRI), and intrathoracic blood volume] remained nearly unaffected, as measured with a continuous cardiac output monitoring (PiCCO) system via a femoral artery catheter (Meininger et al., 2008). Similarly, in the steep (40°) Trendelenburg position during robotic prostatectomy, HR, MAP, CVP, oxygen saturation via pulse oximeter (SpO_2), and end-tidal carbon dioxide ($EtCO_2$) remained within a clinically acceptable range (Kalmar et al., 2010).

The Trendelenburg position changes hemodynamic parameters and moves intraabdominal organs cephalad due to gravity. The head-down position causes an increase in central blood volume in adult patients, with a resulting increase in cardiac output and systolic blood pressure. However, an immediate systemic vasodilatation secondary to reflex barostimulation also occurs, which leads to decreased stroke volume, reduced cardiac output, and diminished perfusion of vital organs. The physiology of a patient in the lithotomy position includes the physiologic consequences of leg elevation on central blood volume and a decrease in tissue perfusion in the elevated legs due to gravity. The lithotomy position and pneumoperitoneum during laparoscopic surgery increase preload, probably as a result of blood shifting from the abdomen to the thorax by compression of splanchnic vessels caused by the pneumoperitoneum (Joris, 2005).

The increased intra-abdominal pressure created in the head-up tilt position would be expected to decrease venous return to the heart. In patients undergoing laparoscopic surgery in the head-up tilt (15-20°) position, as measured with a pulmonary artery catheter, HR, CI, stroke index (SI), CVP, and PCWP decreased, systemic vascular resistance increased, and MAP did not change (Hirvonen et al., 2000). Likewise, Alishlai et al., (2000) found that both cardiac output and stroke volume fell, whereas HR, systolic BP, and diastolic BP did not change in ASA I-III patients undergoing laparoscopic surgery (cholecystectomy, fundoplication, liver thermal ablation) during pneumoperitoneum in the 30° head-up tilt position.

The lateral decubitus position has minimal effects on major organ function when the patient is carefully positioned. In the elderly, hypovolemic, and hypertensive patients, blood pressure may not remain stable. The right lateral decubitus position appears to have greater propensity for caval compression and reduced venous return because of the closer proximity of the vena cava to the right flank. In the lateral flexed position, venous return may fall significantly, resulting in low cardiac output and hypotension. The physiological effects of positioning on cardiorespiratory function, particularly in elderly patients with co-morbidities (obesity, COPD, hypertension, coronary artery disease, etc.) may be catastrophic (Gottumukkala et al., 2008).

Cardiovascular
- Decreased left ventricular function
- Decreased cardiac output
- Decreased mean arterial pressure
- Increased systemic vascular resistance
- Increased central venous pressure
- Increased pulmonary artery pressure
- Increased pulmonary capillary wedge pressure

Respiratory
- Reduced vital capacity
- Decreased respiratory plateau pressure
- Decreased compliance
- Hypoxemia

Central nervous system
- Increased intracranial pressure
- Decreased cerebral perfusion pressure

Table 1. Physiologic changes due to Trendelenburg positioning

2.2 Respiratory and ventilatory effects of positioning

The steep head-down position in an anesthetized patient results in atelectasis and sometimes hypoxemia due to decreased functional residual capacity (FRC). With induction of anesthesia, the increased central blood volume, cephalad displacement of the diaphragm, and the weight of the abdominal contents impeding diaphragmatic excursion reduces pulmonary vital capacity. As a result of these changes, impedance of the chest wall and lung increases, an effect which is more pronounced in elderly and obese patients. Inhibition of lung expansion can occur, as well as right mainstem bronchial intubation, both of which are possible causes of hypoxemia in patients placed in the steep head-down position (Kalmar et al., 2010).

During laparoscopy in the Trendelenburg lithotomy position, compared with young patients, elderly patients had an higher $P(a\text{-}ET)CO_2$ in the setting of mechanical ventilation based on the value of $EtCO_2$. $PaCO_2$ increased progressively in both groups. Increasing the tidal volume to keep $P_{ET}CO_2$ within 20% of the pre-insufflation value may not prevent the increase in $P(a\text{-}ET)CO_2$; thus all patients, especially elderly ones, should be followed with caution while in the Trendelenburg lithotomy position (Takahata et al., 2007). Overweight patients (BMI of 25–29.9 kg/m^2) who underwent totally endoscopic robot-assisted radical prostatectomy under general anesthesia in Trendelenburg position had a significantly lower PaO_2 and higher the alveolar–arterial PO_2 difference compared with normal weight patients (Meininger et al., 2006). Similarly, SpO_2, $EtCO_2$, tidal volume, compliance, and minute ventilation remained within a clinically acceptable range in normal weight patients with steep (40°) Trendelenburg positioning during robotic prostatectomy (Kalmar et al., 2010).

2.3 Cerebral effects of positioning

Trendelenburg positioning causes an increase in intracranial pressure (ICP) due to increased venous pressure, which hinders cerebral venous drainage with a consequential increase in the cerebral blood volume (Mavrocordatos et al., 2000). Only a limited number of studies focus on the relationship between Trendelenburg positioning and regional cerebral oxygen saturation (rSO_2). Harrison et al (Harrison et al., 2001) found no difference in rSO_2 when comparing values at the beginning and end of abdominal surgery performed with patients in the Trendelenburg position.

Regional cerebral oxygen saturation did not change in patients undergoing robot-assisted laparoscopic radical prostatectomy in a 30° Trendelenburg position (Park et al., 2009). However, in a study of gynaecologic laparoscopic surgery patients (Lee et al., 2006), the mean rSO_2 was found to fall from 65.5±5.4% (baseline before surgery) to 60.8±5.6% when the patients were initially placed in the Trendelenburg position.

2.4 Patient position and lower extremity hypoperfusion

While in the lithotomy position, particularly when a head-down position is used, general hypoperfusion of the lower extremities may be exacerbated. Lithotomy positions (low, standard, high, and exaggerated) differ primarily from one another by the degree of hip angulation and height of leg placement. The hydrostatic gradient of arterial blood pressure between the ankle and the heart in these positions may decrease lower extremity blood pressure and contribute to lower extremity hypoperfusion. Lower-extremity systolic pressures may be reduced significantly in some patients, so much so that the lower extremities may be at risk for ischemia (Halliwill et al., 1998). Prolonged ischemia during surgical procedures performed on patients in lithotomy positions probably increases the risk of compartment syndrome. Long operation time (466 min), obesity (body mass index (BMI) 29.0 kg/m^2), and hypothermia during the operation (body temperature 34.2°C) also seemed to be risk factors that could have contributed to the symptoms observed in a case of lithotomy position-related compartment syndrome (Ikeya et al., 2006). To minimize the risk of compartment syndrome, surgeons should perform appropriate positioning and repositioning during surgery.

3. Pneumoperitoneum during laparoscopy

3.1 Hemodynamic changes due to pneumoperitoneum

Pneumoperitoneum is associated with altered cardiac and pulmonary physiology which may cause significant complications. The hemodynamic changes due to position are most significant at the initiation of pneumoperitoneum and near the end of the laparoscopic surgery. The adverse effects of pneumoperitoneum on cardiac performance are due to decreased venous return (cardiac preload), increased systemic vascular resistance (afterload), or both. (Alishlai et al., 2001).

The hemodynamic changes associated with pneumoperitoneum depend on a number of factors, including the mean intraabdominal pressure, amount of CO_2 absorbed, the patient's level of hydration, the type of ventilation, and the nature of the surgery. Investigators have found significant interpatient variability regarding the reduction of cardiac output and stroke volume associated with pnuemoperitoneum (Alishlai, 2001; Haxby, 1994). These differences could be at least be partially due to varying postures, arterial CO_2 partial pressures, anesthetic techniques, measurement techniques, and intraoperative fluid regimens.

A variety of patients undergo laparoscopic cholecystectomy, hernia repair, urogenital surgery, and cancer surgery, ranging from young healthy patients to older patients with cardiopulmonary disease. Morbidly obese patients who undergo gastric bypass surgery often have significant comorbid conditions such as coronary artery disease, diabetes mellitus, cerebral vascular disease, restrictive lung disease, sleep apnea, and hypertension. Invasive hemodynamic monitoring may benefit high-risk patients undergoing laparoscopic surgery (Hironen, 2000; Koivusalo, 2008). Extending the scope of laparoscopic techniques to older patients at higher risk of cardiovascular complications requires reappraisal of hemodynamic monitoring during anaesthesia.

During laparoscopy, to evaluate cardiac function, most investigators have used pulmonary artery catheterization which is both invasive and not routine in clinical practice (Hironen et al., 2000). Usually, invasive haemodynamic monitoring is used only in patients undergoing laparoscopic surgery who have pre-existing cardiovascular disease (Artuso, 2005; Koivusalo, 2008). This technique permits more precise calculation of left ventricular preload, afterload, and oxygen delivery. However, these advantages must be weighed against a low but appreciable risk of morbidity, which may not be acceptable in many patients. Noninvasive monitoring of patients at risk for acute hemodynamic changes that may not be readily revealed by conventional intraoperative monitoring techniques is often recommended, usually transoesophageal echocardiography (Alishahi, 2001; Fahy, 1999; Haxby, 1997; Russoa, 2009; Rist, 2001).

Haxby et al (Haxby et al., 1997) measured aortic flow velocity using oesephageal Doppler before, during, and after induction of carbon dioxide pneumoperitoneum in head-down position patients undergoing laparoscopic hernia repair. They found that the insufflation of the abdomen with the carbon dioxide (at 13 mmHg; a relatively low intraabdominal pressure) produced significant effects on the cardiovascular system, but the clinical significance of these changes was uncertain. Likewise, during laparoscopic surgery of the lower abdomen in the head-up tilt position CO was found to fall after abdominal insufflation (peak intra-abdominal pressure: 13-15 mmHg). The CO fell more (30%) in patients with high surgical risk than in patients with low risk (25%), when patients were classified according to ASA physical status classification (Rist et al., 2001).

Patients in the head-down tilt position during laparoscopic hysterectomy were found to have a significant reduction in stroke volume, cardiac output and left ventricular end-diastolic volume and increase in afterload with pneumopericardium, as measured with cardiac apical Doppler echocardiography. The augmented preload resulted in an increase in stroke volume, cardiac output and left ventricular end-diastolic volume in both laparoscopic hysterectomy and conventional open hysterectomy groups. Branche et al (Branche et al., 1998) investigated the effect of intraperitoneal insufflation of carbon dioxide and head up (10°) tilt position on left ventricular afterload by using transaesophageal echocardiography in patients undergoing laparoscopic cholecystectomy. They found that systolic arterial pressure increased at the beginning of the pneumoperitoneum and subsequently decreased gradually during pneumoperitoneum. Significant variation in HR and regional wall motion were not observed, but left ventricular afterload and left ventricular end-systolic wall stress increased.

In morbidly obese laparoscopic gastric bypass surgery patients (Artuso et al., 2005), upon insufflation of the abdomen, systemic blood pressure, pulmonary artery pressure, central venous pressure, and pulmonary artery capillary wedge pressure increased significantly from baseline values, but CI and SVR did not change significantly. These changes were attenuated when the patient was placed in the reverse Trendelenburg position and almost completely corrected when the abdomen was deflated at the completion of the procedure. Laparoscopic gastric bypass surgery candidates who often have significant cardiorespiratory comorbidities, like other high-risk patients undergoing laparoscopic surgery, may benefit from invasive hemodynamic monitoring. Likewise, the head-up position in patients undergoing laparoscopic cholecystectomy, SI decreased, but CI did not change significantly because of the compensatory increase in heart rate (Hirvonen et al., 2000). CO_2 insufflation at the start of laparoscopy increased CVP and PCWP as well as mean systemic and mean pulmonary arterial pressures without significantly changing CI or SI. Toward the end of the laparoscopy, CI decreased by 15%. The hemodynamic values returned to nearly pre-laparoscopic levels after deflation of the gas, and CI increased during the recovery period, whereas systemic vascular resistance was 15% lower in the recovery room compared to preinsufflation values.

Laparoscopy in the lateral flexed position may significantly decrease venous return, causing low cardiac output and hypotension. This condition can be prevented by fluid loading and promptly reversed by deflation and table deflection.

Fahy et al, (Fahy et al., 1999) detected a high incidence of regurgitation in healthy donors in the lateral decubitus position at the mitral, tricuspid, pulmonic, and aortic valves with trans oesephageal echocardiogram (TEE) after CO_2 insufflation during laparoscopic nephrectomy. The consequences of these challenges in patients with preexisting valvular or cardiac disease would be more serious. Patients with cardiovascular disease have responses to laparoscopy that are affected by the extent of cardiac reserve, baseline medications, level of hydration, and their response to the anesthesia medications used (Slodzinski & Merritt, 2008).

For abdominal laparoscopic procedures, IAP is usually not allowed to exceed 15 mm Hg, but during pelvic procedures a higher IAP (approximately 25 mm Hg) is used. An IAP of less than 15 mm Hg is required during laparoscopic cholecystectomy, in so far as it reduces the risks associated with high pressures (Catani et al., 2004). Cardiovascular variables usually return to preinsufflation values after a pneumoperitoneum of short duration.

When a pneumoperitoneum is created for laparoscopic surgery in patients with no known cardiac disease, a decrease in left ventricular function and CO, and an increase in CVP (from redistribution of abdominal blood volume), systemic vascular resistance, and mean arterial pressure occurs, as measured by noninvasive methods (Critchley, 1993; Girardis, 1996; Westerband, 1992), thermodilution catheter (Hirvonen et al, 2000), transoesophageal echocardiography (Gannedahl, 1996; Harris, 1996; Haxby, 1997; Rist, 2001), and transthoracic echocardiography (Russoa et al., 2009).

Cases of sudden intraoperative cardiovascular collapse or severe pulmonary edema requiring ventilation after uneventful laparoscopic cholecystectomy have been reported (Giaquinto et al., 2003). The adverse effects on cardiac performance produced by pneumoperitoneum may increase the risk of cardiac complications in patients with underlying cardiac and pulmonary disease. In addition to the central changes, pneumoperitoneum results in reduced peripheral venous flow (Alishahi, 2001; Schwenk, 1998) and diminished perfusion of intraabdominal organs (Jakimowicz et al., 1998).

Blood flow falls significantly in the renal, hepatic, gastric, and mesenteric beds during laparoscopic surgery with pneumoperitoneum (Ishizaki et al., 1993; Jakimowicz et al., 1998);

resulting in impaired renal function in some patients. In nephrectomy patients with preexisting renal disease, laparoscopy may create additional kidney injury as a result of elevated intraabdominal pressure and kidney manipulation (Crane et al., 2008). In patients undergoing laparoscopic surgery (cholecystectomy, fundoplication, liver thermal ablation) in the reverse Trendelenburg position, common femoral venous flow falls significantly. The application of intermittent sequential pneumatic compression (ISPC) of the lower limbs during laparoscopic surgery reversed that effect, returning peak systolic velocity to normal (Millard, 1993; Alishahiet, 2001).

3.2 Respiratory and ventilatory effects of pneumoperitonium during laparoscopy

The changes with pneumoperitoneum in the mechanical properties of the respiratory system are related to two main factors: shifting of blood flow to the pulmonary circulation and compression of the lung bases by raising the dome of the diaphragm. Increased pressure within the abdomen increases the intrathoracic pressure by pushing the diaphragm upward, thus decreasing respiratory system compliance, which in turn results in reduced lung volumes and increased airway pressures (Hirvonen, 1995; Odeberg, 1994). These changes predispose patients to airway closure and collapse of dependent lung regions (atelectasis) (Andersson, 2005; El-Dawlatly, 2005; Nguyen, 2005). Atelectasis can be prevented by positive end-expiratory pressure or treated by inflation maneuvers (Strang et al., 2009).

Obese patients have a greater risk of atelectasis than non-obese patients. Preventing atelectasis is important for all patients, but is especially important when caring for obese patients.The use of high positive end-expiratory pressure (10 cm H_2O) in patients undergo laparoscopic bariatric surgery resulted in improved respiratory function and oxygenation in obese patients (Talab et al., 2009). When compared to preinsufflation values, abdominal insufflation to 2.26 kPa caused a significant (31%) decrease in respiratory system compliance, a significant (17%) increase in peak and plateau (32%) airway pressures at constant tidal volume with significant hypercapnia, but no change in arterial O_2 saturation in obese patients undergoing laparoscopic gastroplasty. Respiratory system compliance and pulmonary insufflation pressures returned to baseline values after abdominal deflation (Dumont et al., 1997).

Positive end expiratory pressure (PEEP) prevents the upward shift of the diaphragm during laparoscopy, limits the deliterious effects of surgery on respiratory mechanics, and improves oxygenation. However, no consensus has been reached regarding the ideal level of PEEP during laparoscopic surgery. A PEEP of 10 cm H_2O had better oxygenation both intraoperatively and postoperatively in the PACU, lower atelectasis score on chest computed tomographic scan, and less postoperative pulmonary complications than a PEEP of 0 cm H_2O (ZEEP) and 5 cm H_2O in patients undergo undergo laparoscopic bariatric surgery (Talab et al., 2009.) Likewise, a PEEP of 10 cm H_2O produced beneficial effects in the elasticity, as well as in the resistance, of the respiratory system in patients undergoing cholecystectomy video-laparoscopy procedures (Maracaja-Neto et al., 2009).

The use of a recruitment maneuver (RM) re-expanded atelectasis and improved oxygenation in obese patients undergoing laparoscopic procedures (Almarakbi, 2009; Chalhoub, 2007; Whalen, 2006). RMs and PEEP were both required to prevent rapid reoccurrence of atelectasis, especially when a high-inspired oxygen fraction was used. Oxygenation may be a poor indicator of the extent of lung collapse as oxygenation has not been found to correlate with atelectasis formation during pneumoperitoneum (Andersson, 2005; Strang, 2009).

End-expiratory lung volumes are commonly used in clinical practice to denote functional residual capacity during mechanical ventilation. Futierae et al (Futierae et al., 2010) investigated the effects of RM after application of PEEP on changes in end expiratory lung volume (EELV), respiratory mechanics, and oxygenation in healthy weight and obese patients undergoing laparoscopic surgery. They found that pneumoperitoneum worsened the reduction in EELV and respiratory mechanics produced by anesthesia induction, with no major effect on oxygenation. A PEEP of 10 cm H_2O combined with RM induced sustained improvements in EELV, gas exchange, and respiratory mechanics, and may be useful in counteracting the detrimental effects of pneumoperitoneum, especially on lung volume reduction in healthy weight and obese patients (Futier et al., 2010). Both conventional volume-controlled ventilation and pressure-controlled ventilation (PCV) were found to be equally suited for patients undergoing laparoscopic gynaecologic surgery. However, a higher lung compliance and lower peak airway pressures, plateau pressures, and airway resistance were observed with PCV in laparoscopic gynaecologic surgery patients (Oğurlu et al., 2010).

Patients with pulmonary dysfunction are at high risk for complications; pre-op screening with pulmonary function tests is of the utmost importance for these patients. In morbidly obese patients, compared with open gastric bypass procedure (GBP), laparoscopic gastric bypass resulted in higher $EtCO_2$, peak inspiratory pressure, total exhaled CO_2 per minute, and a lower respiratory compliance. Arterial blood gas analysis demonstrated higher $PaCO_2$ and lower pH during laparoscopic GBP than during open. Laparoscopic GBP alters intraoperative pulmonary mechanics and acid-base balance but does not significantly affect pulmonary oxygen exchange. Changes in pulmonary mechanics are well tolerated in morbidly obese patients when proper ventilator adjustments are maintained (Nguyen et al., 2004). Sprung et al (Sprung et al., 2003) showed that arterial oxygenation during laparoscopy could not be improved by increasing either the tidal volume or respiratory rate. In morbidly obese patients with chronic obstructive pulmonary disease and hypertension, the 20° reverse Trendelenburg position during laparoscopic gastric banding surgery improved respiratory mechanics (respiratory compliance, airway resistance and peak inspiratory pressure) and oxygenation without any apparent adverse effects on haemodynamics (Salihoglu et al., 2003). On the other hand, PaO_2 was significantly lower and the alveolar-arterial oxygen difference (A-aDO_2) was higher in overweight (BMI 25–29.9 kg/m^2) and normal weight (BMI 18.5–24.9 kg/m^2) patients who underwent totally endoscopic robot-assisted radical prostatectomy in the Trendelenburg position (Meininger et al., 2006). Whereas pneumoperitoneum did not have any significant effect in normal weight patients, A-aDO_2 decreased to below baselines values in overweight patients after prolonged (1.5 hours) pneumoperitoneum.

The kidney position can lower the vital capacity by another 5–10%. Most of this decrease is thought to result from reduced movement of the ribs and diaphragm. Although vital capacity and FRC are reduced in the lateral decubitus position, better ventilation–perfusion matching results from increased perfusion in the dependent lung and corresponding increase in ventilation from the stretched dependent hemidiaphragm. However, general anesthesia in the lateral decubitus position causes an increased mismatch in ventilation–perfusion ratios compared to that in awake subjects. Complications from the lateral decubitus position include pressure injuries (ischemic), muscular and ligamentous strain, whiplash-like injury to the cervical spine, neurologic injuries, and ocular complications (corneal abrasions, pressure effects, dependent edema, and blindness) (Gottumukkala, 2008).

3.3 Hypercarbia-induced pneumoperitonium

Laparoscopic procedures use carbon dioxide, a highly diffusable gas, for insufflation. CO_2 insufflated during laparoscopy is soluble in blood, and after transperitoneal absorption is presented to the lungs for excretion. The high solubility of CO_2 in the blood stream minimizes the risk of gas emboli. $ETCO_2$ increases from 0–30% when minute ventilation is held constant, but increasing respiratory rate, tidal volume, or both by as much as 30% may be necessary to keep the $ETCO_2$ in the mid-30s (mm Hg) range. This almost always means general anesthesia with endotracheal intubation to maintain adequate ventilation, which tends to be impaired by surgical positioning and abdominal distension. Higher intraabdominal pressures are associated with faster CO_2 absorption and gas embolism. These effects are further influenced by the intraoperative position of the patient and duration of procedure, and whether the patients have pre-existing cardiovascular disease. (Slodzinski & Merritt, 2008).

Patients with preoperative cardiopulmonary disease demonstrated significantly higher Pa CO_2 levels and lower pH during carbon dioxide insufflation compared to patients without underlying disease. During laparoscopic cholecystectomy, patients with chronic cardiopulmonary disease may require careful intraoperative arterial blood gas monitoring of absorbed carbon dioxide (Catherine et al., 1991). The physiological effects of intraperitoneal carbon dioxide insufflation on cardiorespiratory function, particularly in elderly patients with co-morbidities (obesity, COPD, hypertension, coronary artery disease, etc.), may be catastrophic.

Carbon dioxide levels are easily measured at the end of exhalation and the anesthesiologist should constantly measure these levels and adjust the ventilator to prevent hypercarbia and acidosis. Patients who have pulmonary airway disease compromising the ability to exhale CO_2 might require surgery via another technique. Because pulmonary compliance is decreased and functional residual capacity is impaired by pneumoperitoneum and patient positioning, minute volume may need to be increased in order to correct the ventilation-perfusion mismatch to avoid hypercarbia and acidosis. The retroperitoneal approach for laparoscopic surgery has a greater risk of hypercarbia than the transperitoneal approach.

3.4 Effects of pneumoperitonium on the central nervous system

Pneumoperitoneum during laparoscopic surgery also has the potential to increase cerebral blood flow (CBF), intracranial pressure, and intraocular pressure due to the increased $PaCO_2$ caused by absorption of CO_2 from the peritoneal cavity. The creation of pneumoperitoneum during laparoscopic surgery elevates ICP because increased the abdominal pressure obstructs venous return from the lumbar venous plexus (Halverson et al., 1998). Pneumoperitoneum also increases cerebral blood flow due to an increase in $PaCO_2$ and an increase in catecholamine release independent of $PaCO_2$. The rate of cerebral blood flow changes proportionally to the change in $PaCO_2$ within the range of 2.7–8.0 kPa (Huettemann, 2002; Fujii, 1999).

Regional cerebral oxygen saturation (rSO_2), as measured by near-infrared spectroscopy cerebral oximetry which allows for continuous and noninvasive monitoring of rSO_2, decreased when cerebral perfusion pressure declined as a result of increased ICP (Dunham, 2002; Lee, 2006). Lee et al (Lee et al., 2006) also reported that rSO_2 decreased significantly in the Trendelenburg position. They reported that although no additional effect was seen with pneumoperitoneum, the rSO_2 was further decreased in the setting of hypercapnea, which increased the blood volume with a consequential increase in ICP. In contrast, Park et al

(Park et al., 2009) during robot-assisted laparoscopic radical prostatectomy, in patients in the Trendelenburg position, found that cerebral oxygenation, as assessed by rSO_2, increased slightly, which suggested that the procedure itself did not induce cerebral ischemia. While in the steep (40°) Trendelenburg position, regional cerebral oxygenation was well preserved and CPP remained within the normal limits of cerebral autoregulation, as measured by near-infrared spectroscopy (Kalmar et al., 2010).

Respiratory changes
- Decreased total volume of the lungs
- Decreased pulmonary compliance
- Hypoxemia (secondary to a ventilation-perfusion mismatch and intrapulmonary shunting)
- Hypercapnia and acidosis (secondary to CO_2 absorption)
- Increased $PaCO_2$ and $EtCO_2$

Cardiovascular changes
- Decreased stroke index, cardiac index
- Decreased peripheral venous flow
- Direct and indirect sympatho-adrenal stimulation (caused by hypercarbia)
  - Myocardial depression
  - Direct vasodilation
- Increased SVR, PVR

Renal changes
- Oliguria, decreased renal blood flow
- Increased ADH, renin, and aldosterone
- Intraoperative increase in serum creatinine

Abdominal changes
- Increased intra-abdominal pressure
- Decreased perfusion of intraabdominal organs (kidney, liver, stomach, mesentery) and spinal cord

Table 2. Pathophysiologic changes during pneumoperitoneum

Cerebral blood flow–carbon dioxide (CBF–CO_2) reactivity is one marker of the ability of the cerebral vasculature to respond to cerebral metabolic demands. CBF–CO_2 reactivity did not change significantly in one study of patients undergoing robot-assisted laparoscopic radical prostatectomy (with pneumoperitoneum) while in the Trendelenburg position (Choi et al., 2009). During pneumoperitoneum in the head-down position, the resulting changes in venous pressures, together with hypercapnia, can lead to significant increases in intracranial pressure. These changes can result in brain injury in selected patients, causing postoperative neurological deficits (Fujii, 1994; Huettemann, 2002). Laparoscopic procedures in the head-down position are to be avoided in patients with space-occupying intracranial lesions because of the excessive increase in ICP (Alishahi, 2001; Dunham, 2002).

3.5 Other complications of induced pneumoperitonium

Venous CO_2 embolism may occur intraoperatively and in the early postoperative period. Abnormal gastroesophageal junction competence from high intraabdominal pressure may lead to pneumomediastinum, subcutaneous emphysema, pneumothorax, and retroperitoneal CO_2.

In hand-assisted laparoscopic donor nephrectomy patients, ocular complications and corneal abrasions were reported. These may result from increased fluid intake, flank positioning, and potential increased venous compression resulting from the effects of the pneumoperitoneum. The fact that the dependent eye was involved in all patients suggests conjunctival edema as a potential common pathway (Koning et al., 2011).

Rhabdomyolysis after prolonged laparoscopic nephrectomy in the lateral decubitus position has been reported, but is thought to be rare. Its myoglobinuria may result in kidney dysfunction (Kuang et al., 2002).

4. Intraoperative anesthesia management

Laparoscopy patients should undergo a preoperative evaluation identical to that for patients undergoing the equivalent open procedure. Depending on the surgeon's experience with these procedures, the anesthetic plan should anticipate the possibilities of significant bleeding and conversion to an open procedure. Routine intraoperative monitoring ($EtCO_2$, pulse oximetry, BP, airway pressure) should be adequate for the expected physiologic changes encountered in most patients. The anesthesiologist should continually monitor the insufflating pressure being used and should be alerted if an unusual amount of CO_2 is required.

Noninvasive methods of assessing changes in partial arterial pressures of carbon dioxide (eg. $EtCO_2$ measured with mass spectrography) may be misleading because changes in partial arterial pressures of carbon dioxide are typically much smaller than changes in arterial blood levels and, unlike arterial gas measurements, do not indicate the true level of arterial hypercarbia. During laparoscopic cholecystectomy, patients with chronic cardiopulmonary disease may require careful intraoperative arterial blood gas monitoring of absorbed carbon dioxide (Wittgen et al., 1991). With extended periods of insufflation and higher pressures, faster CO_2 absorption occurs and arterial carbon dioxide levels may reach harmful levels. Measurement of $EtCO_2$ allows the physician to manipulate ventilation as needed (Nguyen & Wolfe, 2005).

Cardiovascular monitoring should be appropriate for the planned procedure, based on the patient's clinical status. Central venous and pulmonary arterial wedge pressure measurements are biased during laparoscopy because of transmission of intraabdominal pressure to the mediastinal space. Use of TEE in high-risk patients allows for more accurate assessment of cardiac volumes. TEE for hemodynamic monitoring may be useful in the prevention and recognition of cardiovascular complications. Femoral venous flow augmentation with intermittent sequential pneumatic compression reverses perioperative cardiac depression and overcompensates for the state of peripheral venous stasis induced by pneumoperitoneum during laparoscopic surgery in the head-up tilt position (Alishahi, 2001; Schwenk, 1998).

When laparoscopic procedures are performed in an ambulatory setting, the choice of induction and maintenance anesthetic agents reflects the need for prompt awakening and rapid recovery. The anesthetic management of laparoscopic surgery includes minimizing hemodynamic changes which may occur due to the pneumoperitoneum and patient's position (Colombo et al., 2001). In laparoscopic surgery, nitrous oxide (N_2O) is often avoided, to prevent bowel distension if the procedure becomes prolonged. Nitrous oxide accumulates in the CO_2 pneumoperitoneum during laparoscopy when N_2O is used as an adjuvant for inhaled anesthesia. Accumulated N_2O in a CO_2 atmosphere may be dangerous because it can lead to excessive dilatation of the bowel.

The risk of CO_2 and N_2O gas embolism is also a concern because the consequences of such embolization may differ from those with the same volume of CO_2 alone. N_2O diffuses into the abdominal cavity and will diffuse into CO_2 bubbles and emboli, increasing their size and potential for an obstructive event. (Diemunsch et al., 2002). Adequate muscle relaxation is required during laparoscopy so that spontaneous respiratory efforts do not impair the surgical procedure or increase the gradient for embolic gas to enter the central circulation. Despite the limited surgical incision(s) of laparoscopic procedures, postoperative muscle pain remains a problem. These problems have not been eliminated by avoiding succinylcholine or by using other anesthetic regimens.

$PaCO_2$ should be maintained within its normal range during pneumoperitoneum in the Trendelenburg position. For example, rSO_2 increased in conjunction with the increase in $PaCO_2$ during pneumoperitoneum in a steep Trendelenburg position in patients undergoing daVinci robot-assisted laparoscopic prostatectomy (Park et al., 2009).

Watanabe et al. found that remifentanil (0.2 μg/kg/min) may suppress the cardiovascular changes caused by pneumoperitoneum in laparoscopic cholecystectomy patients. Through an epidural catheter placed between T_{10-12}, 0.2% ropivacaine was infused continuously at 6 mL/hr. With a pneumoperitoneum, as opposed to an epidural anesthetic, remifentanil significantly suppressed the tachycardia, but not the hypertension caused by the pneumoperitoneum (Watanabe et al., 2009). Esmolol infusion can also be used to provide hemodynamic stability during laparoscopy (Coloma, 2001; Junghans, 2006).

No ventilation technique for laparoscopic surgery has proved to be clinically superior to any other. Both conventional volume-controlled ventilation and pressure-controlled ventilation were found to be equally suited for use in patients undergoing laparoscopic gynaecologic surgery (Oğurlu et al., 2010).

Stationary positioning of the patient over long periods of time during laparoscıpic surgery may place the patient at risk for neuropraxia, rhabdomyolysis, compartment syndrome, and pressure ulcers. Neuromuscular and pressure injury becomes more likely with increasing surgical duration, hence the need for appropriate padding and support, especially during laparoscopic nephrectomies (Elsamra & Pareek, 2010).

Hypotension, decreased cardiac output
Hemorrhage
Acidosis
Pneumothorax
Pneumomediastinum
Endobronchial intubation
Subcutaneous emphysema
Airway obstruction
Retroperitoneal CO_2
Venous stasis
Venous CO_2 embolism
Increased sympathetic activity secondary to increased CO_2
Bradycardia, increased vagal tone
Cardiac arrest
Regurgitation and aspiration

Table 3. Complications during laparoscopy

5. Intraoperative surgical complications

During laparoscopy, positional changes may significantly decrease venous return, causing low cardiac output and hypotension. This condition can be prevented by fluid loading and promptly reversed by deflation and table deflection. The changes listed above may lead to myocardial ischemia in patients at risk. In the rare event of catastrophic hemodynamic collapse during laparoscopy, several possible causes should be considered: bleeding, subcutaneous emphysema, pneumothorax, pneumomediastinum, diaphragmatic tears, and gas embolism. Although the use of CO_2 for pneumoperitoneum reduces the probability of a massive pulmonary embolism, it is a potentially fatal complication and should be considered in case of intraoperative hemodynamic deterioration (Slodzinski & Merritt, 2008).

Initial therapy during a catastrophic event includes releasing the pressurized pneumoperitoneum (i.e., conversion to an open procedure). For pneumothorax, a thoracentesis should be performed. If massive embolization occurs, N_2O, if employed, should be discontinued immediately and cardiopulmonary resuscitation should be performed. The patient should be placed in the left lateral position. Attempts at embolus retrieval should be made through central venous access, if available. If these measures are not sufficient, cardiopulmonary bypass may be necessary (Joris, 2005; Leonard, 2002).

During laparoscopy, hemorrhage can be obvious or occult (e.g., retroperitoneal), and may be encountered intra-operatively or in the postoperative period. Bleeding complications are an important subset of 'non-biliary' injuries, and can cause death on the operating table if not recognized and treated in time. Bleeding complications are the most frequent cause of procedure-related mortality in laparoscopic cholecystectomy (after anaesthesia-related deaths) (Buttenschoen, 2007; Phillips, 2001).

Intra-operative bleeding usually falls into one of the following four patterns: vessel injury, slippage of clips/ligatures of the cystic artery, liver bed bleeding, and miscellaneous. Vessel injuries are usually the most dramatic and occur either during insertion of the first trocar or during dissection/retraction, and were rarely seen before the advent of laparoscopic surgery. The insertion of the pneumoperitoneum needle and the first trocar is considered by many to be the most dangerous step in laparoscopic cholecystectomy, as it is essentially a 'blind' step. As this initial step is common to all laparoscopic operations, it has been reviewed extensively by various authors. As mentioned earlier, the majority of bleeding complications occur in this phase of the operation. Although the most commonly injured vessels are the epigastric vessels, injury can also occur to the major intra-abdominal vessels (aorta, vena cava, iliac vessels), in 0.04% to 0.18% of patients (Geraci et al., 2006). None of the "no entry" techniques for laparoscopy (trocar entry after creation of pneumoperitoneum, trocar entry without prior insufflation, or various modifications of the open technique of port placement) are free from the risk of complications (Kaushik et al., 2010).

Bleeding complications are divided into major and minor depending on the need for conversion, additional surgical procedures, or blood transfusions. Thus, any bleeding that requires a laparotomy is considered major, irrespective of the vessel injured or the timing (intra-operative or postoperative). Similarly, any bleeding that needs an additional surgical procedure (wound exploration and ligation of bleeder) or blood transfusion is also considered to be major, whereas bleeds controllable by pressure or packing, or abdominal wall haematomas that do not require any additional manoeuvres, can be classified as minor bleeds (Kaushik et al., 2010).

Major and minor complication rates for laparoscopic renal surgery have ranged from 1-6% and 6-17%, respectively. Vascular, bowel, and ureteral injuries are reported as the most commonly encountered intraoperative complications. A key component to decreasing the incidence of surgical complications is proper patient selection and identification of preoperative risk factors. Potential preoperative risk factors, such as prior operations, increased age, increased body mass index, poor renal function, and anomalies in renal vasculature, are of crucial importance to proper preoperative risk stratification. Also, the urologist must be facile with current laparoscopic techniques in order to minimize complications (Elsamra & Pareek, 2010). In a study (Colombo et al., 2008) of patients who underwent laparoscopic nephrectomy, nephroureterectomy, laparoscopic partial nephrectomy, and adrenalectomy, age greater than 65 years predicted a longer hospital stay, but was not an independent risk factor for complications. In addition, patients with baseline elevated creatinine were at higher risk of postoperative renal deficiency. Recently, in patients with a BMI less than 25 kg/m^2 and greater than 40 kg/m^2 who underwent laparoscopic radical nephrectomy or laparoscopic partial nephrectomy, no statistically significant difference was found for estimated blood loss, operative time, hospital stay, number of open conversions, or complications. However, a trend toward increased operative time and intra-operative complications (not statistically significant) was noted in patients with increased BMI (Gong et al., 2007). Surgical experience appears to be directly related to the complication rate, with at least 50 laparoscopic cases required to achieve proficiency (Vallancien et al., 2002). In addition, 80% of all major complications of laparoscopic surgery occurred among the surgeon's first 100 cases. Short intensive courses may increase the surgeon's experience, confidence, and competency in advanced laparoscopic procedures (Pareek et al., 2005).

6. Postoperative risks

Postoperative nausea and vomiting (PONV) occurs in 40–70% of patients undergoing laparoscopic cholecystectomy. Female patients have a 1.5-3 times greater incidence of PONV than males, due to increased plasma progesterone levels during their menstrual cycles. Antiemetics used to prevent PONV after laparoscopic cholecystectomy include antihistamines (dimenhydrinate), phenothiazines (perphenazine), butyrophenones (droperidol), benzamides (metoclopramide), dexamethasone, and serotonin-receptor antagonists (ondansetron, granisetron, tropisetron, dolasetron, and ramosetron). Knowledge regarding prophylactic antiemetic therapy is necessary to effectively manage PONV in female patients (Fujii 2005; 2009 and 2010).

In laparoscopic cholecystectomy, before or following induction of anesthesia, dexamethasone alone or in combination with a serotonergic antagonist (granisetron, ondansetron) to prevent nausea and vomiting is well established (Dabbous, 2010; Fujii, 2010; Erhan, 2008). Dexamethasone alone was found as effective as 4 mg ondansetron and 3 mg granisetron (Erhan et al., 2008). Dexamethasone, in combination with a serotonergic antagonist, significantly reduced the incidence of PONV more than promethazine and granisetron monotherapy (Dabbous, 2010; Fujii, 2010). In women undergoing ambulatory gynaecological laparoscopy, prophylactic low-dose granisetron and promethazine together were more effective in reducing PONV than promethazine or granisetron alone (Gan et al., 2009) Risk factors for postoperative PONV after laparoscopic cholecystectomy include pain, dizziness, ambulation, oral intake, and analgesics (opioids). Avoiding these risk factors would result in less PONV for patients undergoing LC (Fujii et al., 2010).

In recent years, mini-laparoscopic cholecystectomy (trocar incision <25 mm) has been increasingly advocated for the removal of the gallbladder, due to better surgical and postoperative outcomes (e.g., better cosmetic result, reduced pain, shorter hospital stay, and quicker return to activity). Although mini-laparoscopy is feasibile and safe, it does require a longer surgical time and has a reasonably high risk for conversion to standard laparoscopic cholecystectomy. Furthermore, mini-laparoscopy has not been found to have any additional clinical benefit compared to standard laparoscopic cholecystectomy (Huang, 2003; McCloy, 2008).

To manage the pain associated with increasingly complex surgical procedures on an ambulatory or short-stay basis, anesthesiologists and surgeons should prescribe multimodal analgesic regimens that use non-opioid analgesics (eg. local anesthetics, nonsteroidal antiinflammatory drugs, cyclooxygenase inhibitors, acetaminophen, ketamine, alpha 2-agonists) to supplement opioid analgesics. The opioid-sparing effects of these compounds may lead to reduced nausea, vomiting, constipation, urinary retention, respiratory depression and sedation. Therefore, use of non-opioid analgesic techniques can lead to an improved quality of recovery for surgical patients (White, 2008). Tramadol and paracetamol cause no respiratory depression while providing analgesia and sedation after operative procedures. Oral tramadol (1 $mg.kg^{-1}$) with IV paracetamol (1 g) decreased the incidence of side effects of tramadol alone without reducing its analgesic efficacy in a day-care laparoscopic surgery setting (Ali & Khan, 2009).

IV tramadol after insufflation of the pneumoperitoneum and again before removal of the trocars was used provided superior postoperative analgesia to IP tramadol in the early postoperative period after laparoscopic cholecystectomy (Akıncı et al., 2008). Epidural analgesia with a bupivacaine/fentanyl combination provided significant improvement in postoperative pain control compared with IV fentanyl during the first 24 hours following laparoscopic cholecystectomy (Erol et al., 2008).

In patients undergoing laparoscopic cholecystectomy, the combination of 0.25% IP bupivacaine and IV morphine was more effective than IP morphine plus IP 0.25% bupivacaine for reducing postoperative analgesic requirements (Hernández-Palazón et al., 2003). Another study in LC patients found pre-operative 50 mg/kg magnesium sulphate IV to be more effective in reducing post-operative pain than saline (Menteş et al., 2008).

Intraoperative and postoperative analgesia usually is performed with a combination of opioids and NSAIDs. While IV or epidural opioids remain the mainstay for postoperative analgesia, their use can be associated with adverse effects, such as ileus, which can prolong hospital stay, especially after colorectal surgery. Thoracic epidural analgesia provides better postoperative analgesia than intraoperative and postoperative IV lidocaine infusion (Wongyingsinn et al., 2011), and spinal anaesthesia using intrathecal morphine in addition to local anaesthetic, and the use of nonsteroidal anti-inflammatory agents (Levy et al., 2010). But thoracic epidural analgesia patients had similar length of hospital stay, time to tolerate a normal diet, and bowel function parameters compared to others under general anesthesia after laparoscopic colorectal surgery (Levy, 2010; Wongyingsinn, 2011). In contrast, when a traditional perioperative care program is used for laparoscopic colectomy, thoracic epidural analgesia is superior to PCA in accelerating the return of bowel function and dietary intake, while providing better pain relief compared to PCA morphine (Taqi et al., 2007).

In patients undergoing ambulatory totally extra-peritoneal laparoscopic inguinal hernioplasty under local anaesthesia, pain and analgesic consumption was less and recovery of daily life activities more rapid compared to those patients undergoing ambulatory

Lichtenstein hernioplasty with local anaesthesia (Planells et al., 2011). Additionally, for patients with recurrent inguinal hernia, or bilateral inguinal hernia, laparoscopic repair offers significant advantages over open techniques with regard to recurrence risk, pain, and recovery (Carter & Duh., 2011). Donors undergoing laparoscopic nephrectomy reported less bodily pain postdonation; this was associated with an improved mental health component of quality of life compared with open nephrectomy patients (Nicholson et al., 2011).

When respiratory functions of patients after open and laparoscopic cholecystectomy were compared, pulmonary function tests were better in patients subjected to LC (Osman et al., 2009). On the first post-operative day, FEV_1, FVC and FEV_1/FVC values in the open cholecystectomy group were significantly lower than those in the laparoscopic cholecystectomy group. The respiratory function tests returned to normal by the 6th postoperative day in both groups. LC resulted in an overall better postoperative respiratory function than open cholecystectomy (Bablekos, 2003; Hendolin, 2000).

Perioperative neurologic complications related to prolonged surgery in the steep head-down position include neurological deterioration after extubation, probably due to cerebral edema. The duration and positioning should be optimized for such prolonged surgery in the steep head-down position to minimize complications (Pandey et al., 2010). Bilateral upper extremity paresis caused by overstretching of the neck with the head was reported in two patients undergoing laparoscopic colectomy in a combined lithotomy and Trendelenburg position with arms abducted to 80° and flexed slightly on padded armboards (Imamura et al., 2010). They developed bilateral numbness of the first, second, and third digits, and the radial side of fourth digit in one patient's right hand, which subsided gradually over three days after physical training in both patients. In a report by Mizuno et al (Mizuno et al., 2008), right median nerve injury was caused by compression and stretching of the brachial plexus after laparoscopic sigmoidectomy in a patient who was operated upon while in the head-down position, with right lateral tilt table, use of shoulder brace, abduction of the upper arm, and extension of the elbow. His findings disappeared completely within one week. In laparoscopic operations in the head-down position, a shoulder brace should not be used to minimize the risk of brachial plexus injury. The arms should be placed at the patient's side, and the elbows should be gently flexed to unload the median nerve and relieve tension on the brachial plexus. Irreversible femoral nerve injury caused by trocar insertion was reported after gynaecologic laparoscopy by Porzionato et al (Porzionato et al, 2008). The patient complained of left thigh weakness and paresthesias, from the site of the left trocar insertion to the anteromedial aspect of the thigh and medial aspect of the leg and foot. Peritoneal adhesions and inadequate pneumoperitoneum may increase the risk of nerve injury. Physicians should be aware of the possibility of this complication, and should avoid too caudal a trocar insertion in the iliac fossa.

7. Conclusion

Laparoscopic surgical procedures aim to minimize the trauma of the interventional process. Advantages of these procedures include smaller incisional sites, lower risks of wound complications, reduced postoperative pain and complications, improved recovery, shorter hospital stays, more rapid return to normal activities, and significant cost savings.

Cardiorespiratory changes associated with laparoscopy include those associated with tilting the patient to facilitate instrumentation and surgical exposure, and pressure effects of the instilled gas into peritoneum. Endoscopic surgery also involves complications, especially when extended periods of carbon dioxide insufflation are used, and especially with the patient in the steep head-down position. In such circumstances, adverse haemodynamic and respiratory effects are more prone to occur. Traumatic injuries associated with blind trocar insertion may injury viscera and blood vessels, leading to severe hemorrhage and morbidity.

Depending on the surgeon's experience, the anesthesiologist should anticipate the possibility of significant bleeding and/or conversion to an open procedure. Laparoscopy patients should undergo a preoperative evaluation identical to that of patients undergoing the comparable open procedure.

When laparoscopic procedures are performed in an ambulatory setting, the choice of induction and maintenance anesthetic agents reflects the need for prompt awakening and rapid recovery. In the anesthetic management of laparoscopic surgery, hemodynamic changes may occur due to the pneumoperitoneum and/or patient's position. In laparoscopic surgery, N_2O is often avoided, to prevent bowel distension if the procedure becomes prolonged. A continuous infusion of bupivicaine via epidural catheter or IV remifentanil or esmolol may suppress the cardiovascular changes caused by the pneumoperitoneum during laparoscopic surgery.

In laparoscopic surgery, no ventilation technique has proved to be clinically superior to any other. Both conventional volume-controlled ventilation and pressure-controlled ventilation have been found to be equally suited for use in patients undergoing laparoscopic gynaecologic surgery. Prophylactic antiemetics should be used to prevent PONV after LC, especially in female patients.

The death rate during operative laparoscopy is 0.1 to 1 per 1000 cases and the incidence of hemorrhage and visceral injury (the most lethal complications of laparoscopic surgery) is 2 to 5 per 1000 cases. Good surgical technique and early recognition and management of such cases are keys to prevent complications due to laparoscopy. Experience and skill of the anaesthesia and surgical teams continue to be key factors to ensure optimal results.

8. References

Andersson, LE; Baath, M; Thorne A; Aspelin, P. & Odeberg- Wernerman, S. (2005). Effect of carbon dioxide pneumoperitoneum on development of atelectasis during anesthesia, examined by spiral computed tomography. *Anesthesiology,* Vol.102, No.2, (February 2005), pp. 293–9, ISSN 0003-3022

Akinci, SB; Ayhan, B; Aycan, IO; Tirnaksiz, B; Basgul, E; Abbasoglu, O; Aypar, U. & Sayek, I. (2008). The postoperative analgesic efficacy of intraperitoneal tramadol compared to normal saline or intravenous tramadol in laparoscopic cholecystectomy. *Eur J Anaesthesiol,* Vol. 25, No. 5, (May 2008) , pp. 375-81. ISSN 0265-0215

Ali, M. & Khan, FA. (2009). Comparison of analgesic effect of tramadol alone and a combination of tramadol and paracetamol in day-care laparoscopic surgery. *Eur J Anaesthesiol.* Vol.26, No 6, (June 2009), pp. 475-9, ISSN 0265-0215

Alishahi, S; Francis, N; Crofts, S; Duncan, L; Bickel, A.& Cuschieri, A. (2001). Central and Peripheral Adverse Hemodynamic Changes During Laparoscopic Surgery and Their Reversal with a Novel Intermittent Sequential Pneumatic Compression Device. *Annals of Surgery.* Vol. 233, No. 2, (February 2001), pp.176–182, ISSN 0003-4932

Almarakbi, WA; Fawzi, HM. & Alhashemi, JA. (2009). Effects of four intraoperative ventilatory strategies on respiratory compliance and gas exchange during laparoscopic gastric banding in obese patients. *Br J Anaesth,* Vol. 102, No. 6, (Jun 2009), pp. 862- 8, ISSN 0007-0912

Artuso, D; Wayne, M; Cassaro, S; Cerabona, T; Teixeira, J. & Grossi, R. (2005). Hemodynamic changes during laparoscopic gastric bypass procedures. *Arch Surg.* Vol.140, No.3, (Mar 2005), pp. 289-92, ISSN 0004-0010

Bablekos GD, Roussou T, Rasmussen T, Vassiliou MP, Behrakis PK. (2003). Postoperative changes on pulmonary function after laparoscopic and open cholecystectomy. *Hepatogastroenterology,* Vol. 50, No.53, pp. 1193-200. ISSN 0172-6390

Branche, PE; Duperret, SL; Sagnard, PE; Boulez, JL; Petit, PL. & Viale, JP. (1998). Left ventricular loading modifications induced by pneumoperitoneum: a time course echocardiography study. *Anesth Analg* . Vol: 86, No. 3, (Mar 1998), pp. 482–87, ISSN 0003-2999

Buttenschoen, K; Tsokos, M. & Schulz, F. (2007). Laparoscopic Cholecystectomy Associated Lethal Hemorrhage. JSLS. Vol.11, No. 1, (Jan–Mar, 2007), pp.101–105, ISSN 1086-8089

Carter, J. & Duh, QY. (2011). Laparoscopic Repair of Inguinal Hernias. *World J Surg.* Mar 12 (2011) [Epub ahead of print]

Catani, M; Guerricchio, R; De Milito, R; Capitano, S; Chiaretti, M; Guerricchio, A; Manili, G. & Simi, M. (2004). Low pressure laparoscopic cholecystectomy in high risk patients - (ASA III and IV): our experience. *Chir Ital.* Vol.56, No.1, (Feb 2004), pp. 71-80, ISSN 0009-4773

Chalhoub, V; Yazigi, A, Sleilaty, G; Haddad, F; Noun, R; Madi-Jebara, S. &Yazbeck, P. (2007). Effect of vital capacity manoeuvres on arterial oxygenation in morbidly obese patients undergoing open bariatric surgery. *Eur J Anaesthesiol;* Vol. 24, No. 3, (Mar 2007), pp. 283- 8, ISSN 0265-0215

Choi, SH; Lee, SJ; Rha, KH; Shin, SK. & Oh, YJ. (2008). The effect of pneumoperitoneum and Trendelenburg position on acute cerebral blood flow–carbon dioxide reactivity under sevoflurane anaesthesia. *Anaesthesia,* Vol: 63, No.12, (Dec 2008), pp. 1314–18, ISSN 0003-2409

Clavien, PA; Sanabria JR. & Strasberg, SM. (1992). Proposed classification of complications of surgery with examples of utility in cholecystectomy. *Surgery;* Vol. 111, No.5, (May 1992), pp. 518–26. ISSN 0039-6060

Coloma, M; Chiu, JW; White, PF. & Armbruster, SC. (2001). The use of esmolol as an alternative to remifentanil during desflurane anesthesiafor fast tract outpatient gynecologic laparoscopic surgery. *Anesth Anal;* Vol. 92, No.2, (Feb 2001), pp. 352- 7, ISSN 0003-2999

Colombo, JR., Haber, GP., & Gill, IS. (2008). Laparoscopic partial nephrectomy in patients with compromised renal function. *Urology.* Vol. 71, No.6, (Jun 2008), pp.1043–8, ISSN 0090-4295

Crane, NJ; Pinto, PA; Hale, D; Gage, FA; Tadaki, D; Kirk, AD; Levin, IW. & Elster EA. (2008). Non-invasive monitoring of tissue oxygenation during laparoscopic donor nephrectomy. *BMC Surg.* Vol. 17, (April 2008), pp.8, ISSN 1471-2482

Critchley, L; Critchley, J. & Gin, T. (1993). Hemodynamic changes in patients undergoing laparoscopic cholecystectomy: measurement by transthoracic electrical bioimpedance. *Br J Anaesth.* Vol: 70, No. 6, (jun 1993), pp. 681–83, ISSN 0007-0912

Dabbous, AS; Jabbour-Khoury, SI; Nasr, VG; Moussa, AA; Zbeidy, RA; Khouzam, NE; El-Khatib, MF. & Baraka, AS. (2010) Dexamethasone with either granisetron or ondansetron for postoperative nausea and vomiting in laparoscopic surgery. *Middle East J Anesthesiol.* Vol.20 , No. 4. (Feb 2010), pp.565-70, ISSN 0544-0440.

Diemunsch, PA; Van Dorsselaer, T; Torp, KD; Schaeffer, R. & Geny, B. (2002). Calibrated pneumoperitoneal venting to prevent N2O accumulation in the CO2 pneumoperitoneum during laparoscopy with inhaled anesthesia: an experimental study in pigs. *Anesth Analg.* Vol. 94, No.4, (Feb 2002), pp. 1014-8, ISSN 0003-2999

Dindo, D; Demartines, N. & Clavien, PA. (2004). Classification of surgical complications: a new proposal with evaluation in a cohort of 6336 patients and results of a survey. *Ann. Surg, Vol.* 240, No. 2, (Aug 2004), pp. 205–13, ISSN 0003-4932

Dumont, L; Mattys, M; Mardirosoff, C; Vervloesem, N; Allé, JL. & Massaut, J. (1997) Changes in pulmonary mechanics during laparoscopic gastroplasty in morbidly obese patients. *Acta Anaesthesiol Scand* Vol. 41, No.3, (Mar 1997), pp. 408 –13, ISSN 0001-5172

Dunham, CM; Sosnowski, C; Porter, JM; Siegal, J. & Kohli, C. (2002). Correlation of noninvasive cerebral oximetry with cerebral perfusion in the severe head injured patients: a pilot study. *J Traum,* Vol: 52, No. 1, (Jan 2002), pp. 225–8, ISSN 1529-8809

El-Dawlatly, AA; Al-Dohayan, A; Abdel-Meguid, ME; El-Bakry, A. & Manaa, EM. (2004). The effects of pneumoperitoneum on respiratory mechanics during general anesthesia for bariatric surgery. *Obes Surg;* Vol.14, No.2, (Feb 2004), pp.212–5, ISSN 1708-0428

Elsamra, S. & Pareek, G. (2010). Complications of laparoscopic renal surgery *International Journal of Urology* Vol.17, No.3, (Mar 2010), pp. 206–14, ISSN 1442-2042

Erhan, Y; Erhan, E; Aydede, H; Yumus, O. & Yentur, A. (2008). Ondansetron, granisetron, and dexamethasone compared for the prevention of postoperative nausea and vomiting in patients undergoing laparoscopic cholecystectomy: A randomized placebo-controlled study. *Surg Endosc.* Vol.22, No. 6, (Jun 2008), pp.1487-92, ISSN 0930-2794

Erol, DD; Yılmaz, S; Polat, C. & Arıkan, Y. (2008). Efficacy of thoracic epidural analgesia for laparoscopic cholecystectomy. *Adv Ther.* Vol.25, No.1, (Jan 2008), pp.45-52, ISSN 0741-238X

Fahy, BG; Hasnain, JU; Flowers, JL; Plotkin, JS. & Odonkor, P. (1999). Transesophageal Echocardiographic Detection of Gas Embolism and Cardiac Valvular Dysfunction During Laparoscopic Nephrectomy. *Anesth Analg,* Vol:88, No.3, (Mar 1999), pp. 500 –4, ISSN 0003-2999

Fujii, Y; Tanaka, H; Tsuruoka, S; Toyooka, H. & Amaha, K. (1994). Middle cerebral arterial blood flow velocity increases during laparoscopic cholecystectomy. *Anesth Analg,* Vol. 78, No.1, (Jan 1994), pp.80–3, ISSN 0003-2999

Fujii, Y. (2011). Management of postoperative nausea and vomiting in patients undergoing laparoscopic cholecystectomy. *Surg Endosc,* Vol. 25, No.3, (Mar 2011), pp. 691-5, ISSN 0930-2794

Fujii, Y. & Itakura, M. (2010). Reduction of postoperative nausea, vomiting, and analgesic requirement with dexamethasone for patients undergoing laparoscopic cholecystectomy. *Surg Endosc,* Vol. 24, No.3, (Mar 2010), pp. 692-6, ISSN 0930-2794

Fujii, Y. (2009). Postoperative nausea and vomiting and their sex differences. *Masui.* Vol. 58, No. 1, (Jan 2009), pp. 59-66 . ISSN:0021-4892

Fujii, Y. (2005). The utility of antiemetics in the prevention and treatment of postoperative nausea and vomiting in patients scheduled for laparoscopic cholecystectomy. *Curr Pharm Des.*Vol. 11, No. 24, pp. 3173-83, ISSN 1381-6128

Futier, E; Constantin, JM; Pelosi, P; Chanques, G; Kwiatkoskwi, F; Jaber, S. & Bazin JE. 2010. Intraoperative Recruitment Maneuver Reverses Detrimental Pneumoperitoneum-induced Respiratory Effects in Healthy Weight and Obese Patients Undergoing Laparoscopy. *Anesthesiology,* Vol. 113, No. 6, (Dec 2010), pp. 1310 -9, ISSN 0003-3022

Gan, TJ; Candiotti, KA; Klein, SM; Rodriguez, Y; Nielsen, KC; White, WD. & Habib, AS. (2009). Double-blind comparison of granisetron, promethazine, or a combination of both for the prevention of postoperative nausea and vomiting in females undergoing outpatient laparoscopies. *Can J Anaesth.* Vol. 56, No. 11, (Nov 2009), pp. 829-36, ISSN 0832-610X

Gannedahl, P; Odeberg, S; Brodin, L. & Sollevi, A. (1996). Effects of posture and pneumoperitoneum during anaesthesia on the indices of left ventricular filling. *Acta Anaesthesiol Scand.* Vol:40, No.2, (Feb 1996), pp.160–166, ISSN 0001-5172

Geraci, G; Sciume, C; Pisello, F; Li Volsi, F; Facella, T. & Modica, G. (2006). Trocar-related abdominal wall bleeding in 200 patients after laparoscopic cholecystectomy: Personal experience. *World J Gastroenterol* Vol.28, No.12, (Dec 2006), pp.7165-7, ISSN 1007-9327

Giaquinto, D; Swigar, K. & Johnson, MD. (2003). Acute congestive heart failure after laparoscopic cholecystectomy: a case report. *AANA J.* Vol.71, No.1, (Feb 2003), pp. 17-22, ISSN 0094-6354

Girardis, M; Broi, U; Antonutto, G. & Pasetto, A. (1996). The effect of laparoscopic cholecystectomy on cardiovascular function and pulmonary gas exchange. *Anesth Analg,* Vol:83, No. 1, (Jul 1996), pp. 134–140, ISSN 0003-2999

Gong, EM; Orvieto, MA; Lyon, MB;, Lucioni, A; Gerber, GS. & Shalhav AL. (2007). Analysis of impact of body mass index on outcomes of laparoscopic renal surgery. *Urology Vol.* 69, No. 1, (Jan 2007), pp. 38–43, ISSN 0090-4295

Gottumukkala, V. (2008). Positioning of Patients for Operation, In *Anesthesiology,* Longnecker DE, 1314-38, The McGrawHill Companies, 0-07-145984-7, New York

Halliwill, JR; Hewitt, SA; Joyner, MJ. & Warner, MA. (1998). Effect of Various Lithotomy Positions on Lower-extremity Blood Pressure. *Anesthesiology,* Vol. 89, No.6, (Dec 1998), pp.1373–76, ISSN 0003-3022

Halverson, A; Buchanan, R; Jacobs, L; Shavani, V; Hunt, T; Riedel, C. & Sackier, J. (1998). Evaluation of mechanism of increased intracranial pressure with insufflation. *Surg Endosc.* Vol: 12, No.3 (Mar 1998), pp. 266–9, ISSN 0930-2794

Harris, S; Ballantyne, G; Luther, M. & Perrino, A. (1996). Alterations of cardiovascular performance during laparoscopic colectomy: a combined hemodynamic and echocardiographic analysis. *Anesth Analg,* Vol: 83, No.3, (Sep 1996), pp.482–487, ISSN 0003-2999

Harrison, GR. (2001). The effect of posture on cerebral oxygenation during abdominal surgery. *Anaesthesia,* Vol.56, No.12, (Dec 2001), pp. 1181–4, ISSN 0003-3022

Haxby, EJ ;Gray, MR; Rodriguez, C; Nott, D; Springall, M. & Mythen M; (1997). Assessment of cardiovascular changes during laparoscopic hernia repair using oesophageal Doppler. *British Journal of Anaesthesia.* Vol :78, No. 5, (may 1997), pp.515-19, ISSN 0007-0912

Hendolin, HI; Pääkönen, ME; Alhava, EM; Tarvainen, R, Kemppinen, T. & Lahtinen, P. (2000). Laparoscopic or open cholecystectomy: a prospective randomised trial to compare postoperative pain, pulmonary function, and stress response. *Eur J Surg.* Vol. 166, No. 5, (May 2000), pp. 394-9, ISSN 1365 -2168

Hernández-Palazón, J; Tortosa, JA; Nuño de la Rosa, V. Gimenez –ViudezJ; Ramirez, G. & Robles R. (2003). Intraperitoneal application of bupivacaine plus morphine for pain relief after laparoscopic cholecystectomy. *Eur J Anaesthesiol.* Vol.20, No.11, (Nov 2003), pp. 891-6, ISSN 0265-0215

Hirvonen, EA; Poikolainen, EO; Pääkkönen, ME. & Nuutinen, LS. (2000). The adverse hemodynamic effects of anesthesia, head-up tilt, and carbon dioxide pneumoperitoneum during laparoscopic cholecystectomy. *Surg Endosc.* Vol. 14, No. 3, (Mar 200), pp.272-7, ISSN 0930-2794

Hirvonen, EA., Nuutinen, LS. & Kauko, M. (1995). Haemodynamic due to Trendelenburg positioning and pneumoperitoneum during laparoscopic hysterectomy. *Acta Anaesthesiol Scand* Vol.39, No.7, (Oct 1995), pp.949–55, ISSN 0001-5172

Huang, MT; Wang, W; Wei, PL; Chen, RJ. & Lee, WJ. (2003) Minilaparoscopic and laparoscopic cholecystectomy: a comparative study. *Arch Surg,* Vol.138, No.9, (Sep 2003), pp. 1017-23, ISSN 0004-0010

Huettemann, E; Terborg, C; Sakka, SG, Petrat, G; Schier, F. & Reinhart, K. (2002). Preserved CO_2 reactivity and increase in middle cerebral arterial blood flow velocity during laparoscopic surgery in children. *Anesth Analg,* Vol. 94, No.2, (Feb 2002), pp. 255–8, ISSN 0003-2999

Ikeya, E; Taguchi, J; Ohta, K; Miyazaki, Y; Hashimoto, O; Yagi1,K; Yamaguchi, M; Inamura S. & Makuuchi, H. (2006). Compartment Syndrome of Bilateral Lower Extremities Following Laparoscopic Surgery of Rectal Cancer in Lithotomy Position: Report of a Case. *Surg Today,* Vol. 36, No.12, (2006), pp.1122–25, ISSN 0941-1291

Ishizaki, Y; Bandai, Y; Shimomura, K; Abe, H ; Ohtoma, H. & Idezuki, Y. (1993). Changes in splanchnic blood flow and cardiovascular effects following peritoneal insufflation of carbon dioxide. *Surg Endosc,* Vol.7, No.3, (Sep 1993), pp. 420–23, ISSN 0930-2794

Imamura, S; Chinzei, M. & Yamada, Y. (2010). Two cases of bilateral upper extremity pareses during laparoscopic colectomy. *Masui*, Vol.59, No.12, (Dec 2010), pp.1494-7, ISSN 0021-4892

Jakimowicz, J; Stultiëns, G. & Smulders, F. (1998). Laparoscopic insufflation of abdomen reduces portal venous flow. *Surg Endosc.* Vol.12, No.2. (Feb 1998), pp.129–132, ISSN 0930-2794

Joris, JL. (2005) Anesthesia for Laparoscopic Surgery , In: *Miller's Anesthesia,* R.D. Miller, (Ed.), 2285-2306, Elsevier, ISBN 0-443-06618-3, Philadephia, USA

Junghans, T; Modersohn, D; Dörner, F; Neudecker, J; Haase, O. & Schwenk, W. (2006). Systematic evaluation of different approaches for minimizing hemodynamic changes during pneumoperitoneum. *Surg Endosc.* (2006), Vol.20, No.5, (May 2006), pp. 763-9, ISSN 0930-2794

Kalmar, AF; Foubert, L; Hendrickx, JF; Mottrie, A; Absalom, A; Mortier, EP. & Struys, MMRF. (2010). Influence of steep Trendelenburg position and CO(2) pneumoperitoneum on cardiovascular, cerebrovascular, and respiratory homeostasis during robotic prostatectomy. *Br J Anaesth.* Vol. 104, No. 4, (Apr 2010), pp. 433-9, ISSN 0007-0912

Kaushik, R. (2010). Bleeding complications in laparoscopic cholecystectomy: Incidence, mechanisms, prevention and management. *J Minim Access Surg.* Vol.6, No.3, (Jul 2010), pp. 59–65, ISSN 0972-9941

Kehlet, H; Gray, AW; Bonnet, F; Camu, F; Fischer, HB; McCloy, RF; Neugebauer, EA; Puig, MM; Rawal, N. & Simanski CJ. (2005). A procedure-specific systematic review and consensus recommendations for postoperative analgesia following laparoscopic cholecystectomy. *Surg Endosc* Vol.19, No.10, (Oct 2005), pp. 1396-415, ISSN 0930-2794

Koivusalo, AM; Pere, P; Valjus, M. & Scheinin T. (2008). Laparoscopic cholecystectomy with carbon dioxide pneumoperitoneum is safe even for high-risk patients. *Surg Endosc.* 2008, Volume. 22, Number 1, (Jan 2008), pp. 61- 7, ISSN 0930-2794

Koning, JL; Nicolay, LI; Jellison, F; Heldt, JP; Dunbar, JA. & Baldwin. DD. (2011). Ocular complications after open and hand-assisted laparoscopic donor nephrectomy. *Urology,* Vol.77, No.1, (Jan 2011), pp. 92-6, ISSN 0090-4295

Kuang, W; Ng, CS; Matin, S; Kaouk, JH; El-Jack, M. & Gill, IS. (2002). Rhabdomyolysis after laparoscopic donor nephrectomy. *Urology,* Vol.60, No.5, (Nov 2002), pp. 911, ISSN 0090-4295

Lee, JR; Lee, PB; Do, SH; Jeon, YT; Lee, JM; Hwang, JY. & Han, SH. (2006). The effect of gynaecological laparoscopic surgery on cerebral oxygenation. *J Int Med Res,* Vol. 34, No.5, (Sep- Oct 2006), pp. 531-6, ISSN 1473-2300

Leonard, IE. & Cunningham, AJ.(2002). Anaesthetic considerations for laparoscopic cholecystectomy. *Best Pract Res Clin Anaesthesiol,* Vol.16, No.1, (Mar 2002), pp. 1-20, ISSN 1521-6896.

Levy, BF; Tilney, HS; Dowson, HM. & Rockall, TA. (2010). A systematic review of postoperative analgesia following laparoscopic colorectal surgery. *Colorectal Dis.* Vol.12, No.1, (Jan 2010), pp. 5-15, ISSN 1462-8910

Maracaja-Neto, LF; Verçosa, N; Roncally, AC; Giannella, A; Bozza, FA. & Lessa, MA. (2009). Beneficial effects of high positiveend-expiratory pressure in lung respiratory mechanics during laparoscopic surgery. *Acta Anaesthesiol Scand,* Vol. 53, No.2, (Feb 2009), pp. 210 -7, ISSN 0001-5172

Mavrocordatos, P; Bissonnette, B. & Ravussin, P. (2000). Effects of neck position and head elevation on intracranial pressure in anesthetized neurosurgical patients. *J Neurosurg Anesthesiol,* Vol.12, No.1, (Jan 2000), pp. 10–4, ISSN 0898- 4921

McCloy, R; Randall, D; Schug, SA; Kehlet, H; Simanski, C; Bonnet, F; Camu, F; Fischer, B; Joshi, G; Rawal, N. & Neugebauer, EA. (2008). Is smaller necessarily better? A systematic review comparing the effects of minilaparoscopic and conventional laparoscopic cholecystectomy on patient outcomes. *Surg Endosc,* Vol.22, No.12, (Dec 2008), pp. 2541-53, ISSN 0930-2794

Meininger,. D; Westphal, K; Bremerich, DH; Runkel, H; Probst, M; Zwissler, B. & Byhahn, C. (2008). Effects of posture and prolonged pneumoperitoneum on hemodynamic parameters during laparoscopy. *World J Surg,* Vol.32, No.7, (Jul 2008), pp.1400-5, ISSN 0364-2313

Meininger, D; Zwissler, B; Byhahn, C; Probst, M; Westphal, K. & Bremerich, DH. (2006). Impact of overweight and pneumoperitoneum on hemodynamics and oxygenation during prolonged laparoscopic surgery. *World J Surg,* Vol.30, No. 4, (Apr 2006), pp. 520-6, ISSN 0364-2313

Meininger, D; Byhahn, C; Mierdl, S; Westphal, K. & Zwissler, B. (2005). Positive end-expiratory pressure improves arterial oxygenation during prolonged pneumoperitoneum. *Acta Anaesthesiol Scand,* Vol. 49, No.6, (Jul 2005), pp. 778–83, ISSN 0001-5172

Mentes, O; Harlak, A; Yigit, T; Balkan, A; Balkan, M; Cosar, A; Savaser, A; Kozak, O. & Tufan, T. (2008). Effect of intraoperative magnesium sulphate infusion on pain relief after laparoscopic cholecystectomy. *Acta Anaesthesiol Scand,* Vol.52, No.10, (Nov 2008), pp. 1353-9, ISSN 0001-5172

Millard, JA; Hill, BB; Cook, PS; Fenoglio, ME. & Stahlgren, LH. (1993). Intermittent sequential pneumatic compression in prevention of venous stasis associated with pneumoperitoneum during laparoscopic cholecystectomy. *Arch Surg,* Vol:28, No.8, (Aug 1993), pp. 914-8, ISSN 0004-0010

Mizuno, J; Yonenaga, K; Arita, H. & Hanaoka, K. (2008). Right median nerve injury following laparoscopic sigmoidectomy. *Masui.* Vol.57, No.6, (Jun 2008), pp. 752-5, ISSN 0021-4892

Morgan, M; Smith, N; Thomas, K. & Murphy, DG. (2009). Is Clavien the new standard for reporting urological complications? *Br. J. Urol,* Vol.104, No.4, (Aug 2009), pp. 436–6, ISSN 1365-2176

Nguyen, NT. & Wolfe, BM. (2005). The physiologic effects of pneumoperitoneum in the morbidly obese. *Ann Surg,* Vol. 241, No. 2, (Feb 2005), pp. 219 -26, ISSN 0003-4932

Nguyen, NT; Anderson, JT; Budd, M; Fleming, NW; Ho, HS; Jahr, J; Stevens, CM. &Wolfe, BM. (2004). Effects of pneumoperitoneum on intraoperative pulmonary mechanics and gas exchange during laparoscopic gastric bypass. *Surg Endosc,* Vol. 18, No.1, (Jan 2004), pp. 64-71, ISSN 0930-2794

Nicholson, ML., Elwell, R., Kaushik, M., Bagul, A. & Hosgood, SA. (2011) Health-related quality of life after living donor nephrectomy: a randomized controlled trial of laparoscopic versus open nephrectomy. *Transplantation.* Vol.91, No.4, (Feb 2011), pp. 457-61, ISSN 1534-0608

Odeberg, S; Ljungqvist, O; Svenberg, T; Gannedahl, P; Bäckdahl, M; von Rosen, A. & Sollevi, A. (1994). Haemodynamic effects of pneumoperitoneum and the influence of posture during anaesthesia for laparoscopic surgery. *Acta Anaesthesiol Scand,* Vol:38. No. 3, (Apr 1994), pp. 276–83, ISSN 0001-5172

Oğurlu, M; Küçük, M; Bilgin, F; Sizlan, A; Yanarateş, O; Eksert, S; Karaşahin, E & Coşar A. (2010). Pressure-controlled vs volume- controlled ventilation during laparoscopic gynecologic surgery. *J Minim Invasive Gynecol.* Vol.17, No.3, (May- Jun 2010), pp.295-300, ISSN 1553-4650

Osman, Y; Fusun, A; Serpil, A; Umit, T; Ebru, M; Bulent, U; Mete, D. & Omer, C. (2009).The comparison of pulmonary functions in open versus laparoscopic cholecystectomy. *J Pak Med Assoc,* Vol.59, No.4, (Apr 2009), pp. 201-4, ISSN 0030-9982

Pandey, R; Garg, R; Darlong, V; Punj, J; Chandralekha, & Kumar A. (2010). Unpredicted neurological complications after robotic laparoscopic radical cystectomy and ileal conduit formation in steep trendelenburg position: two case reports. *Acta Anaesthesiol Belg,* Vol.61, No.3, pp.163-6, ISSN 0001-5164

Pareek, G; Hedican, SP; Bishoff, JT; Shichman, SJ; Wolf, JS Jr. & Nakada, SY. (2005). Survey from skills-based hands on learning courses demonstrates increased laparoscopic caseload and clinical laparoscopic suturing. *Urology,* Vol.66, No.3, pp. 271–3. ISSN 0090-4295

Park, EY; Koo, BN; Mın, KT. & Nam, SH. (2009). The effect of pneumoperitoneum in the steep Trendelenburg position on cerebral oxygenation. *Acta Anaesthesiol Scand,* Vol.53, No.7, (Aug 2009), pp. 895–899, ISSN 0001-5172

Porzionato, A; Macchi, V; Fenato, F; Parenti, A. & De Caro, RJ. (2008). Femoral nerve injury after gynecologic laparoscopy *Minim Invasive Gynecol,* Vol.15, No.1, (Jan- Feb 2008), pp. 105-7, ISSN 1553-4650

Phillips, PA. & Amaral, JF. (2001). Abdominal access complications in laparoscopic surgery. *J Am Coll Surg,* Vol.192, No.4, (April 2001), pp.525–36, ISSN 1072-7515

Planells Roig, M; Arnal Bertomeu, C; Cervera Delgado, M; Garcia Espinosa, R; Sanahuja Santafé, A. & Carrau Giner, M. (2011). Pain, analgesic consumption and daily life activities recovery in patients undergoing ambulatory totally extra-peritoneal laparoscopic inguinal hernioplasty versus ambulatory Lichtenstein hernioplasty. *Cir Esp,* Apr 8. Epub ahead of print. ISSN 1131-0898

Rist, M; Hemmerling, TM; Rauh, R; Siebzehnrübl, E. & Jacobi, KE. (2001) Influence of pneumoperitoneum and patient positioning on preload and splanchnic blood volume in laparoscopic surgery of the lower abdomen. *J Clin Anesth.* Vol. 13, No.4, (Jun 2001), pp. 244-9, ISSN 1873-4529

Russoa, A; Maranaa ,E; Vivianib, D, Polidoria, L; Coliccia, S; Mettimanob, M; Proiettia, R. & Di Stasioc, E. (2009). Diastolic function: the influence of pneumoperitoneum and Trendelenburg positioning during laparoscopic hysterectomy. *Eur J Anaesth,* Vol.26, No.11, pp. 923–927, ISSN 0265-0215

Salihoglu, Z; Demiroluk, S. & Dikmen, Y. (2003). Respiratory mechanics in morbid obese patients with chronic obstructive pulmonary disease and hypertension during pneumoperitoneum. *Eur J Anaesthesiol,* Vol.20, No.8, (Aug 2003), pp. 658-61, ISSN 0265-0215

Schwenk, W; Böhn, B; Fügener, A. & Müller, JM. (1998). Intermittent pneumatic sequential compression (ISC) of the lower extremities prevents venous stasis during laparoscopic cholecystectomy. *Surg Endosc,* Vol:12, No.1, (Jan 1998), pp. 7–1, ISSN 0930-2794

Slodzinski, M. & Merritt, WT. (2008). Anesthesia for Gastrointestinal Surgery, In *Anesthesiology,* D.E. Longnecker, (Ed.), 1314-38, The McGrawHill Companies, ISBN 0-07-145984-7, New York, USA

Sprung, J; Whalley, DG; Falcone, T; Wilks, W; Navratil, JE. & Bourke, DL. (2003). The effects of tidal volume and respiratory rate on oxygenation and respiratory mechanics during laparoscopy in morbidly obese patients. *Anesth Analg,* Vol.97, No.1, (Jul 2003), pp. 268-74, ISSN 0003-2999

Strang, CM; Hachenberg, T; Frede´n, F. & Hedenstierna, G. (2009). Development of atelectasis and arterial to end-tidal PCO2- difference in a porcine model of pneumoperitoneum. *Br J Anaesth,* Vol.103, No.2, (Aug 2009), pp. 298–303, ISSN 0007-0912

Takahata, O; Kunisawa, T; Nagashima, M; Mamiya, K; Sakurai, K; Fujita, S; Fujimoto, K. & Iwasaki, H. (2007). Effect of age on pulmonary gas exchange during laparoscopy in the Trendelenburg lithotomy position. *Acta Anaesthesiol Scand,* Vol.51, No.6, (Jul 2007), pp. 687-92, ISSN 0001-5172

Talab, HF; Zabani, IA; Abdelrahman, HS; Bukhari, WL; Mamoun, I; Ashour, MA; Sadeq, BB. & El Sayed, SI. (2009). Intraoperative ventilatory strategies for prevention of pulmonary atelectasis in obese patients undergoing laparoscopic bariatric surgery. *Anesth Analg,* Vol. 109, No. 5, (Nov 2009), pp. 1511–6, ISSN 0003-2999

Taqi, A; Hong, X; Mistraletti, G; Stein, B; Charlebois, P. & Carli, F. (2007). Thoracic epidural analgesia facilitates the restoration of bowel function and dietary intake in patients undergoing laparoscopic colon resection using a traditional, nonaccelerated, perioperative care program. *Surg Endosc.* Vol. 21, No.2, (Feb 2009), pp. 247-52, ISSN 0930-2794

Vallancien, G; Cathelineau, X; Baumert, H; Doublet, JD. & Guillonneau, B. (2002). Complications of transperitoneal laparoscopic surgery in urology: review of 1,311 procedures at a single center. *J. Urol,* Vol. 168, No. 1, (Jul 2002), pp. 23–6, ISSN 0022-5347

Volpino, P; Cangemi, V; D'Andrea, N; Cangemi, B. & Piat, G. (1998). Hemodynamic and pulmonary changes during and after laparoscopic cholecystectomy. *SurgEndosc,* Vol.12, No. 2, (Feb 1998), pp. 119–123, ISSN 0930-2794

Watanabe M, Shimizu H & Kikuchi C. (2009). Anesthetic management with remifentanil infusion during laparoscopic cholecystectomy. *Masui, The Japanese journal of anesthesiology,* Vol.58, No.10, (Oct 2009), pp.1232-5, ISSN 0021-4892

Whalen, FX; Gajic, O; Thompson, GB; Kendrick, ML; Que, FL; Williams, BA; Joyner, MJ; Hubmayr, RD; Warner, DO. & Sprung, J. (2006). The effects of the alveolar recruitment maneuver and positive end-expiratory pressure on arterial oxygenation during laparoscopic bariatric surgery. *Anesth Analg,* Vol.102, No.1, (Jan 2006), pp. 298–305, ISSN 0003-2999

White PF. (2008). Multimodal analgesia: its role in preventing postoperative pain. *Curr Opin Investig Drugs.* Vol. 9, No.1, (Jan 2008), pp. 76-82, ISSN 2040-3429

Westerband, A; Van De Water, J; Amzallag, M; Lebowitz, PW; Nwasokwa, ON; Chardavoyne, R; Abou-Taleb, A; Wang, X. & Wise, L. (1992). Cardiovascular changes during laparoscopic cholecystecotmy. *Surg Gynecol Obstet,* Vol.175, No.6, (Dec 1992), pp. 535–538, ISSN 0039-6087.

Wittgen, CM; Andrus, CH; Fitzgerald, SD; Baudendistel, LJ. & Dahms, TE. (1991). Analysis of the Hemodynamic and Ventilatory Effects of Laparoscopic Cholecystectomy *Arch Surg.* Vol.26, No.8, (Aug 1991), pp. 997-1001, ISSN 0004-0010

Wongyingsinn, M; Baldini, G; Charlebois, P; Liberman, S; Stein, B. & Carli, F. (2011). Intravenous lidocaine versus thoracic epidural analgesia: a randomized controlled trial in patients undergoing laparoscopic colorectal surgery using an enhanced recovery program. *Reg Anesth Pain Med,* Vol.36, No.3, (May-Jun 2011), pp. 241-8, ISSN 1098-7339

2

Laparoscopy in Children and Infants

Ngozi Joy Nwokoma[1] and Thomas Tsang[2]
[1]Addenbrooke's Hospital, Cambridge
[2]Norfolk and Norwich University Hospital
United Kingdom

1. Introduction

The *"first do no harm"* ethics of medical care has its age-long influence manifested in the continual search for the least invasive method of administering treatment to the patient. The advancement of the minimally invasive surgery has therefore been a very welcome development in surgical specialities with paediatric surgery not left behind in this quest.

Laparoscopy is the visual inspection of the peritoneal cavity aided by a telescope and facilitated by the creation of a pneumoperitoneum. The earliest description of diagnostic laparoscopy was by Cortesi et al., (1976). However, diagnostic laparoscopy was originally introduced in 1910 by the Swedish physician - Hans Christian Jacobeus who published his results from diagnostic laparoscopy and thoracoscopic procedures (Badani et al., 2006). Therapeutic laparoscopy was made popular following the description of laparoscopic appendicectomy by a German gynaecologist - Kurt Semm in 1983 (Semm, 1983) and of laparoscopic cholecysytectomy by the German surgeon - Erich Muhe in 1985 (Badani et al., 2006). Advancements in development of instrument components particularly illumination, optics, fiberoptic transmission, insufflation and video-apparatus have progressed alongside development of techniques for minimal access into the abdominal cavity. Development of paediatric laparoscopy was marked by Gans in his contribution to the development of paediatric instruments in 1970 (Tantoco et al., 2005).

Laparoscopy offers the surgeon the option of achieving high standard surgical treatment while keeping tissue trauma to a minimum. Since the early 20th century, laparoscopic approach to surgical treatment has gained increasing popularity. However, the paediatric surgical subspecialty has lagged behind adult surgery in exploring the advances offered by laparoscopy. This is largely because some common conditions in adults like cholelithiasis which opened the gateway to the explosion in the application of laparoscopic surgery are uncommon in the paediatric age group. In addition, the low volume of corresponding conditions in the paediatric population has made it unattractive to companies involved in manufacturing and developing the paediatric laparoscopic equipment. For example, laparoscopic cholecystectomy which is a relatively non-complex procedure developed faster in the adult population than in children because of the lower case volume in the latter. Higher case volume equates to higher demand which attracts investors. The converse being the case in the paediatric population has hindered enthusiasm among product developers.

Development of laparoscopy in the paediatric population has followed the same course as the development and modification of the laparoscopic apparatus to fit this patient group. Advances in paediatric anaesthetic monitoring and support equipment have also made a huge contribution to this development. The result is an increasingly wider application to the use of laparoscopy in children. Jen and Shew (2010) observed an increase in the utilization of laparoscopy for the management of appendicitis in children from 18.6% in 1999 to 52.4% in 2006. Several diagnostic and therapeutic procedures have been demonstrated to be safely and efficiently undertaken with laparoscopy with several advantages over traditional methods of approach.

The development of 3mm instruments has pushed the boundaries of diagnostic, as well as therapeutic laparoscopy into the infant and neonatal population. In the investigation of the neonate with abdominal distension, free gas on plain abdominal radiograph in the absence of corresponding clinical or physiological signs of peritonism, laparoscopy has been used to evaluate the condition and arrive at more focused specific management decisions with improved outcome. In our experience an uncommon case of neonatal perforated appendicitis was diagnosed and treated at laparoscopy with quick recovery and discharge home within 48hours. Should the same neonate have had laparotomy for presumed bowel perforation from unknown cause with the consequent greater degree of bowel handling, resultant postoperative ileus and high doses of opiate, recovery would have been slower with longer duration of hospitalisation.

Many procedures can be performed safely in children through small incisions, for example the repair of inguinal hernia. This has contributed to the reluctance of paediatric surgeons to embrace the laparoscopic approach. However, better access, panoramic visual field, quick recovery and reduced complication rates still put laparoscopy ahead in these procedures.

2. Advantages of paediatric laparoscopy

There is growing evidence that laparoscopy has more advantages and benefits to offer children than was earlier presumed to be the case. These benefits have been widely reported (Table 1) and significantly outweigh any concerns regarding the technical difficulties (Table 2) which are largely overcome with increasing experience and further developments in the laparoscopic equipment.

Reduced wound size
Reduced wound trauma
Less wound infection
Less incisional hernia
Less wound dehiscence
Less wound pain
Early mobilisation
Less bleeding
Less heat loss from tissue
Wider field of vision
Less postoperative adhesions
Less postoperative ileus
Earlier return to usual activities
Earlier commencement of chemotherapy
Less respiratory complications
Less risk of thromboembolism
Reduction in nerve entrapment

Table 1. Advantages of laparoscopy

Loss of tactile sensation
Loss of spatial and depth orientation
Two-dimensional imaging
Difficulty with control of bleeding
Difficulty with extraction of resected tissue

Table 2. Technical difficulties of laparoscopy

Some of these benefits have been published in our publications (Rehman et al., 2010; Panteli et al., 2009; Nwokoma et al., 2009a, Nwokoma et al., 2009b). The age-long principles of safe surgery include adequate access, adequate target organ visualisation and minimal tissue trauma. In children, access can be quite a challenge because of the smaller height/width ratio of the abdomen particularly observed in those under 7 years of age. In many cases, however long the incision, gaining access to the target organ, or indeed to the four quadrants of the abdomen and pelvis, can be very difficult. Laparoscopy offers the paediatric surgeon the advantage of been able to visualise these areas while reducing the trauma usually consequent upon use of large abdominal wall incisions. In conventional or open surgery, access is also facilitated by the use of retractors. The purpose built retractors for the abdominal wall have meant the junior trainees can be spared the arduous task of holding retractors for prolonged periods of time. Despite these, quite often a trainee or two are required to further improve access by using less heavy retractors at different stages of an abdominal operation. In children, particularly infants, this challenge is heightened by the fact that the small size precludes access and space for more than one surgeon to be actively involved from any one side of the patient.

In the repair of paediatric inguinal hernia, laparoscopy offers significant advantage over conventional methods. There is a clear visualisation of the vas deferens and testicular vessels with reduction in the risk of injury to these structures. Following reduction of an incarcerated hernia when the cord tissues are oedematous and friable with higher risk of complications, laparoscopic approach offers a safer alternative with the added benefit of inspection of reduced structures. The senior author's experience of recurrence following laparoscopic repair of inguinal hernia is less than 1%. On the other hand, the reported overall recurrence rate in children following open hernia repair is 0.3 – 3.8% and up to 8.6% in neonates (Morecroft et al., 1993; Nagraj et al., 2006; Parkinson & Pierro, 2006). Laparoscopic approach to inguinal hernia repair also allows the assessment of the contralateral side and closure of any patent processus vaginalis. This is particularly important for infants in whom the rate of synchronous hernia discovered during laparoscopy is up to 40%. Though there is no clear evidence on how many of these will eventually manifest as clinical hernia, repair of a patent processus vaginalis discovered intra-operatively is highly recommended. This is due to the fact that documented risk of metachronous hernia is 10% in children under 2years and up to 68% in infants (Parkinson & Pierro, 2006). Some cases of hernia can present unusual challenges which are best tackled laparoscopically. Interestingly, Lee and Dubois (2000) noted a case of recurrent inguinal hernia following laparoscopic herniotomy to be due to a direct hernia. The laparoscopic approach facilitated appropriate diagnosis and treatment, avoiding the unnecessary exploration for a presumed recurrent patent processus vaginalis. In another case, we found a male infant with bilateral inguinal hernia to have rudimentary female internal sex organs; in such cases, laparoscopy is highly valuable. In addition, the senior author reported the first case of emergency laparoscopic repair of Amyand's hernia in an 8-week-old infant (Rehman et al., 2010).

For many years paediatric surgeons argued about the safety, efficiency and cost implications of laparoscopy. With the development of experience and equipment, the laparoscopic

approach has been demonstrated to be a safe, cost-effective and efficient way of managing increasingly complex procedures in children. We demonstrated that laparoscopic approach offered significant advantages with better outcomes than open approach in paediatric advanced appendicitis with less wound-related complications: 8.6% versus 17.6% (Nwokoma et al., 2009a). In a different study, we also demonstrated that the risk of developing post-operative adhesions was much less following laparoscopic procedures than open approach, with a rate of adhesions comparable to those who have never had any abdominal surgery; 10% versus 10-28% (Nwokoma et al., 2009b).
Trauma resulting from establishing access to the abdominal cavity contributes greatly to postoperative pain, delayed recovery, delayed discharge, respiratory complications and delayed return to usual activity. This is minimised by laparoscopy with corresponding advantages. The old assumption that neonates had impaired perception of pain and physiological response has been set aside in light of evidence to the contrary (Anand et al., 1985; Anand & Hickey, 1987; Anand & Aynsley-Green, 1988). As in older children neonatal post-operative pain is also minimised by laparoscopy while the children are spared the need for strong analgesia, risk of over sedation and respiratory depression to which younger infants are particularly susceptible.

3. Laparoscopic procedures in children

Some surgical procedures that have been safely and efficiently accomplished through laparoscopic approach in children are enumerated in anatomical and regional groups below.

3.1 Upper gastrointestinal tract

Ladd's procedure for intestinal malrotation
Pylomyotomy
Fundoplication
Reduction of intussusception
Gastrostomy tube insertion
Jejunostomy
Heller myotomy
Treatment of duodenal atresia
Treatment of Jejunal atresia
Intestinal duplication cyst
Torsion of appendix epiploicae
Adhesiolysis
Mesenteric cyst resection
Resection of Meckel's diverticulum
Inflammatory bowel
Repair of post-traumatic gastric perforation
Repair of post-traumatic duodenal perforation

3.2 Lower gastrointestinal tract

Appendicectomy
Antegrade continence enema
Laparoscopy assisted endorectal pullthrough procedure

3.3 Abdominal wall defects
Egigastric hernia repair
Umbilical hernia repair
Inguinal hernia repair
Femoral hernia repair

3.4 Solid Intra-abdominal organs
Splenectomy
Deroofing of liver cyst
Laparoscopic Kasai portoenterostomy
Pancreatic biopsy
Liver biopsy
Abdominal cystic masses
Adrenal gland biopsy
Adrenal gland excision
Excision of intra-abdominal neuroblastoma
Excision of hepatoblastoma
Excision of intra-abdominal extralobar pulmonary sequestration
Partial pancreatectomy
Splenic cyst resection
Cholecystectomy
Cholecystotomy

3.5 Gynaecologic
Ovarian cystectomy
Ovarian detorsion
Oophorectomy
Diagnostic laparoscopy for chronic abdominal pain

3.6 Urology
Laparoscopy for impalpable testis
Fowler Stephen's stage 1 orchidopexy
Ligation of varicocele
Renal biopsy
Ureteral implanatation,
Mitrofanoff appendicovesicostomy,
Bladder augmentation
Pyeloplasty
Nephroureterectomy
Heminephrectomy
Placement of dialysis catheter

4. Physiological considerations

4.1 The cardiovascular system
Potentially, pneumoperitoneum could result in reduction in cardiac filling with resultant reduction in cardiac output by compression of the veins running across the abdominal

cavity. This may result in increase in systemic vascular resistance with reduction in blood flow to the renal vasculature. Gómez et al (2005) noted anuria in 88% of children less than 1 year-old during laparoscopic procedure and oliguria in 32% of those above 1 year of age. This was found to be completely reversible within 5 to 6 hours after the surgery with no significant associated reduction in renal blood flow or rise in serum creatinine and urea levels. For this reason, intra-operative urine output in children undergoing laparoscopic procedures is not a reliable indicator of intravascular volume or need for intravenous therapy until 5 hours after surgery.

With good cardiac reserve in the absence of underlying cardiac or coronary artery or vascular disease, children respond well to the stress of pneumoperitoneum on the circulatory system. Therefore problematic rise in heart rate and blood pressure changes in this population are rare. To keep these physiological changes to a minimum, the lowest intra-abdominal pressure required to carry out the procedure safely is recommended: between 5 - 8mmHg in the newborn, 10 - 12mmHg in infants and less than 15mmHg in older children. Flow rate for insufflation of carbon dioxide ranges from 1 to 5L/min.

The longer operating times associated with many laparoscopic procedures, means longer period of cardiovascular stress. The reverse Trendelenburg position of 10-15degrees often used to facilitate laparoscopy of the upper abdomen may also reduce venous return and preload with consequent reduction in cardiac output and tissue perfusion. Applying the minimal intra-abdominal pressure required for adequate access and visualisation of the target organ and operating field avoids the reduced cardiac output, impairment of distal limb perfusion, tissue hypopefusion and resultant reperfusion injury.

4.2 Respiratory system

Pneumoperitoneum leads to diaphragmatic splinting and upward displacement into the thoracic cavity. This in turn leads to a reduction in compliance of the thoracic cage and lung tissue, reduction in the functional residual capacity and tidal volume as well as a rise in the peak pressure required to aerate the bronchoalveolar system. The carbon dioxide used for pneumoperitoneum is cheap, non-combustible, highly soluble with little risk of causing gas embolism. It diffuses easily into the general circulation and needs to be eliminated via the lungs. There are concerns about other gases which could be used for insufflation. Nitrous oxide may cause explosion while helium is linked with a higher risk of gas embolism and subcutaneous emphysema and argon may cause cardiac depression (Fingerhut et al., 2005). The pressure on ventilation from the pneumoperitoneum as stated above may make the respiratory system inefficient at this resulting in hypercarbia and respiratory acidosis. The Trendelenburg position often used to facilitate laparoscopy of the lower abdomen/pelvis further contributes to diaphragmatic elevation.

The elimination of carbon dioxide during and immediately after insufflation with carbon dioxide in children is age and size dependent with the younger and smaller children eliminating more carbon dioxide than older children. The reason for this is not clear but is thought to be because of the different characteristics of their peritoneal surface (McHoney et al, 2003). However, this did not result in any clinically evident effect on the cardiovascular or respiratory system. For this reason, more careful observation is recommended in smaller children during and immediately following laparoscopic procedures. Pacilli et al (2006) demonstrated that in children after 10 -12mins of laparoscopy, 10-20% of expired carbondioxide derived from absorption of exogenous carbon dioxide and continues to be eliminated for up to 30minutes after the end of insufflation. Minute ventilation needs to be

adjusted in order to avoid hypercarbia.. McHoney et al (2003) observed the elimination of carbon dioxide in children to be age-dependent.
The short trachea in children increases the risk of endobronchial intubation. The tip of the tracheal tube has been observed to have a tendency to be displaced caudally with the cranial displacement of lung tissue and carina during the establishment of pneumoperitoneum. This risk is greater when the head up Trendelenburg tilt is employed to facilitate laparoscopy of the upper aspect of the abdominal cavity (Böttcher-Haberzeth et al, 2007). Prior discussion with the anaesthetic team will enable appropriate choice of tube, depth of endotracheal tube placement and degree of neck extension required to prevent this complication.

5. Anatomic considerations

Safe and efficient laparoscopy relies heavily on good apparatus and expertise but also on appropriate placement of telescope and instruments. Infants have a relatively shorter and wider abdominal cavity than do older children. This anatomic variation usually exists up to the age of seven years. In addition, the abdominal wall thickness is often moderate and requires careful choice of placement of ports to allow as much space as possible for safe and effective laparoscopy. The urinary bladder is often an abdominal organ in infants and young children. It will need to be emptied by expression with gentle compression pressure on the lower abdomen or by use of a urethral catheter. To maximise the space, a nasogastric tube is often inserted and intermittently aspirated to decompress the stomach. Some surgeons give aperients to the children to empty intestinal contents 24 to 48hours before laparoscopic surgery to minimise interference with surgery and optimise the space within the abdominal cavity. The relatively higher body surface/ mass ratio in infants means they have a delicate fluid balance which is easily stressed and put under pressure by evaporation of body fluids from exposure of abdominal contents at laparotomy. This is minimized by the laparoscopic approach and modification of laparoscopic equipment is on-going to further limit any drying effect the gas and light may exert on abdominal viscera. As mentioned above, the short trachea in children, particularly in young infants, needs careful consideration during the entire length of the procedure especially where special positioning is required.

6. Anaesthetic considerations

Laparoscopic procedures commonly take longer to perform than their conventional open counterparts. This means prolonged neuromuscular blockade/paralysis. The intubation of the patient has to be skilfully administered to avoid intraluminal gaseous distension and the consequent impairment of visualisation. To minimise this, limited use of the bag and mask is recommended as well as immediate decompression of the stomach by use of a nasogastric tube. The positioning of the patient may require the patient being at the end of the bed and far from the anaesthetic machine. This will need long length apparatus and connectors to intravenous access lines to facilitate management of anaesthetic requirements intraoperatively. The endotracheal tube is preferable to the laryngeal mask or facial mask ventilation as it leads to less risk of distension of stomach and bowel which would limit view and make surgery more difficult. The orientation and length of tubing should allow appropriate patient positioning. Adequate patient relaxation through out the duration of surgery is required to allow lower pressures to be used for adequate pneumoperitoneum.

Communication between team members is crucial to enable the anaesthetist interpret haemodynamic changes appropriately.

7. Surgical planning

7.1 Preoperative assessment

This is crucial in all children in preparation for a laparoscopic procedure. This can be as a formal assessment in a dedicated preoperative assessment clinic led by experienced paediatric surgeons with easy access to paediatric anaesthetist and paediatrician or informally in the outpatients' clinic when the decision to undertake the procedure is made. The anaesthetic team would need to be informed if any potential cardiovascular/ respiratory problems are anticipated. The child's suitability for laparoscopy by way of respiratory and cardiovascular status as well as suitability regarding skin condition at proposed site of access and situations which may make access to the abdominal cavity greatly limited. For example severe kyphoscoliosis may make laparoscopy quite challenging or impossible, and this needs to be addressed during the preoperative assessment.

7.2 Informed consent

Parents or carers with parental responsibility for the child need to be appropriately informed in the relevant aspects of the laparoscopic procedure. The indication for surgery as well as other treatment options, risks and complications - both general and specific to the child's condition and expected outcome need to be discussed. The possible risk of conversion to an open procedure needs to be discussed in most cases to deal with complications or to facilitate safe undertaking of the procedure.

7.3 Equipment

Availability of essential equipment should be checked before the day of surgery. In our institute, this is usually done by way of distributing the operating list to theatre coordinating department who would then arrange for the appropriate equipment to be available on the day. Some special apparatus may need to be ordered several weeks ahead. On the day of the surgery, every equipment required must be carefully checked by the surgeon with the support of the theatre staff. A set of equipment required for open approach for the procedure must also be available for use in the event of need for conversion.

7.4 Positioning

Careful positioning of the equipment and staff to achieve optimal access to the patient is crucial to successful laparoscopy. Examples are given in Figures 1 and 2. The position must allow adequate exposure of the patient and safe access to the operating field. The recommended alignment is to have the monitor, operating surgeon and the patient or target organ in a straight line.

It is preferable to have two monitors to serve the operating surgeon and his or her assistant separately; this is standard for most operating rooms today. The position of other staff members including the surgeon's assistant, scrub nurse and anaesthetist depends on where the operating surgeon is positioned. The position of the patient depends on the target organ for the procedure. Supine position can be applied to a good number of the procedures. A Trendelenburg position may be preferred for pelvic laparoscopy and a reverse Trendelenburg position for upper abdominal laparoscopy to visualise the diaphragm and its

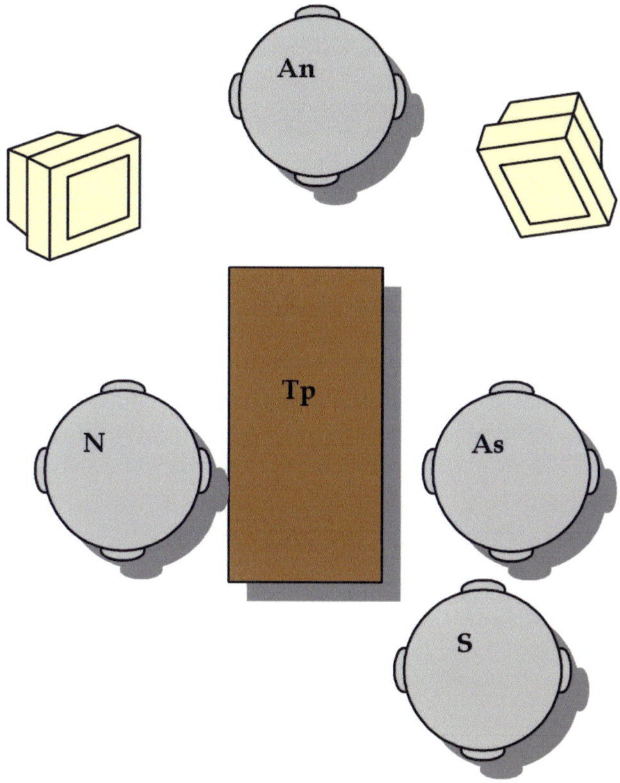

Fig. 1. Operative positioning for laparoscopic appendicectomy. S: surgeon, As: surgeon's assistant, N: scrub nurse, An: anaesthetist, Tp: table with patient. Two monitors are shown on either side of the anaesthetist.

apertures or any hernia present, stomach and liver. A lateral tilt position may be required for splenic or renal and retroperitoneal organs. In all cases, appropriate care must be taken to avoid pressure area injury to the patient and the use of gel-filled flexible or rigid moulds or support apparatus needs to be considered. Adhesive material may be needed to further secure the patient in the desired position.

7.5 Port insertion

The open Hasson's technique for the insertion of the primary port is almost exclusively applied by most paediatric surgeons having been shown to be associated with fewer complications than the Veress' needle. The centre of the umbilicus is commonly used for this purpose. Particular care should be taken if there is a history of previous abdominal surgery. Secondary ports should be inserted under direct visual control with the camera. The 5mm port is often used in most cases; the 10mm port may be suitable for older children whose periumbilical region can accommodate this without excessive scarring. Secondary port size would vary according to nature of procedure. For repair of inguinal hernia, the instrument may be introduced directly through a 2-3mm opening in the skin. The depth of insertion of the port should be such as allows space for the instrument to be inserted and manoeuvred while allowing for the port to be anchored to the abdominal wall. Various methods are used

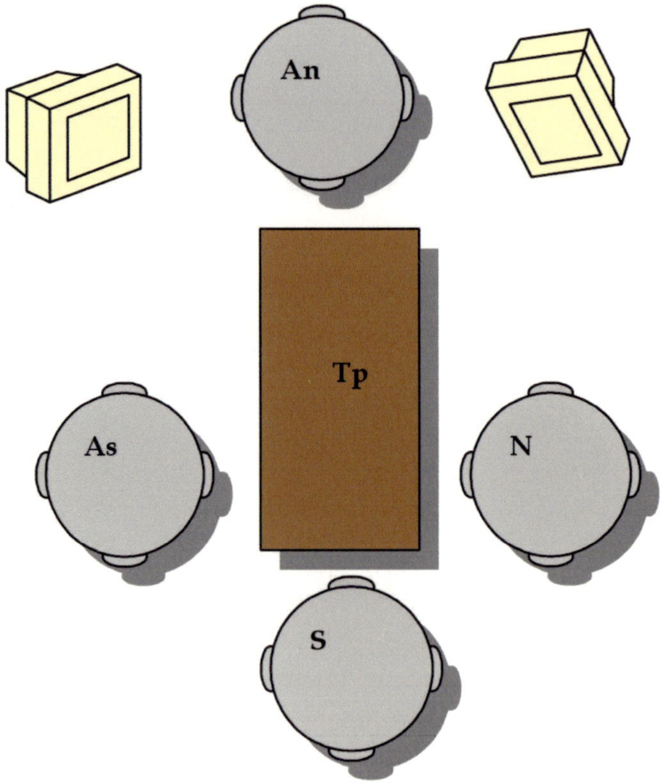

Fig. 2. Operative positioning for laparoscopic fundoplication. S: surgeon, As: surgeon's assistant, N: scrub nurse, An: anaesthetist, Tp: table with patient. Two monitors are shown on either side of the anaesthetist.

to secure the port to the abdominal wall. A common practice is to insert a purse string to the deep fascia at the point of port insertion and tie this to the sides of the port. Care should be taken to plan port insertion appropriately and keep the number of ports to the number required for safe laparoscopy. We demonstrated that the risk of port site adhesions though low, is further reduced by using less ports (Nwokoma et al., 2009b).

7.6 Closure

At the end of the procedure, all incisions of 5mm and above should be closed with standard sutures at deep fascia and skin level as these may still result in incisional hernia if not closed appropriately. Tissue glue or adhesive strips can be used to close incisions of less than 5mm size.

8. Contraindications

Experience in paediatric laparoscopy has advanced supported by advances in paediatric anaesthetic care as well as improvement and adaptability of instruments and equipment. This has led to a shift in classification of certain clinical conditions from *absolute* to *relative* contraindications to laparoscopy. The contraindications are listed in Table 3.

Patient unsuitable for open surgery
Uncontrolled bleeding or coagulation problems
Multiple previous abdominal surgery

Table 3. Contraindications to paediatric laparoscopy

Infants less than six months old respond to challenges to their circulatory system by compensatory increase in their heart rate, their relatively immature cardiac muscles being unable to increase contractility in such situations. Consequently, children in this age group need to be carefully selected when significant congenital cardiac disease is present. In the presence of coagulopathy or haemoglobinopathies, laparoscopic cholecystectomy and splenectomy have been carried out safely. In these cases, safety has not been compromised by the theoretical diminution in visibility caused by the absorption of light consequent upon blood in the operating field. Careful medical management of these conditions compliment surgical technique to make laparoscopic approach safe in these patients. The early mobilisation, smaller scars needing less opiate analgesics give added benefit in these situations. Children with respiratory difficulties also benefit from the benefits of smaller scar and less opiate analgesia, early mobilisation which leads to reduction of hospital stay, reduced risk of atelectasis or exacerbation of respiratory problems (Nagraj et al., 2006). Complication rate is higher in children who weigh less than 5kg. This was observed by Iwanaka et al (2004) following Nissen's fundoplication. The little intra-abdominal space in this group of patients limits surgeon's movement and efficiency, and may contribute to a higher complication rate. Several urologic procedures have been safely performed by laparoscopic approach in children. However, Lee DJ et al., advocate that ureteric reimplantation is contraindicated in children less than 4years of age, in the presence of concomitant ureterocele or megaureter requiring tapering.

9. Controversies

9.1 Laparoscopy and intra-abdominal tumours

Laparoscopy has contributed significantly to the management of paediatric abdominal tumours. Similar to other medical conditions, the usefulness of laparoscopy in paediatric oncology can be broadly viewed as diagnostic or therapeutic.

Diagnostic laparoscopy is a valuable tool for visualising and obtaining tissue for diagnosis from intra-abdominal masses. It offers the advantage of the biopsy being done under direct vision, being less invasive than open biopsy, less post-operative pain and fewer problems with adhesion of tissue to the abdominal wall. Unlike ultrasound-guided or CT-guided percutaneous biopsy which also requires a general anaesthetic, it offers the operator visual appreciation of the biopsy site and opportunity to control any resultant bleed. It also allows a deeper reach than the percutaneous approach. The risk of collateral tissue injury and inadequate sampling is also reduced. The extent of the tissue or mass lesion and its resectability can also be evaluated while planning of definitive surgery can be undertaken including best mode and site of access, if required at a later date. Its applicability relies on there being enough space and optimal site for introduction of camera and instruments with safe creation of pneumoperitoneum. For these reasons, large tumours may present a challenge and require careful evaluation and case selection. Peritoneal washings can also be obtained at laparoscopy. Despite these advantages, many advocate that its use in diagnosis for malignancy be complimentary to and not a replacement for other non-invasive diagnostic tools (Conlon & Toomey, 2003).

The surgeon and oncologist continually face the challenge of obtaining adequate tissue for immunohistochemcal, karyotyping and molecular analysis. Incorrect diagnosis leads to inappropriate management and therefore must be avoided as much as possible. Laparoscopy has been demonstrated to be safe in various childhood tumours such as neuroblastoma, rhabdomyosarcoma and liver tumours. The combination with ultrasonography adds information regarding the status of the tissue beneath the surface and increasing the diagnostic yield by 14% to 25%; core biopsies can be obtained and Doppler flow may add information about vessels and tumour-vessel interface (Conlon & Toomey, 2003).

The development of coagulative equipment such as the bipolar and harmonic scalpel, coagulative gels and tissue glue have contributed significantly to the reduction in risk of bleeding as well as the safe management of bleeding complications in laparoscopy. Concerns regarding tumour spillage and port site secondaries have limited the use of laparoscopy in oncology. Sandoval et al (2004) found tumour spillage in a therapeutic biopsy of a thoracic paraspinal Wilm's tumour and recommend open biopsy in these cases. They however found laparoscopic biopsy to have benefit in other intra-abdominal tumours.

Iwanaka et al (2003) reported port site recurrence to be rare in children. It is noteworthy that 64% of the patients in their report had neuroblastoma diagnosed following mass screening using levels of urinary Vanillylmandelic acid and homovanillic acid. Some have suggested that port-site recurrence is related to surgeon's inexperience (Bailey & Love, 2008) while others reported no difference in rate of port site or incisional recurrence in open or laparoscopic tumour surgery (Conlon & Toomey, 2003). Tumour rupture or spillage, implant and metastasis (including port site metastasis) were observed to be significantly higher in laparoscopic surgery than in open surgery following laparoscopy for gynaecological cancers and its use is limited to a clinically presumed benign diagnosis with normal levels of tumour markers (Medeiros LRF et al., 2010).

Iwanaka et al (2001) in their review of laparoscopic versus open adrenalectomy noted that there was reduced duration of hospital stay, time to post-operative feeding and commencement of chemotherapy in the laparoscopic group. Early post-operative high dose adjuvant chemotherapy has been found to reduce port site recurrence in abdominal neuroblastoma. Care should be taken with heat-operated instruments to avoid heat damage to tumour and surrounding organs. The transperitoneal approach is recommended as this offers the advantage of inspection of the contralateral adrenal gland and biopsy of regional para-aortic lymph nodes which is a requirement for the International Neuroblastoma Staging System to facilitate accurate staging of abdominal neuroblastoma (Iwanaka, 2008).

Laparoscopy was found to offer less blood loss, decreased time of postoperative feeding, decreased time to start chemotherapy, reduced hospital stay, better prognosis and quality of life to children (Iwanaka et al., 2007). Bax and van der Zee (2004) reported improved outcome from laparoscopy assisted interruption of the median sacral artery and dissection of the internal component of sacrococcygeal teratomas. Desai et al (2009) reported the ligation of median sacral artery in a premature neonate with a giant sacrococcygeal teratoma achieving minimal blood loss in the remaining part of the surgery.

9.2 Laparoscopy in trauma

Diagnostic laparoscopy is gaining increasing application in paediatric trauma in the stable patient with equivocal clinical parameters not requiring immediate laparotomy but not symptom-free. It has a sensitivity of 88% for liver and spleen injuries; 83% for diaphragm, 57% for pancreas and kidney and 25% for hollow viscus. It is not recommended in penetrating injuries because distension of the anterior abdominal wall by pneumoperitoneum risks disruption of injured tissues which may aggravate bleeding (O'Neill et al., 2003). Laparoscopy in paediatric trauma still has limited application and evidence available is mostly case reports. With a sensitivity of less than 50% for identification of perforation of hollow viscera and difficulty in interpreting haemodynamic changes, more evidence is required to clearly delineate its use in this patient group. It has been successfully used to evaluate abdominal trauma in children who are haemodynamically stable but with clinical suspicion of injury with normal imaging (Goldstein and Stylianos, 2005). Tytgat et al (2010) reported successful treatment of gastric and duodenal perforation following blunt abdominal trauma in children.

9.3 Sceptics

Opposers to the claim of the supremacy of the laparoscopic approach to open surgery cite the need for endotracheal general anaesthesia rather than regional block for procedures such as ingunal herniotomy as additional needless trauma, stress and cost (Raveenthiran V. 2010). This argument fails in the paediatric population where regional anaesthetic is of limited application as children do not tolerate this like the adults. Moreover, the pathology of hernia in adults is different from that in children this difference dictating different modes of treatment. In addition, concomitant contralateral inguinal hernia may not be apparent in children without laparoscopy. Raveenthiran (2010) argues that laparoscopy should not be a preferred option in children as they have nothing to benefit from early return home, having no loss of wages to account for. However, the cost of hospital admission and also early return to work for parents counters this stance. The psychologic trauma of separation from usual environment, siblings, play toys or equipment has been documented and may be enough to delay a child's recovery. Problems such as nocturnal enuresis and disrupted sleep patterns have been noted to be decreased with reduction in hospital stay (Brennan & Prabhu, 2003).

10. Complications of laparoscopy

The challenges facing the paediatric surgeons with regards to the use of to laparoscopic approach for treatment in children are often peculiar to the particular condition in question and also to the age and size of the patient. The experience of the surgeon may also be a contributory factor. Complication rates are therefore variable; from 2% in elective procedures (Chen et al., 1996) to 17.4% in emergency procedures (Nwokoma et al., 2009a). Panteli et al, (2008) observed an overall complication rate of 6.9% among trainee paediatric surgeons. A list of possible complications is presented in Table 4.

Rigorus pursuit of haemostasis is essential for success in laparoscopic surgery as blood in the operating field significantly reduces visibility. Adequate control of blood vessels of target organ must be achieved to minimise risk of uncontrollable blood loss this often being the reason for conversion to an open approach. Vascular injury can affect the primary target organ or secondary intra-abdominal organs. This can have dire consequences for the devascularised organ. Vascular injury to the mesenteric vessels can result in bowel ischaemia and loss resulting in feeding problems commensurate with the length of bowel

Prolonged operative time
Visceral injury
Bladder injury
Bleeding
Shoulder tip pain
Vascular injury
Conversion to open procedure
Pneumothorax
Wound infection
Port site hernia
Renal impairment
Adhesive Intestinal obstruction
Intra-abdominal abscesses
Port site recurrence of malignancy
Gas embolism
Gastric volvulus

Table 4. Complications of laparoscopy

affected. Direct perforation of the bowel by instrumentation or diathermy heat injury is a well-documented complication. If noted at the time of surgery, repair can usually be achieved with minimal disruption to the procedure and without significant increase in morbidity. If missed, this can lead to delayed presentation with peritonitis or sepsis with possible bowel loss which may require the formation of a diverting stoma in emergency surgery. Shoulder tip pain is common following laparoscopy with a rate of 35% reported by Lejus et al., (1996).

Intra-abdominal abscess may complicate surgery particularly in the presence of peritoneal contamination or ischaemic tissues. Jen and Shew (2010) reported intra-abdominal abscess rate of 4.9% in perforated appendicitis versus 0.6% in non-perforated appendicitis. Due to the relatively new techniques of laparoscopic surgery as compared to conventional open approach surgical expertise is still developing in this area leading to increased operating time. Panteli et al., (2008) demonstrated an increased operating time for laparoscopic procedures among trainees which reduced with time and experience. This can be facilitated with the use of simulators for training surgeons. Many of the available simulators are easy to set up and can be modified to suit training needs. Jaffer et al., (2009) developed a low cost simulator to aid training in laparoscopic paediatric hernia repair. In addition, operating room staff may not be fully aware of alternative instruments which may be required intra-operatively to deal with challenges or conditions that were not apparent before the start of the procedure. Ure et al (2000) noted that problems with instruments and devices led to a mean time loss of 15.1 minutes in 15.6% of the laparoscopic procedures in their series.

The rate of conversion is related to the complexity of the procedure as indicated by target organ position in the abdominal cavity, adherence to neighbouring or surrounding structures, malignant tendency, inflammation, presence of pus or peritoneal soiling, presence of adhesions between the abdominal wall and intra-abdominal structures as well as surgeon's expertise. Hazzan et al (2001) reported a conversion rate of 7% in laparoscopic excision for benign adrenal neoplasm. In our report of laparoscopy for advanced appendicitis in children (Nwokoma et al., 2009a), we had a conversion rate of 0%.

Port site hernia is not common but is more likely with port site incisions of more than 5mm length. Chen et al, (1996) reported a port site hernia rate of 0.003%.
Gastric volvulus complicating inappropriate placement of gastrostomy tube is rare. Jen and Shew (2010) reported other uncommon complications as follows: cardiac 0.1%, respiratory 0.2 - 1%, renal 0.1-0.2% and intestinal obstruction 0.5 -2.0%. Gas embolism from carbon dioxide is very rare with reported incidences of between 0.0016% and 0.013% (Fingerhut et al., 2005).

11. Economic considerations

Macarulla E et al., (1997) found the laparoscopic approach to appendicectomy to have an average cost of $394 while the open approach had an average cost pf $508. The laparoscopic equipment and instruments are continually being modified. Many of them are single use. These factors contribute to their cost being above their open surgery equivalents, many of which are reusable after sterilisation. As already stated above, the advantage of reduced hospital stay makes for enough savings to cover the extra operative time and cost of equipment and instruments. This cost advantage is more evident when the duration of hospital stay for the open approach would normally be 4 days or more (Morris and Wood, 2000).

12. On-going developments

Single site laparoscopy was introduced in 1992 (Pelosi and Pelosi 1992). Since then it has continued to gain wide acceptance among paediatric surgeons. Limitations to its practical application include the relatively small size of periumbilical region or skin fold in children, the single incision multiport system still being between 15 - 20mm size. This potentially increases the risk of long unsightly scars, infection and incisional hernia. Also, the angle of instrumentation for the single port system limits movement, hindering dexterity which leads to prolonged operating time and higher risk of complications including collateral injury to tissues in and near the operating field. This problem is of course compounded by the smaller intra-abdominal cavity space in children. Further development of the single incision or single port system to suit the paediatric population is needed to extend its use and benefits to this patient group. Nevertheless, there are reports of some procedures that have been successfully performed using the single incision multi-port system and they include cholecystectomy, appendicectomy, intussusception reduction, splenectomy, inguinal hernia repair, Nissen's fundoplication, insertion of gastrostomy tube, pyloromyotomy, ovarian detorsion, gastric sleeve resection and gastric band placement (Ponsky & Krpata, 2011).
The 3-dimensional imaging system is also getting increasingly available and will improve the spatial and depth perception of target organ. The use of heated humidified carbon dioxide for the creation of pneumoperitoneum is gaining increasing popularity but is not yet common practice. Some studies have demonstrated that it can lead to even less post-operative pain, hypothermia and analgesic requirement but no difference in length of hospital stay or less fogging rates. (Sajid et al., 2008). Peng et al., (2008) further observed that it caused less peritoneal damage and less post-operative adhesions. Further studies are needed to confirm these findings.

13. Conclusion

An increasingly wider range of surgical procedures are now being safely undertaken using the laparoscopic approach. In spite of the paucity of randomised clinical trials in the paediatric population, many studies in this patient group have demonstrated a clear advantage of the laparoscopic approach over the open approach in different clinical situations. We believe that, *'What is worth doing, is worth doing well'*. We advocate that as laparoscopy certainly gives an undeniable edge over the conventional approach to the treatment of several surgical conditions in children, it merits increased focus and advancement.

14. Acknowledgment

The authors would like to express their appreciation to their colleagues who have worked with them in various studies evaluating the clinical application of laparoscopy in children; some of the published work are included in the text.

15. References

Anand, K.J.; Brown, M.J.; Causon, R.C.; Christofides, N.D.; Bloom, S.R. & Ainsley-Green, A. (1985). Can the human neonate mount an endocrine and metabolic response to surgery? *Journal of Pediatric Surgery,* Vol.20, No.1, (February 1985), pp. 41-48, ISSN 0022-3468

Anand, K.J. & Hickey, P.R. (1987). Pain and its effects in the human neonate and fetus. *New England Journal of Medicine,* Vol.317, No.21, (November 1987), pp. 1321-1329, ISSN 0028-4793

Anand, K.J. & Aynsley-Green, A. (1988). Measuring the severity of surgical stress in newborn infants. *Journal of Pediatric Surgery,* Vol.23, No.4, (April 1988), pp. 297-305, ISSN 0022-3468

Badani, K.K.; Patel, H.R.H. & Hemal, A.K. (2006). Historical development of keyhole surgery, In: *Minimally Invasive Surgery: Looking through the keyhole,* H. Patel, J. Joseph, (Eds.), 2-3, MA Healthcare Ltd, ISBN 1-85642-296-8, London, United Kingdom

Bailey and Love's Short Practice of Surgery, (2008). Twenty-fifth edition. N.S. Williams, C.J.K. Bulstrode, P.R. O'Connell, (Eds.), 247-249, Hodder Arnold, ISBN 9780340939321, London, United Kingdom

Bax, N.M.A. & van der Zee, D.C. (1998). Trocar fixation during endoscopic surgery in infants and children. *Surgical Endoscopy,* Vol.12, No.2, pp. 181-182, 0930-2794

Bax, N.M. & van der Zee, D.C. (2004). The laparoscopic approach to sacrococcygeal teratomas. *Surgical Endoscopy,* Vol.18, No.1, (January 2004), pp. 128-130, ISSN 0930-2794

Böttcher-Habberzeth, S.; Dullenkoff, A.; Gitzelmann, A. & Weiss, M. (2007). Tracheal tube tip displacement during laparoscopy in children. *Anaesthesia,* Vol.62. No.2, (February 2007), pp. 131-134, ISSN 0003-2409

Chen, M.K.; Schropp, K.P. & Lobe, T.E. (1996). Complications of minimal-access surgery in children. Journal of Pediatric Surgery, Vol.31, No.8, (August 1996). pp. 1161-1165, ISSN 0022-3468

Conlon, K.C. & Toomey, D. (2007). Diagnostic Laparoscopy, In: *Mastery of Surgery, Volume 1.* Fifth edition, J.E. Fischer, K.I. Bland, (Eds.), 251-258, Wolters Kluwer/Lippincott Williams & Wilkins, ISBN 9780781771658, Philadelphia, USA

Desai, A.P.; Wragg, R.; kulkarni, M. & Tsang, T. (2009). Sacrococcygeal teratoma: Excision aided by laparoscopic ligation of the median sacral artery in a premature neonate. *Journal of IndianAssociation of Pediatric Surgeons,* Vol.14, No.1, (January 2009), p. 39, ISSN 0971-9261

Fingerhut, A.; Millat, B. & Borie, F. (2005). Prevention of complications in laparoscopic surgery, In: *Mastery of Endoscopic and Laparoscopic Surgery,* N.J. Soper, L.L. Swanström, W.S. Eubanks, (Eds.), 57-58, Lippincott Williams & Wilkins, ISBN 0-7817-4445-8, Philadelphia, USA

Goldstein, A.M. & Stylianos, S. (2005). The role of minimal access surgery in pediatric trauma, In: *Pediatric Minimal Access Surgery.* Edited by J.C. Lange, C.T. Albanese, (Eds.), 81-88, Taylor and Francis Group, ISBN 0-8247-5447-6, Florida, USA

Gómez, D.B.H.; Karanik, E.; Glüer, S.; Jesch, N.K.; Kübler, J.; Latta, K.; Sümpelmann, R. & Ure, B.M. (2005). Anuria during pneumoperitoneum in infants and children: a prospective study. *Journal of Pediatric Surgery,* Vol.40, No.9, (September 2005), pp. 1454-1458, ISSN 0022-3468

Hazzan, D.; Shiloni, E.; Golijanin, D.; Jurim, O.; Gross, D. & Reissman, P. (2001). Laparoscopic versus open adrenalectomy for benign adrenal neoplasm. A comparative study. *Surgical Endoscopy,* Vol.15, No.11, (November 2001), pp. 1356-1358, ISSN 0930-2794

Iwanaka, T.; Arai, M.; Ito, M,; Kawashima, H.; Yamamoto, K.; Hanada, R. & Imaizumi S. (2001). Surgical treatment for abdominal neuroblastoma in the laparoscopic era. *Surgical Endoscopy,* Vol.15, No.7, (July 2001), pp. 751-754, ISSN 0930-2794

Iwanaka, T.; Arai, M.; Yamamoto, H.; Fukuzawa, M.; Kubota, A.; Kouchi, K.; Nio, M.; Satomi, A.; Sasaki, F.; Yoneda, A.; Ohhana, Y.; Takehara, H.; Morikawa, Y. & Miyano, T. (2003). No incidence of port-site recurrence after endosurgical procedure for pedaitric malignancies. *Pediatric Surgery International,* Vol.19, No.3, (May 2003), pp. 200-203, ISSN 0179-0358

Iwanaka, T.; Uchida, H.; Kawashima, H.; Nishi, A.; Kudou, S. & Satake, R. (2004). Complications of laparoscopic surgery in neonates and small children. *Journal of Pediatric Surgery,* Vol.39, No.12, (December 2004), pp. 1838-1841, ISSN 0022-3468

Iwanaka, T.; Kawashima, H. & Uchida, H. (2007). The laparoscopic approach to neuroblastoma. *Seminars in Pediatric Surgery,* Vol.16, No.4, (November 2007), pp. 259-265, ISSN 1055-8586

Iwanaka, T. (2008). Laparoscopic approach to abdominal neuroblastoma, In: *Endoscopic Surgery in Infants and Children.* Edited by N.M.A. Bax, K.E. Georgeson, S.S. Rothenberg, V. Jean-Stěphane, C.K. Yeung, (Eds.), 617-627, Springer, ISBN 978-3-540-00115-7, Berlin Heidelberg, Germany

Jaffer, U.; Manoharan, S. & Tsang, T. (2009). Low cost laparoscopic paediatric inguinal hernia repair simulator. *Annals of the Royal college of Surgeons of England,* Vol.91, No.6, (September 2009), p. 515, ISSN 0035-8843

Jen, H.C. & Shew, S.B. (2010). Laparoscopic versus open appendectomy in children: outcomes comparison based on a state wide analysis. *Journal of Surgical Research,* Vol.161, No.1, (June 2010), pp. 17-19, ISSN 0022-4804

Lee, D.J.; Kim, P.H. & Koh, C.J. (2010). Current trends in pediatric minimally invasive urologic surgery. *Korean Journal of Urology,* Vol.51. No.2, (February 2010), pp. 80-87, ISSN 2005-6737

Lee, S.L. & DuBois, J.J. (2000). Laparoscopic diagnosis and repair of pediatric femoral hernia. Initial experience of four cases. *Surgical Endoscopy,* Vol.14, No.12, (December 2000), pp. 1110-1113, ISSN 0930-2794

Lejus, C.; Delile, L.; Plattner, V.; Guillou, S.; Héloury, Y. & Souron, R. (1996). Randomised, single-blinded trial of laparoscopic versus open appendectomy in children: effects on post-operative analgesia. *Anesthesiology,* Vol.84, No.4, (April 1996), pp. 801-806, ISSN 0003-3022

Macarulla, E.; Vallet, J.; Abad, J.M.; Hussein, H.; Fernandez, E. & Nieto, B. (1997). Laparoscopic versus open appendectomy: a prospective randomized trial. *Surgical Laparoscopy & Endoscopy,* Vol.7, No.4, (August 1997), pp. 335-339, 1051-7200

McHoney, M.; Corizia, L.; Eaton, S.; Kiely, E.M.; Drake, D.P.; Tan, H.L.; Spitz, L. & Pierro A. (2003). Carbon dioxide elimination during laparoscopy in children is age dependent. *Journal of Pediatric Surgery,* Vol.38, No.1, (January 2003), pp. 105-110, 0022-3468

Medeiros, L.R.F.; Rosa, D.D.; Bozzetti, M.C.; Mines, R.; Edelweiss, M.I.; Stein, A.T.; Zelmanowicz, A.; Ethur, A.B. & Zanini, R.R. (2010). Laparoscopy versus laparotomy for FIGO (International Federation of Gynaecology and Obstetrics) Stage 1 ovarian cancer (Review), The Cochrane Collaboration, The Cochrane Library 2010 (on line), Issue 12, ISSN 1469-493X

Meehan, J.J. & Georgeson, K.E. (1997). Laparoscopic fundoplication yields low postoperative complications in neurologically impaired children. *Pediatric Endosurgery & Innovative Techniques,* Vol.1, No.1, (January 1997), pp. 11-14, ISSN 1092-6410

Morecroft, J.A.; Stringer, M.D.; Higgins, M.; Holmes, S.J. & Capps, S.N. (1993). Follow up after inguinal herniotomy or surgery for hydrocele in boys. *British Journal of Surgery,* Vol.80, No.12, (December 1993), pp. 1613-1614, ISSN 0007-1323

Morris, P.J. & Wood W.C. (2000). Endoscopic surgery, In: *Oxford Textbook of Surgery,* Second edition. Volume 1. p. 603, Oxford University Press Inc. ISBN 0-19-262884-4, New York, USA

Nagraj, S.; Sinha, S.; Grant, H.; Lakhoo, K.; Hitchcock, R. & Johnson, P. (2006). The incidence of complications following primary inguinal herniotomy in babies weighing 5kg or less. *Pediatric Surgery International,* Vol. 22, No.6, (June 2006), pp. 500-502, ISSN 0179-0358

Nwokoma, N.J.; Swindells, M.G.; Pahl, K.; Mathur, A.B.; Minocha, A.; Kulkarni, M. & Tsang TT. Pediatric advanced appendicitis: open versus laparoscopic approach. *Surgical Laparoscopy, Endoscopy & Percutaneous Techniques,* Vol.19, No.2, (April 2009), pp. 110-113, ISSN 1530-4515

Nwokoma, N.J.; Hassett, S. & Tsang TT. (2009). Trocar site adhesions following laparoscopic surgery in children. *Surgical Laparoscopy, Endoscopy & Percutaneous Techniques,* Vol.19, No.6, (December 2009), pp. 511-513, ISSN 1530-4515

O'Neill Jr., J.A.; Grosfeld J.L.; Fonkalsrud E.W.; Coran A.G.; Caldamone, A.A. (2004). Diagnostic Laparoscopy, In: *Principles of Pediatric Surgery,* Second edition, (Eds.), 163, Mosby, ISBN 0323-01827-0, St. louis, Missouri, USA

Pacilli, M.; Pierro, A.; Kingsley, C.; Curry, J.I.; Herod, J. & Eaton S. (2006). Absorption of carbon dioxide during laparoscopy in children measured using a novel mass spectrometric technique. *British Journal of Anaesthesia,* Vol.97, No.2, (August 2006), pp. 215-219, ISSN 0007-0912

Panteli, C.; Desai, A.; Manoharan, S.; Bouhadiba, N.; Singh, S. & Tsang, T. (2008). Emergency laparoscopic appendicectomy: the results in the hands of trainees. *Journal of Pediatric Surgical Specialties,* Vol.2, No.3, (December 2008), pp. 14-17, ISSN 2066-2009

Panteli, C.; Minocha, A.; Kulkarni, M.S. & Tsang, T. (2009). The role of laparoscopy in the management of adnexal lesions in children. *Surgical Laparoscopy, Endoscopy & Percutaneous Techniques,* Vol.19, No.6, (December 2009), pp. 514-517, ISSN 1530-4515

Parkinson, E.J. & Pierro, A. (2006). Inguinal and umbilical hernias, In: *Pediatric Surgery and Urology – Long Term Outcomes,* M.D. Stringer, K.T. Oldham KT, P.D.E. Mouriquand PDE, (Eds.), Second edition, 286-288, Cambridge University Press, ISBN 0-521-83902-5, New York, USA

Pelosi, M.A. & Pelosi, M.A. 3rd (1992). Laparoscopic appendectomy using a single umbilical puncture (minilaparoscopy). *Journal of Reproductive Medicine,* Vol.37, No.7, pp. 588-594, ISSN 0024-7758

Peng, Y.; Zheng, M.; Ye, Q.; Chen, X.; Yu, B. & Liu, B. (2008). Heated and humidified CO2 prevents hypothermia, peritoneal injury and intra-abdominal adhesions during prolonged laparoscopic insufflations. *Journal of Surgical Research,* Vol.XX, No.X, (October 2008), pp.1-8, ISSN 0022-4804

Ponsky, T.A. & Krpata, D.M. (2011). Single-port laparoscopy: considerations in children. *Journal of Minimal Access Surgery,* Vol.7, No.1, (January-March 2011), pp. 96-98, ISSN 0972-9941

Raveenthiran, V. (2010). Pediatric laparoscopy: facts and factitious claims. *Journal of Indian Association of Pediatric Surgeons,* Vol.15, No.4, (October-December 2010), pp. 122-128, ISSN 0971-9261

Rehman, M.R.; Panteli, C. & Tsang, T. (2010). Laparoscopic repair of Amyand hernia in an 8-week-old infant. *Hernia,* Vol.14, No.4, (August 2010), pp. 443-445, ISSN 1265-4906

Sajid, M.S.; Mallick, A.S.; Rimpel,J. Bokari, S.A.; Cheek, E. & Baig, M.K. Effect of heated and humidified carbon dioxide on patients after laparoscopic procedures: a meta-analysis. *Surgical Laparoscopy, Endoscopy & Percutaneous Techniques,* Vol.18, No.6, (December 2008), pp. 539-546, ISSN 1530-4515

Sandoval, C.; Strom, K. & Stringel, G. (2004). Laparoscopy in the management of pediatric intra-abdominal tumors. *Journal of the Society of Laparoendoscopic Surgeons,* Vol.8, No.2, (April-June 2004), pp. 115-118, ISSN 1086-8089

Semm, K. (1983). Endoscopic appendectomy. *Endoscopy,*Vol.15, No.2, (March 1983), pp. 59-64, ISSN 0013726X

Tantoco, J.G.; Glick, P.L. & Levitt, M.A. (2005). History of pediatric minimal access surgery, In: *Pediatric Minimal Access Surgery*, J.C. Langer, C. T. Albanese, (Eds.), 12, Taylor & Francis Group, ISBN 0-8247-5447-6, Florida, USA

Tytgat, S.H.; Zwaveling, S.; Kramer, W.L. & van der Zee, D.C. (2010). Laparoscopic treatment of gastric and duodenal perforation in children after blunt abdominal trauma. *Injury*, December 1 2010 (Epub) PMID: 21129741

Ure, B.M.; Bax, N.M.A. & van der Zee, D.C. (2000). Laparoscopy in infants and children: a prospective study on feasibilty and the impact on routine surgery. *Journal of Pediatric Surgery*, Vol.35, No.8, (August 2000), pp. 1170-1173, ISSN 0022-3468

van der Zee, D.C. & Bax, N.M.A. (1999). Laparoscopic approach to intestinal obstruction in children, In: *Endoscopic Surgery in Children*, N.M.A. Bax, K.E. Georgeson, A. Najmaldin, J.S. Valla. (Eds.), 215 -219, Springer, ISBN 3540640738, Verlag, Berlin. Germany

3

Laparoscopic Hernia Repair in Neonates, Infants and Children

Yaron Armon and Dan Arbell
Department of Pediatric Surgery, Hadassah-Hebrew University Hospital, Jerusalem Israel

1. Introduction

Inguinal hernia is a very common condition in children 1-3 and adults and is the most common operation performed on children 4 (other than ritual circumcision). Since the "classic" open repair was introduced, it has become the standard operation for hernias, with very few controversies: whether the surgeon should perform only a herniotomy or reinforce the repair, whether a contralateral groin exploration be performed, and so forth. The operation is quick, safe, 5 and can be done in an outpatient setting with anesthesia via a laryngeal mask. The recurrence rate is acceptable, 1%-5%6-8, depending on the expertise of the surgeon, the child's' age and concomitant diseases.
The advent of laparoscopy has changed many dogmas in all fields of surgery, pediatric hernia repair included. Many operations that were considered as "gold standard" are being challenged by the laparoscopic approach and the new technologies it has brought with it. In the specific case of pediatric hernia repair, another challenge on the open technique was introduced by the development of fertility clinics and the higher than expected incidence of azoospermia due to an injury to the vas deferens during bilateral hernia repairs 9-10,14. Therefore, two major applications of laparoscopy were introduced to hernia repair in children. The first, performing an intra-operative diagnostic laparoscopy for diagnosing a non-symptomatic contralateral hernia during open hernia surgery. The second, performing a laparoscopic repair. During the forthcoming chapter, the merits, disadvantages and techniques of both procedures will be reviewed.

2. Diagnostic laparoscopy during open pediatric hernia repair

The incidence of a contralateral, asymptomatic groin hernia in children is not well defined. Reports vary from 10% to 60%, depending on prematurity of the child, gendre and side 11-12. Also, there is no consensus on whether a patent processus vaginalis is considered a hernia for practical purposes, i.e. whether it should be repaired or not.
It is established that the premature have a higher incidence of bilateral hernias 13, and that bilateral hernias are commoner in females with a left sided hernia 11-12. Until laparoscopy developed, there was controversy regarding whether a contralateral groin exploration should be performed and to whom. On the one hand, an exploration ensured a diagnosis during one operation and anesthesia, an option that carries many advantages to the patient

and the parents. On the other hand, most of these explorations performed on children above the age of 1 year were negative, doubling the operating and anesthetic time and risking a bilateral vas deferens injury with future infertility 14. Therefore, most surgeons had loosely based criteria on whom the exploration was performed. Since a hernia can be very easily and accurately diagnosed from within the peritoneum, introduction of a laparoscope during the operation seemed like a natural answer for the question.

3. Technique

During the operation for a hernia, the hernia sac is separated from the spermatic cord and isolated. Before ligating the sac, a 5 mm port is introduced through the sac and a 70^0 scope is passed into the peritoneum. The patient is put head down and most times there is need for mild insufflation up to pressure of 6-8mmHg of the abdominal cavity in order view the contralateral inguinal area. Care must be taken to avoid injury to the hernia sac while introducing the port, and the sac opening has to be secured to the port in order to avoid air escaping around it. We recommend placing vessel loops or other markers around the elements of the cord in order to ease their identification after the laparoscopy and continue with the hernia repair. It is also helpful to ensure an empty bladder before the laparoscopy, as it may be difficult to pass a full bladder from this approach, certainly in a small child. If a synchronous hernia is identified, a contralateral open repair is performed after finishing the original side. Our custom is to treat a patent processus as a hernia.

4. Results

In our experience, diagnostic trans-inguinal laparoscopy has been accurate in 97% of the cases. In 2% there was failure to identify a hernia due to tear of the hernia sac, or inadequate visualization. There were no cases of false positive examinations. In 1% of the patients the laparoscopy was aborted because the pneumoperitoneum compromised the anesthesia. These results are similar to those reported in the literature.15,16

5. Advantages

Diagnostic trans-inguinal laparoscopy provides definite advantages in the accurate diagnosis of a contralateral synchronous hernia during a single anesthesia 15,16. It is easy to learn and is very comfortable for a surgeon that is proficient in the open hernia repair technique. Usually, the pneumoperitoneum required does not preclude anesthesia via a laryngeal mask and does not require paralytic agents.

6. Disadvantages

The major disadvantage of this approach is when dealing with a very young or premature baby with a very delicate hernia sac. This is true also for a hernia accompanying an undescended testicle. In these cases, the insertion of the port may easily tear the hernia sac and compromise the ipsilateral repair. Another disadvantage is that in the case of a synchronous hernia, a bilateral open repair is performed with the concomitant risk of bilateral damage to the spermatic cord and infertility.

7. Laparoscopic hernia repair

When challenging a time honored technique in surgery, it is necessary to convince that are major advantages in the newer one. This is certainly true for laparoscopic repair of pediatric hernias, as the open repair is very common, safe, quick and the surgeon is very familiar with the procedure. Therefore, prior to describing the laparoscopic repair, we shall examine the pitfalls of the open one.

1. The subject of synchronous or metachronous contralateral hernia has been discussed in the previous paragraph.
2. Damage to the spermatic cord during hernia repair is an under evaluated topic in surgery. Recent reports in adult surgical literature have enhanced the awareness of spermatic cord injury during hernia repair, mostly those using a mesh graft. Of higher consequence to our discussion are the reports of an increased rate of male infertility following a bilateral hernia repair during early childhood. It is hard to assess the true rate of cord injury during hernia surgery, since the operation is very common, and there has to be a complete bilateral blockade in the vas deferens in order to cause infertility. Yet, the rate of damage is probably higher than previous assessments.
3. Testicular atrophy may be a consequence of an incarcerated hernia with compromised testicular blood supply and may also be due to vascular damage during hernia repair. It is hard for the surgeon to assess the viability of a compromised testicle during a repair, as well as to assess the possibility of vascular damage during the handling of the cord.
4. An open repair during an incarcerated hernia is sometimes cumbersome and tedious. It is often difficult to assess the viability of the organs that were incarcerated, as they tend to spontaneously reduce during anesthesia or at the beginning of surgery. In cases of necrotic bowel, omentum or severe edematous tissues, it becomes a challenge to correctly identify the anatomy to allow for a good repair.
5. Recurrent hernias are rare in the pediatric population, with reports ranging from 0.5% to 5%, depending on the child's age and maturity. Although rare, every surgeon has to face this challenge every once in a while, and is familiar with the problem of dissecting through scar tissue in order to discern the anatomy.
6. A symptomatic hernia in an undescended testicle is a complex problem. Whilst it is better to wait for 6-12 months before performing orchipexy, sometimes surgical intervention is needed sooner than that. This, of course, may compromise either the hernia repair or the orchipexy.

The laparoscopic approach is supposed to provide an answer to all these issues. First, as discussed previously, laparoscopy provides an excellent visualization of the groin from within the peritoneum, adequately diagnosing a synchronous hernia 15,17 or patent processus vaginalis. Second, since the vas and blood vessels are visualized with precision and are not handled in most laparoscopic repairs, the possibility of cord damage during surgery is reduced. The same goes for vascular compromise of a borderline testicle that suffered from incarceration. When dealing with an incarcerated hernia, laparoscopy allows direct visualization of the reduced incarcerated contents and their viability. It also circumnavigates the problem of anatomical precision in edematous or scarred areas (such as in a recurrent hernia) with a lower complication rate 4. Last, laparoscopy can allow a hernia closure in an undescended testicle without compromising the forthcoming orchipexy.

8. Technique

The child requires endotracheal intubation and anesthesia with paralytic agents in order to allow adequate pneumoperitoneum. A camera port is introduced above the umbilicus, since in very small infants one gains a small but significant space for working in the abdomen. We advocate using the open "Hasson" technique for accessing the peritoneum. After insufflation according to the patient's weight, the patient is put head down and the groin area inspected. The surgeon places himself at the patient's head and his assistant next to him on the side opposite the hernia. Two needle holders are placed on each flank of the patient, about the level of the camera port. Usually, there is no need for a port and the instruments are placed directly into the abdomen. One of the needle holders is inserted with the suture held just above the needle in order to facilitate it's navigation into the abdomen. We utilize non-absorbable sutures, usually a prolene 0-4 for reasons that will be discussed later. Shortening the suture to 10-11cm with a not at the end may facilitate identification of the suture end, a maneuver that is helpful in small infants where the space is very limited and the suture end might stay outside the abdomen or slip while pulling the strings. A purse string is sutured around and proximal to the hernia opening and tied intra-corporeally, closing the opening. Care should be taken to identify precisely the vas deferens and blood vessels, in order to pass the suture above them and not through or under them. We routinely reinforce the suture with another "Z" suture above the repair. If there is a synchronous hernia, the procedure is repeated on the other side using a new suture. Attention should be given to needle extraction under vision, as the suture may break during the extraction leaving the needle in the abdomen. Performing the operation without the ports reduces the risk of this happening. After completion, the umbilicus is closed along with a concomitant umbilical hernia if there is one. The side entries do not usually require closure.

9. Technical pitfalls

In the technique described, there are several technical pitfalls that became apparent as experience grew, and the major problem of the operation became apparent - an increased rate of recurrence, 4%-10% of the cases. Before discussing the proposed solutions for decreasing the recurrence rate, there are several points that should be stressed in the technique.

1. Suture material. Since the hernia sac is not dissected or cut in the aforementioned procedure, care must be taken to use non-absorbable sutures. Part of the recurrence is due to the suture material being absorbed after several months, leaving the hernia sac widely opened as if there was no operation at all. This is indeed the view seen when operating a recurrence either laparoscopically or open. We utilize a prolene suture as it is non-absorbable, has a variety of needle sizes and is very easy to handle. Intra-corporeal suturing of prolene requires experience, as the suture material tends to break if improperly handled, and we put a knot at the end to facilitate identification before the suture slips into the tissues.
2. Placement of suture. Many of the patients are small infants that continue to grow after the operation. If the repair is made inside the opening of the hernia sac, the minute residual opening may grow to become a hernia. Care should be taken to place the suture just inside the inguinal ream. This complication is more common in small infants with large inguino-scrotal hernias.

3. Needle retrieval. When operating small children, it is advisable not to use operating ports but rather to introduce the instruments directly into the abdomen. Three mm ports do not allow insertion and retrieval of the regular curved needle. The needle tends to lodge in the port opening and disconnect, causing a search for it in the abdomen, sometimes requiring a conversion to a laparotomy for the retrieval. When the instruments are directly inserted, the abdominal wall closes snugly around the instrument with little or no escape of gas. Needle retrieval is easily done by manipulating the needle through the wound. It is always advisable to follow the retrieval with the camera to ensure safety.
4. Pneumoperitoneum and anesthesia. It is very helpful for the surgeon to stand at the head of the operating table when dealing with small children. It is our experience that only with this stance he may achieve the necessary movements in the small space the pediatric abdomen allows. By doing that, he compromises the control the anesthetist has on patient airway and venous lines, which may be critical in infants. It is very important to have the endotracheal tube and venous lines well secured and approachable before starting to prepare the patient, since dislodgement of these may have hazardous consequences.
5. Hernia in an undescended testicle. Infants with a symptomatic hernia in an undescended testicle are always small, less than 6 months of age; otherwise an orchipexy would be performed. In this age group, the testicle may migrate downwards naturally during the months after the repair. This migration may include the repair itself "en block". The parents should be advised that the hernia repair may be a temporary measure for the symptoms until a definite orchipexy is performed at a later age.
6. Direct hernia. A direct hernia is very rare in the pediatric population but should be actively sought after when visualizing the groins. This is easily done when thought of beforehand.

In view of all these pitfalls, it is appropriate to mention that a laparoscopic hernia repair does not greatly compromise a subsequent open repair, as the area is virtually untouched, avoiding the anatomical confusion of the scar tissue when doing a repeat open repair.

10. Proposed technical improvements

In view of the higher recurrence rate, several technical improvements have been proposed. These include dissection of the hernia sac with or without disconnection of the distal part, 18 different suture techniques such as percutaneous suturing or "flip-flap" modifications 19,20. There is consensus that the approach in infants should be intra-peritoneal and that there is no need for reinforcement of the repair with foreign materials such as meshes. Most of these modifications are performed in single centers and have not yet passed the time required to prove a definite improvement, though the early reports carry a promise for minimizing recurrence while not significantly augmenting the risks for cord injury or operative time.

11. Advantages

There are definite advantages to the laparoscopic hernia repair in children. This approach offers excellent diagnosis of a synchronous hernia or patent processus vaginalis 15,17,21 and the repair is performed with minimal handling and potential damage to the spermatic cord. It is very useful for treating incarcerated or recurrent hernias, bypassing the anatomical challenges in these cases 22. After a necessary learning curve, most technical pitfalls can be avoided and operating times shortened to those of the open hernia repair.

12. Disadvantages

The laparoscopic approach does require a learning curve 23. Most surgeons feel very comfortable with the open technique and would rather face the challenges of a difficult case such as the incarcerated, recurrent or undescended testicle hernia than learn a completely new technique. Laparoscopy in infants requires a more complex anesthetic setting with facilities and personnel that may be not available in outpatient clinics. Undoubtedly, for the time being, laparoscopic repairs carry a higher recurrence rate 24,25. Although recurrence after laparoscopy is not as challenging as after open repair, this should be weighed against the potential benefits of the approach.

13. Conclusions

The advent of laparoscopy has widely changed the scope of pediatric hernia repairs. Whether as a diagnostic or operative tool, the use of laparoscopy is widely gaining popularity as it provides an answer to many dilemmas. Since there are advantages and disadvantages to all approaches, a consensus as to the best approach has not been reached. It seems logical that there is no dogmatic "best" approach for all cases, each case requiring a specific tailoring of the care required. It is still up to the parent to decide what risks are preferred: a metachronous hernia, the risk of future infertility or the increased rate of recurrence. Therefore, it seems wise at this time that a pediatric surgical team be well versed in all approaches in order to combine the advantages to the benefit of the patient.

14. Reference

[1] Grosfeld, JL. Current concepts in inguinal hernia in infants and children. World J Surg 1989; 13:506.

[2] Cox J. Inguinal hernia of childhood. Surg Clin North Am 1985; 65:1331-1342.

[3] Hamey M, Johnstone M, Fossard D. Inguinal herniotomy in children: A five year survey. Br J Surg 1985; 72:485-487.

[4] Kapur, P, Caty, MG, Glick, PL. Pediatric hernias and hydroceles. Pediatr Clin North Am 1998; 45:773.

[5] Nagar H. Stitch granulomas following inguinal herniotomy: a 10-year review. J Pediatr Surg 1993;28:1505- 7.

[6] Levitt MA, Ferraraccio D, Arbesman MC, Brisseau GF, Caty MG, Glick PL. Variability of inguinal hernia surgical technique: a survey of North American pediatric surgeons. J Pediatr Surg 2002; 37:745–751

[7] Antonoff MB, Kreykes NS, Saltzman DA, Acton RD American academy of pediatrics section on surgery hernia survey revisited. J Pediatr Surg 2005; 40:1009–1014

[8] Ein SH, Njere I, Ein A Six thousand three hundred sixty one pediatric inguinal hernias; a 35-year review. J Pediatr Surg 2006; 41:980–986

[9] Sandhu DPS., Osborn DE, and Munson KW. Relationship of azoospermia to inguinal surgery. International Journal of Andrology. 1992;15: 504–506.

[10] Zendejas B, Zarroug AE, Erben YM, Holley CT, Farley DR.Impact of childhood inguinal hernia repair in adulthood: 50 years of follow-up. J Am Coll Surg. 2010 Dec;211(6):762-8

[11] Tackett, LD, Breuer, CK, Luks, FI, et al. Incidence of contralateral inguinal hernia: a prospective analysis. J Pediatr Surg 1999; 34:684.

[12] Miltenburg, DM, Nuchtern, JG, Jaksic, T, et al. Meta-analysis of the risk of metachronous hernia in infants and children. Am J Surg 1997; 174:741.

[13] Rescorla FJ, Grosfeld JL. Inguinal hernia repair in the perinatal period and early infancy: clinical considerations. J Pediatr Surg 1984;19:832 - 7.

[14] Sheynkin YR, Hendin BN, Schlel PN, et al. Microsurgical repair of iatrogenic injury to the vas deferens. J Urol 1998;159:139- 41.

[15] Lipskar AM, Soffer SZ, Glick RD, Rosen NG, Levitt MA, Hong AR. Laparoscopic inguinal hernia inversion and ligation in female children: a review of 173 consecutive cases at a single institution. J Pediatr Surg. 2010 ;45(6):1370-4.

[16] Klin B, Efrati Y, Abu-Kishk I, Stolero S, Lotan G. The contribution of intraoperative transinguinal laparoscopic examination of the contralateral side to the repair of inguinal hernias in children. World J Pediatr. 2010 ;6(2):119-24

[17] Parelkar SV, Oak S, Gupta R, Sanghvi B, Shimoga PH, Kaltari D, Prakash A, Shekhar R, Gupta A, Bachani M. Laparoscopic inguinal hernia repair in the pediatric age group-experience with 437 children. J Pediatr Surg. 2010 ;45(4):789-92.

[18] Aaron M. Lipskar, Samuel Z. Soffera, Richard D. Glicka, Nelson G. Rosena, Marc A. Levittb and Andrew R. Hong. Laparoscopic inguinal hernia inversion and ligation in female children: a review of 173 consecutive cases at a single institution. J Pediatr Surg. 2010;45(6):1370-1374.

[19] Shalaby R, Ismail M, Dorgham A, Hefny K, Alsaied G, Gabr K, Abdelaziz M. Laparoscopic hernia repair in infancy and childhood: evaluation of 2 different techniques.J Pediatr Surg. 2010 Nov;45(11):2210-6.

[20] Hassan ME, Mustafawi AR.Laparoscopic flip-flap technique versus conventional inguinal hernia repair in children. JSLS. 2007 Jan-Mar;11(1):90-3.

[21] Esposito C, Montinaro L, Alicchio F, Savanelli A, Armenise T, Settimi A. Laparoscopic treatment of inguinal hernia in the first year of life. J Laparoendosc Adv Surg Tech A. 2010 ;20(5):473-6.

[22] Nah SA, Giacomello L, Eaton S, Coppi PD, Curry JI, Drake DP, Kiely EM, Pierro A. Surgical Repair of Incarcerated Inguinal Hernia in Children: Laparoscopic or Open? Eur J Pediatr Surg. 2010 Oct 11. [Epub ahead of print]

[23] Sneider EB, Jones S, Danielson PD. Refinements in selection criteria for pediatric laparoscopic inguinal hernia repair. J Laparoendosc Adv Surg Tech A. 2009 Apr;19(2):237-40.

[24] F. Schier, Laparoscopic inguinal hernia repair—a prospective personal series of 542 children, J Pediatr Surg. 2006;41: 1081–1084

[25] F.Schier, P.Montupet and C.Esposito et al. Laparoscopic inguinal herniorrhaphy in children: a 3 centre experience with 933 repairs, J Pediatr Surg. 2002;37(3): 395-397.

4

Laparoscopy-Assisted One-Stage Trans-Scrotal Orchiopexy Applicable to All Types of Maldescended Testes

Masao Endo, Miwako Nakano, Toshihiko Watanabe, Michinobu Ohno, Fumiko Yoshida and Etsuji Ukiyama
Department of Pediatric Surgery, Saitama City Hospital
Japan

1. Introduction

So-called malposition of the testis includes congenital undescended testis (intra-abdominal, canal, and high scrotal), ectopic testis, retractile testis, vanishing testis and so on. An exact preoperative diagnosis has been mandatory for selecting an appropriate therapeutic modality for each type of malposition. Embryologically, undescended testis syndrome should be associated with a patent processus vaginalis (PPV) (Fonkalsrud, 1986). The principle of orchiopexy for undescended testis consists of the closure of the PPV high at its neck (Radmayr C. et al., 1999) and the placement of the pedunculated testis into the dartos pouch. Inguinal exploration has been a standard approach for this aim and Fowler-Stephens' one-stage or two-stage operation has been recommended for intra-abdominal testes (Kogan, 1992).
Laparoscopic PPV closure using an Endoneedle, which we specifically developed for PPV closure (Endo, et al., 2001) conducted us to its application to orchiopexy. And the procedures have been sophisticated to facilitate one-stage orchiopexy that is applicable to all types of malpositioned testes by combining a diagnostic/therapeutic laparoscopy and an orchiopexy through trans-scrotal incision, while rendering most of preoperative diagnostic modalities unnecessary. The purpose of this paper is to introduce our strategy for a systematic approach to cryptorchidism using laparoscopy, and to discuss the detailed operative procedures and its outcomes.

2. Materials and methods

[Surgical strategy]
Diagnostic laparoscopy was initially performed using a 5-mm telescope inserted through the umbilicus and 2-mm grasping forceps placed below the umbilicus to evaluate internal inguinal rings (IIRs). If a PPV was not present, the procedure advanced to pathway 1, 2 or 3, as shown in Fig. 1.
In the case of a mid-canal, low canal or high scrotal testis with or without inguinal hernia or hydrocele, the procedure advanced to pathway 4; in the case of intra-abdominal, peeping or high canal testis, the procedure advanced to pathway 5.

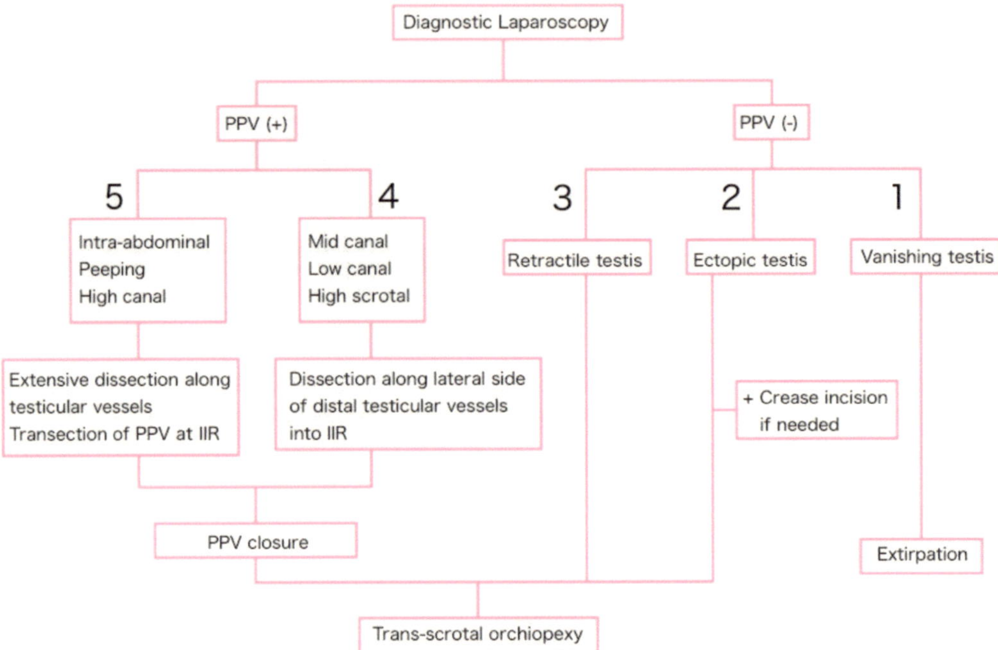

Fig. 1. Flow chart for systematic approach to malpositioned testes. Even in pathway 1, 2 or 3, PPV closure is performed if a concurrent PPV/cPPV is found.
Abbreviations; PPV, patent processus vaginalis; IIR, internal inguinal ring

Laparoscopic procedures: A 14-gauge sheath needle, which can be used as a port, is inserted immediately above the internal inguinal ring (IIR) or in the flank of the affected side at the same level as the umbilicus. For mid-canal, low canal, or high scrotal testes (pathway 4), small electrocautery incisions are made along the distal portion of the testicular vessels to separate the vessels from the peritoneum. Next, the spermatic cord is detached from the peritoneum. Dissection of the peritoneum and retroperitoneal tenacious tissues along the lateral side of the vessels at the IIR level allows the seminal cord to be mobilized (Fig. 2).
These procedures are performed using a 2-mm grasper with monopolar electrocautery device and endo-scissors inserted through the 14-gauge sheath needle.
For intra-abdominal, peeping or high canal testes, the peritoneum overlying the testicular vessels is incised along both sides of the vessels toward the mesentery root using electrocautery and endo-scissors. Thorough stripping of the vessels and cord is performed postero-laterally, and the peritoneal wall of the processus vaginalis is incised circularly at the IIR so as to transect the PPV. The gubernaculum is cut off if it is necessary for further mobilization of the testicular system. After thrusting the testicle into the processus vaginalis (PV) (Fig. 3), the proximal portion of the processus vaginalis is closed using an Endoneedle, placing the testicular vessels and cord outside of the ligature.
In cases of contra-lateral PPV (cPPV), proximal portion of the PV was simultaneously closed using the same procedure. Details of the techniques for PPV closure have been reported previously (Endo, et al., 2009).
Trans-scrotal orchiopexy: A 2 cm incision is made along the uppermost border of the scrotum. A dartos pouch is prepared toward the bottom of the scrotum by separating a layer between the dartos sheath and scrotal skin. The distal portion of the PV is identified and freed from

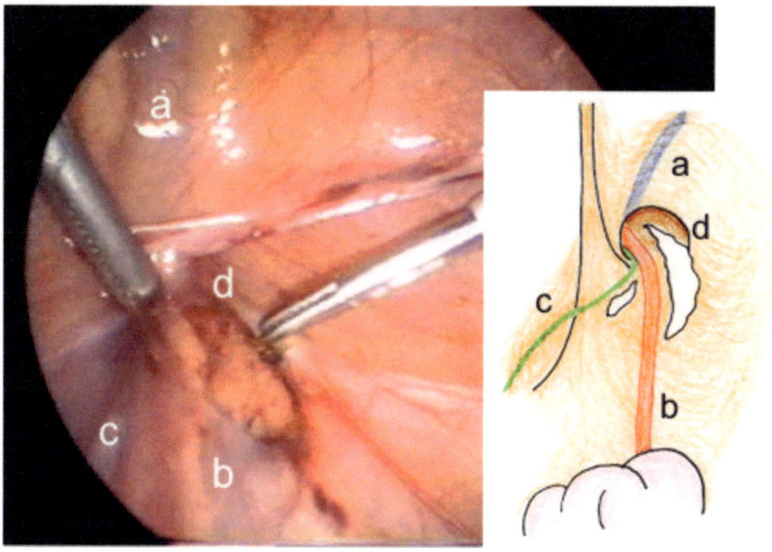

Fig. 2. Preparation of the distal testicular vessels for right sided mid canal testis. Dissection of the peritoneum and retroperitoneal tenacious tissue along the lateral side of the testicular vessels into the IIR so as to allow the medial and downward shift of the vessels.
Abbreviations; a, hypogastric vessels; b, testicular vessels; c, spermatic cord; d, orifice of PPV

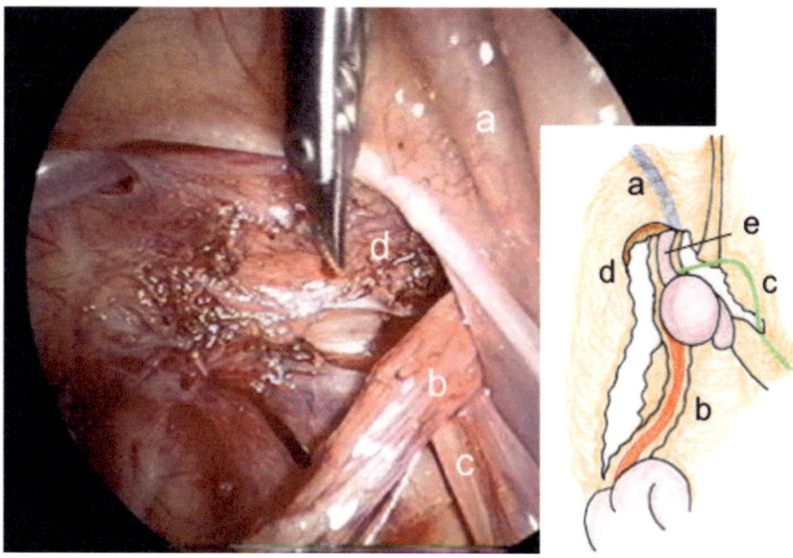

Fig. 3. Extensive dissection along the testicular vessels for left sided peeping testis. Thorough stripping of the vessels and cord from a postero-lateral aspect and transection of the PPV at the level of the IIR. Photograph shows endoscissors cutting off the tenacious tissue at the floor of the inguinal canal to loosen the seminal cord. The testis has been placed in transected PV, waiting for traction from the outside.
Abbreviations; a-d, same as figure 2; e, gubernaculum testis

the surrounding connective tissues high at its neck through the incision. The testis is drawn out through this incision and drawn past the lowest portion of the PPV. The seminal stalk is stitched to the dartos sheath at the cephalad leaf of the incision, which is retracted cranially by a hook while providing a gentle downward traction of the testis so as to place the stitch on the stalk at as high a point as possible. Finally, the pedunculated testis is placed inside the dartos pouch (Fig. 4).

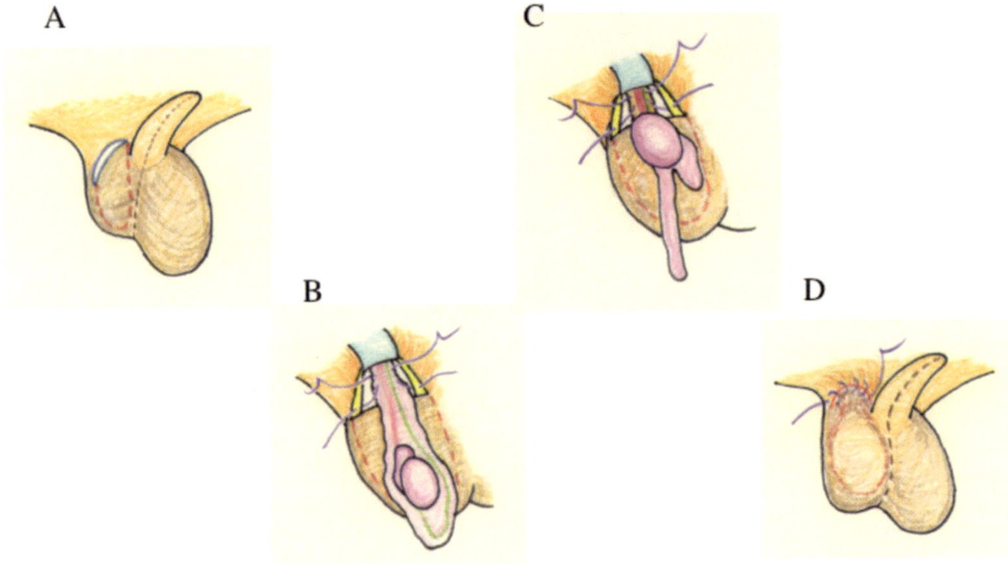

Fig. 4. Schematic drawing of trans-scrotal orchiopexy. A: A 2 cm incision is made along the uppermost line of the scrotum, and a large dartos pouch sufficient to accommodate the testis and attached structures is created. B: In cases of canal testis, the PPV containing the testis is drawn out, freed from tenacious connective tissue high at its neck, and trimmed along the testis and seminal cord, cutting away an excess vaginal tunic containing cremaster muscle fibers. The stalk is stitched to the dartos sheath of the cephalad leaf of the wound at a suitable height to accommodate the testis in the dartos pouch. C: In cases of intra-abdominal or peeping testis, the scrotal wound is retracted with a retractor. Sutures for fixation are applied to the tunica along the cord and vessels as high as possible. D: The scrotal skin is closed with a running suture.

[Study design]

Between May 2000 and December 2007, this procedure was performed in 159 boys with maldescended testes (191 testes). Preoperative diagnosis was conducted at our outpatient department and confirmed upon admission. Patient characteristics with regard to the testicular location and associated hernia/hydrocele are shown in Table 1.

This series included 23 boys with non-palpable testis (NPT) including 1 with hernia and 80 boys with canal testis, in whom 7 had bilateral canal testes, 12 (13.6%) had hernia and 5 (5.7%) with hydrocele. High scrotal testis was observed in 35 boys, in whom 6 had bilateral high scrotal testes, 3 (7.0%) had hernia and 26 (60.5%) had hydrocele. Eight out of 10 boys with retractile testis had bilateral retractile testes, and none of them exhibited hernia or hydrocele. The remaining 11 boys had maldescended testes in combination of varying locations.

Location of testes	Affected side: Right	Left	Bilateral	Total numbers of patients	Total numbers of testes
NPT	14	9		23	23
(with hernia)		(1)		(1, 4.3%)	(1, 4.3%)
Canal	27	46	7	80	87
(with hernia)	(6)	(4)	(right, 2)	(12, 13.6%)	(12, 12.6%)
(with hydrocele)	(2)	(3)		(5, 5.7%)	(5, 5.3%)
High scrotal	22	7	6	35	41
(with hernia)	(1)	(1)		(3, 7.0%)	(3, 6.1%)
(with hydrocele)	(17)	(5)	(right,1; bilateral, 2)	(26, 60.5%)	(28, 57.1%)
Retractile	1	1	8	10	18
Combined			11	11	22
NPT & Canal	NPT	Canal		1	2
NPT & High scrotal	High scrotal	NPT		1	2
Canal & High scrotal	Canal	High scrotal		3	6
(with hydrocele)		(1)			
	High scrotal	Canal		2	4
Canal & Retractile	Retractile	Canal		1	2
	Canal	Retractile		1	2
High scrotal & Retractile	Retractile	High scrotal		2	4
Total				159	191
(with hernia/hydrocele)				(47, 29.6%)	(49, 25.7%)

Table 1. Patient characteristics
Notes; The words in parenthesis indicate numbers and rates of associated hernia/hydrocele. Rates of associated hernia/hydrocele in the total numbers of patients and testes include each testis in combined cases individually.
Abbreviation; NPT, non-palpable testis

Age at operation ranged from 4 months to 13 years, with a median age of 2 years and 0 months. Ages of patients according to the testicular location generally decreased in proportion to a higher position.

Location of testes	Total number of patients	Age: Minimum	Maximum	Median
NPT	25	11m	10y8m	1y4m
Canal	87	9m	12y2m	1y11m
High scrotal	37	4m	13y0m	2y2m
Retractile	10	1y3m	4y7m	3y8m
Total	159	4m	13y0m	3y0m

Table 2. Age distribution according to the location of testes.
Note; In cases of combined locations, the higher location is represented.

Each boy underwent various operative procedures according to the flow chart shown in Fig. 1. Medical records of these children were analyzed to determine detailed location of testis, which was confirmed during the operation; patency of the PV; types of operative procedures used; operation times; and postoperative outcomes. Patients were followed up regularly at our outpatient department by physical examination, including periodical echogram, until 7 months, and once each year until adolescence, when seminal emission begins. Follow-up periods ranged from 3 years and 2 months to 10 years and 9 months.

3. Results

Percentages of associated PPV according to testis location determined during operation are shown in Table 3; overall, PPV was associated with 84.1% of all undescended testes, excluding the retractile and ectopic testes, which are not considered to be true undescended testes.

Location of testes	Affected side		Total numbers of testes	PPV	
	Right	Left		affected side	contralateral side
Intra-abdominal	1	3	4	4(100%)	2(50%)
Peeping	4	11	15	15(100%)	5(33.3%)
High canal	12	12	24	18(75%)	3(12.5%)
Midcanal	6	8	14	11(78.6%)	4(28.6%)
Low canal	26	26	52	41(78.8%)	17(32.7%)
High scrotal	26	16	42	38(90.5%)	22(52.4%)
Retractile	20	18	38	9(23.7%)	11(28.9%)
Ectopic	1	1	2	1(50%)	0(0%)
Total	96	95	191	127/151(84.1%)*	53/151(35.1%)*

Table 3. Location of testes defined from operation and concurrent presence of PPVs. Abbreviation; *, Numbers of retractile and ectopic testis were excluded from denominators.

All intra-abdominal and peeping testes had PPV. High scrotal testes exhibited the second highest rate of PPV (90.5%). Contra-lateral PPV was found in 35.1% of patients. All PPVs and cPPVs were closed in the same session.

Types of procedures performed included extensive dissection along the testicular vessels with transection of the PPV at the IIR (ExtVasDic) + laparoscopic PPV closure (LPC) + trans-scrotal orchiopexy (TSO) in 30 boys (average operation time, 99 +/- 23 minutes); preparation of the distal testicular vessels with peritoneal dissection along the lateral side of the IIR (DistVasPrep) + LPC + TSO in 11 boys (average operation time, 82 +/- 17 minutes), LPC + TSO in 67 boys (average operation time, 70 +/- 15 minutes), and a diagnostic laparoscopy (DiagLap) + TSO in 15 boys (average operation time, 48 +/- 13 minutes; see Table 4).

Operative procedure	Number of patients	Operation Time Mean +/- SD (minutes)
DiagLap + TSO	15	48 +/- 13
LPC + TSO	67	70 +/- 15
DistVasPrep + LPC + TSO	11	82 +/- 17
ExtVasPrep + LPC + TSO	30	99 +/- 23
Crease incision added	4	124 +/- 24
Bilateral TSO*	32	83 +/- 43

Table 4. Operative procedures and operation times.
Abbreviations; DiagLap, diagnostic laparoscopy; LPC, laparoscopic closure of PPV; DistVasPrep, preparation of distal portion of testicular vessels; ExtVasPrep, extensive vascular preparation; *, Bilateral orchiopexy with various combinations of above the procedures (DiagLap+TSO and LPC+TSO occupied 97% of 62 procedures performed in 32 patients).

A crease incision was added in 4 boys: one with an intra-abdominal testis, 2 with high canal testes, and 1 with an ectopic testis. The crease incision was performed in the first case to ensure the anatomical relationship of laparoscopically prepared IIR from outside of the body, as this was the first time this type of procedure had been conducted; in the latter cases, incisions were made due of difficulty in finding the distal sac for the obliterated PV. This occurred near the beginning of the surgeons' learning curve. In all the cases, the testes were successfully repositioned, and they continued to descend toward the bottom of the scrotum after the operation (Fig. 5).

Testicular atrophy or hernia formation did not occur in any of the cases, and cosmesis was excellent in all the patients (Fig. 6).

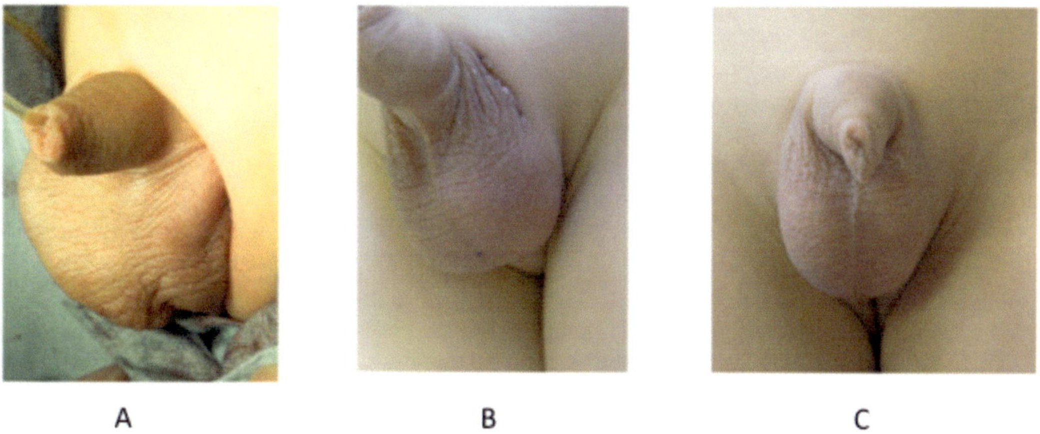

Fig. 5. Follow-up figures of trans-scrotal orchidopexy. A: Immediately after the operation, the closed wound is markedly retracted into the inguinal canal because of the short seminal cord. B: Three months later, the testicle has descended into the scrotum in conjunction with the retracted wound returning to the previous position. C: Six months after the operation, the wound has healed leaving no scar.

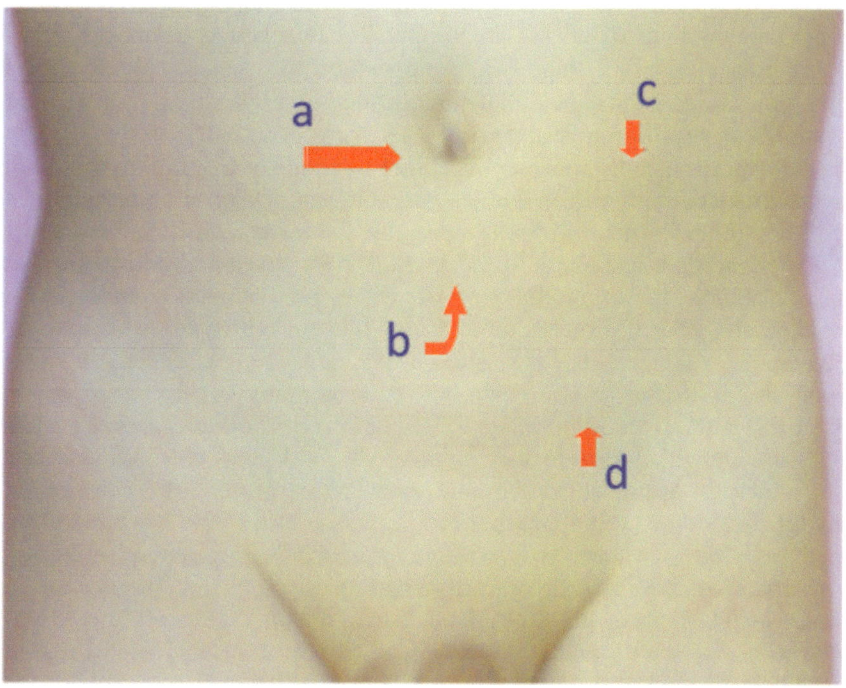

Fig. 6. Wound cosmesis 6 months after the operation in a boy who underwent orchiopexy for left canal testis. Actually invisible surgical wounds for a 5-mm laparoscope inserted through the umbilicus (a), a 2-mm grasping forceps placed below the umbilicus (b), a 14-G sheath needle used as a port for grasping forceps, electrocautery device or endoscissors (c) and 16-G Endoneedle for the closure of the PPV (d).

4. Discussion

The most effective strategy for treating undescended testes remains controversial. Patients with cryptorchidism have their testes in various locations from intra-abdominal region to a high scrotal position. Inguinal exploration has been a standard approach for managing undescended testis. Many surgical procedures have been devised as alternatives to this approach. Diagnostic and therapeutic laparoscopy has flourished as a treatment for nonpalpable testis. Jordan et al. reported a completely endoscopic approach to orchiopexy (Jordan, et al., 1992); since then, laparoscopic orchiopexy for intra-abdominal testis with direct transfer or a Fowler-Stephens (F-S) procedure has been developed, providing better results than the traditional open orchiopexy (success rates of 95% vs. 76%) (Samadi, et al., 2003). Moursy, et al. reported better outcomes using laparoscopic F-S procedures in comparison with laparoscopic direct orchiopexy, with overall success rates of 100% and 88.8%, respectively. Therefore, there is a higher tendency to perform F-S orchiopexy in patients treated laparoscopically, than in patients for which open orchiopexies were performed (Alam, et al., 2003).

A recent strategy for treating intra-abdominal testis under laparoscopic control has been the combination of laparoscopic direct and F-S orchiopexy, depending on the distance of the testis from the internal inguinal ring, in which the F-S orchiopexy occupies approximately 20-30% of total (Samadi, et al., 2003, Kim, et al., 2010). A recent meta-analysis of F-S orchiopexy reported a pooled estimated success rate of 80% for single F-S orchiopexy and 85% for 2-stage F-S orchiopexy. There was no difference in the success rate between laparoscopic and open techniques in either single or 2-stage F-S orchiopexy (Elyas, et al., 2010). On the other hand, laparoscopic procedures exhibit potential complications, including risk of testicular atrophy, with an overall F-S procedure success rate of 85% (Chang, et al, 2001).

Following the experiences of laparoscopic direct orchiopexy in intra-abdominal testis, the application of this technique to canalicular palpable testis has been attempted (Docimo, et al., 1995). Although, procedures for treating canalicular testis require increased laparoscopic skill and experience compared to those required for intra-abdominal testis treatment (Riquelme, et al., 2006), the reported success rates are promising, accounting for more than 95%, in comparison with the report of open method, in which the success rate was 82% (Docimo, 1995).

Trans-scrotal or pre-scrotal orchiopexy has been recently emerging as an alternative approach for testes that can be mobilized into the scrotum under general anesthesia. This procedure is advantageous due to less invasiveness and good cosmesis compared to the standard two-incision approach in selected cases (Yucel, et al., 2011, Dayanc, et al., 2007, Lais, Ferro, 1996). However, for palpable but immobile testes or testes located proximal to the external ring, the standard two-incision approach is recommended because of the difficulty in PV dissection and ligation at a sufficiently high level and shortness of the vascular pedicle (Dayanc, et al., 2007, Lais, Ferro, 1996). Our procedure involved only cutting off a portion of the PV wall, in which cremaster muscle fibers are included, along the spermatic pedicle, instead of the separation of the vas and vessels from the PV and ligation of the PV high at its neck, because the open IIR is closed from inside of the abdomen by the Endoneedle technique (Endo, et al., 2009).

For delivery of the testis, a neo-ring lateral to the bladder and medial to the median umbilical ligament has been widely utilized by employing an additional scrotal trocar for intra-abdominal and high canalicular testes (Poppas, et al., 1996, Docimo, et al., 1995, He, et al., 2008). The presence of PPV is ignored in the description of operation procedures in most reports (Samadi, et al., 2003, Chang, et al., 2001, Kim, et al., 2010, Moursy, et al., 2010), and recent consensus in the literature has been to leave the ring open because of rare occurrence of postoperative inguinal hernia (Riquelme, et al., 2006, Mohta, et al., 2003), although Poppas et al. included closure of the defect using a stapling device if a hernia was present (Poppas, et al., 1996).

However, a potential disadvantage of laparoscopic orchiopexy, compared to the traditional open approach, is the subsequent development of an inguinal hernia or hydrocele (Baker, et al., 2001, Chang, et al., 2001, Metwalli, Cheng, 2002, Al-Mandil, et al., 2008, Palmer, Rastinehad, 2008). Ziylan O, et al. reported that patients requiring reorchiopexy had inadequate repair of inguinal hernia or PPV in 62.5% of cases, which was considered to be an important factor leading to failure after surgical treatment of undescended testis (Ziylan, et al., 2004). Essentially, cryptorchidism is frequently associated with PPV as He D., et al reported associated PPV in 90.3% of ipsilateral side and 15.6% of contralateral side (He, et al., 2008). In our series, 29.6% of patients had associated hernia/hydrocele, and 84.1% of patients had ipsilateral PPV and 35.1% had cPPV. Because second operations for subsequent hernia repair in a scarred wound can cause serious injury to the testicular blood supply, we strongly recommend the closure of the PV during orchiopexy (Metwalli, Cheng, 2002, Yucel, et al., 2011).

Retractile testis is defined as the testis that is usually located outside the scrotum, but can be drawn manually into the bottom of the scrotum, and has no associated PPV. It is considered not to be true undescended testis and does not require therapy (He, et al., 2008). We performed operations on 10 boys with preoperatively diagnosed retractile testis in whom the testis was not found inside the scrotum in more than 50% of occasions during parental observation. These operations were carried out after a period of observation at outpatient clinic and under informed consent. This explains why the averaged ages of this group was high, as indicated in Table 2. Four boys who had retractile testis as one of the combined maldescended testes underwent operation to prevent an expected imbalance of testicular location relative to the opposite side, where the true undescended testis had been relocated. Inan M., et al. observed smaller testicular volume in school age children with retractile testis and estimated some negative effects on the development of testicular volume of retractile testis (Inan, et al., 2008). Patients and their parents were very satisfied that the testes were always in the scrotum.

Our procedures provide a systematic approach using the algorithm shown in Fig. 1 to treat all types of maldescended testis. The primary advantage of our technique is that it can be used as a one-stage diagnostic and therapeutic modality to treat all types of maldescended testes, including routine PPV closures, orchiopexy through the natural embryological route, and trans-scrotal orchiopexy. Our laparoscopy-assisted one-stage trans-scrotal orchiopexy can free patients from many preoperative examinations, such as angiography, radioisotope, CT, and MRI, among others.

Retroperitoneum dissection and preparation of the testicular vessels from the mesentery root into the processus vaginalis in proportion to the testicular position provides the additional length required for proper mobilization of the testis into the dartos pouch. Preparation of the extra-abdominal seminal cord high at its neck can be easily performed through an incision placed in the uppermost region of the scrotum.

It is strongly advised to obtain a completely tension-free pedicle before fixing the testis into the scrotum (Yucel, et al., 2011). In our procedure, the testis does not need to be placed

enough into the scrotum, because during fixing of the seminal cord to the cephalad leaf of the incisional wound, the wound is retracted by a hook in a cranial direction, while the seminal cord is pulled down in a caudal direction. Therefore, the seminal cord can be sutured at its highest position to the dartos sheath of the retracted wound. The testis descends further into the scrotum as the sutured position descends along with the wound, returning to the previous position. Because laparoscopic orchiopexy performed without dividing the spermatic vessels does not affect normal testicular vascularization, the F-S procedure was not required in the present series. Eposito C, et al. successfully performed orchiopexy for intra-abdominal testis without division of the testicular vessels (direct pull-through into the scrotum), through the IIR, if this open, or through the Neo-Ring with subsequent closure of the IIR (Esposito, et al., 2000), which is in accordance with our procedure of pathway 5.
The testes were successfully repositioned and postoperatively continued to descend toward the bottom of the scrotum in all of the patients in this series. No testicular atrophy or hernia formation occurred, and cosmesis was excellent in all the patients.

5. Conclusion

We proposed a systematic approach to cryptorchidism, facilitating one-stage orchiopexy by combining a diagnostic/therapeutic laparoscopy and an orchiopexy through a trans-scrotal incision. This systematic approach was applied to 191 testes in 159 boys. The testes were provided additional length of the vascular stalk by dissecting the retroperitoneum in proportion to the testicular position under laparoscopic control. All concurrent PPVs were closed using the Endoneedle technique. And all the testes were delivered into the scrotum through the natural embryological route from the scrotal incision without necessitating any F-S procedures. This procedure was thought to be a useful one-stage diagnostic and therapeutic maneuver for all nonpalpable and palpable maldescended testes, enabling increased patient privacy owing to virtually invisible scars.

6. References

Al-Mandil, M., Khoury, A. E., El-Hout, Y., Kogon, M., Dave, S. & Farhat, W. A. (2008). Potential complications with the prescrotal approach for the palpable undescended testis? A comparison of single prescrotal incision to the traditional inguinal approach. *J Urol*, 180(2), 686-689.

Alam, S. & Radhakrishnan, J. (2003). Laparoscopy for nonpalpable testes. *J Pediatr Surg*, 38(10), 1534-1536.

Baker, L. A., Docimo, S. G., Surer, I., Peters, C., Cisek, L., Diamond, D. A., Caldamone, A., Koyle, M., Strand, W., Moore, R., Mevorach, R., Brady, J., Jordan, G., Erhard, M. & Franco, I. (2001). A multi-institutional analysis of laparoscopic orchidopexy. *BJU Int*, 87(6), 484-489.

Chang, B., Palmer, L. S. & Franco, I. (2001). Laparoscopic orchidopexy: a review of a large clinical series. *BJU Int*, 87(6), 490-493.

Dayanc, M., Kibar, Y., Irkilata, H. C., Demir, E., Tahmaz, L. & Peker, A. F. (2007). Long-term outcome of scrotal incision orchiopexy for undescended testis. *Urology*, 70(4), 786-788; discussion 788-789.

Docimo, S. G. (1995). The results of surgical therapy for cryptorchidism: a literature review and analysis. *J Urol,* 154(3), 1148-1152.

Docimo, S. G., Moore, R. G., Adams, J. & Kavoussi, L. R. (1995). Laparoscopic orchiopexy for the high palpable undescended testis: preliminary experience. *J Urol,* 154(4), 1513-1515.

Elyas, R., Guerra, L. A., Pike, J., DeCarli, C., Betolli, M., Bass, J., Chou, S., Sweeney, B., Rubin, S., Barrowman, N., Moher, D. & Leonard, M. (2010). Is staging beneficial for Fowler-Stephens orchiopexy? A systematic review. *J Urol,* 183(5), 2012-2018.

Endo, M., Ukiyama, E. (2001). Laparoscopic closure of patent processus vaginalis in girls with inguinal hernia using a specially devised suture needle. *Pediatr Endosurg Innov Techn,* 5(2), 187-191.

Endo, M., Watanabe, T., Nakano, M., Yoshida, F. & Ukiyama, E. (2009). Laparoscopic completely extraperitoneal repair of inguinal hernia in children: a single-institute experience with 1,257 repairs compared with cut-down herniorrhaphy. *Surg Endosc,* 23(8), 1706-1712.

Esposito, C., Vallone, G., Settimi, A., Gonzalez Sabin, M. A., Amici, G. & Cusano, T. (2000). Laparoscopic orchiopexy without division of the spermatic vessels: can it be considered the procedure of choice in cases of intraabdominal testis? *Surg Endosc,* 14(7), 658-660.

Fonkalsrud, E. W. (1986). Undescended testis. In *Pediatric Surgery* ed 4, ed. K. J. Welch, Randolph, J.G., Ravitch, M.M., O'Neil, J.A.Jr., Rowe, M.I., Year Book Medical Publishers Inc. Chicago, London, pp. 793-807.

He, D., Lin, T., Wei, G., Li, X., Liu, J., Hua, Y. & Liu, F. (2008). Laparoscopic orchiopexy for treating inguinal canalicular palpable undescended testis. *J Endourol,* 22(8), 1745-1749.

Inan, M., Aydiner, C. Y., Tokuc, B., Aksu, B., Ayhan, S., Ayvaz, S. & Ceylan, T. (2008). Prevalence of cryptorchidism, retractile testis and orchiopexy in school children. *Urol Int,* 80(2), 166-171.

Jordan, G. H., Robey, E.L., Winslow, B.H. (1992). Laparoendoscopic surgical management of the abdominal/transinguinal undescended testicle. *J Endourol,* 6, 157-161.

Kim, J., Min, G. E. & Kim, K. S. (2010). Laparoscopic orchiopexy for a nonpalpable testis. *Korean J Urol,* 51(2), 106-110.

Kogan, S. (1992). Cryptorchidism. 3 ed. In *Clinical Pediatric Urology,* ed. L. L. King, Belman, A., WB Saunders. Philadelphia, pp. 1050.

Lais, A. & Ferro, F. (1996). Trans-scrotal approach for surgical correction of cryptorchidism and congenital anomalies of the processus vaginalis. *Eur Urol,* 29(2), 235-8; discussion 238-239.

Metwalli, A. R. & Cheng, E. Y. (2002). Inguinal hernia after laparoscopic orchiopexy. *J Urol,* 168(5), 2163.

Mohta, A., Jain, N., Irniraya, K. P., Saluja, S. S., Sharma, S. & Gupta, A. (2003). Non-ligation of the hernial sac during herniotomy: a prospective study. *Pediatr Surg Int,* 19(6), 451-452.

Moursy, E. E., Gamal, W. & Hussein, M. M. (2010). Laparoscopic orchiopexy for non-palpable testes: outcome of two techniques. *J Pediatr Urol.* Epub date, Jun 9.

Palmer, L. S. & Rastinehad, A. (2008). Incidence and concurrent laparoscopic repair of intra-abdominal testis and contralateral patent processus vaginalis. *Urology,* 72(2), 297-299; discussion 299.

Poppas, D. P., Lemack, G. E. & Mininberg, D. T. (1996). Laparoscopic orchiopexy: clinical experience and description of technique. *J Urol,* 155(2), 708-711.

Radmayr, C., Corvin, S., Studen, M., Bartsch, G. & Janetschek, G. (1999). Cryptorchidism, open processus vaginalis, and associated hernia: laparoscopic approach to the internal inguinal ring. *Eur Urol,* 36(6), 631-634.

Riquelme, M., Aranda, A., Rodriguez, C., Villalvazo, H. & Alvarez, G. (2006). Laparoscopic orchiopexy for palpable undescended testes: a five-year experience. *J Laparoendosc Adv Surg Tech A,* 16(3), 321-324.

Samadi, A. A., Palmer, L. S. & Franco, I. (2003). Laparoscopic orchiopexy: report of 203 cases with review of diagnosis, operative technique, and lessons learned. *J Endourol,* 17(6), 365-368.

Yucel, S., Celik, O., Kol, A., Baykara, M. & Guntekin, E. (2011). Initial pre-scrotal approach for palpable cryptorchid testis: results during a 3-year period. *J Urol,* 185(2), 669-672.

Ziylan, O., Oktar, T., Korgali, E., Nane, I. & Ander, H. (2004). Failed orchiopexy. *Urol Int,* 73(4), 313-315.

5

Laparoscopy for the Undescended Testes

Nerli R. B., Reddy M. N. and Hiremath M.B.
Dept of Urology, KLES Kidney Foundation, KLE University's J N Medical College
Belgaum, Karnataka
India

1. Introduction

Cryptorchidism is a term that has been used interchangeably with the term undescended testis. Both terms refer to an abnormally positioned testis, but cryptorchidism literally means "hidden testis". Isolated cryptorchidism is one of the most common congenital anomalies found at birth and affects upward of 3% of full-term male newborns [1-3]. Unilateral cryptorchidism is more common than bilateral cryptorchidism, which occurs in 1.6% to 1.9% of boys. Testicular descent into scrotum is usually complete by the second trimester; however a significantly higher rate of cryptorchidism in premature boys suggests that the process of descent may not be complete until close to term. The cause of cryptorchidism is multifactorial. An undescended testis can be located anywhere between the abdominal cavity and just outside the anatomic scrotum. Approximately 70% to 77% of cryptorchid testes will spontaneously descend, usually by 3 months of age [3]. Factors that predict complete spontaneous descent by 3 months of age include low birth weight, bilateral cryptorchidism, normal scrotal anatomy and testis that are positioned lower along the normal path of descent; boys with a small or poorly rugated scrotum and those with hypospadias are more likely to be cryptorchid at 3 months [2]. By 1 year of age, the incidence of cryptorchidism declines to about 1% and remains constant throughout adulthood.

Normal germ cell development during childhood is a continuous process that is completed at puberty [4]. Undescended testes demonstrate more pronounced impairment in germ cell development the higher the testes are located, although newborns with intrabdominal testes have a normal number of germ cells [4]. The histopathologic hallmarks associated with cryptorchidism are evident between 1 and 2 years of age and include decreased numbers of leydig cells, degeneration of sertoli cells, delayed disappearance of gonocytes, delayed appearance of adult dark (Ad) spermatogonia, failure of primary spermatocytes to develop, and reduced total germ cell counts [5-7]. A decrease in cryptorchid testes volume by 6 months of age has been reported [8]. Similar pathology has been observed in the contralateral descended testis, though to a lesser extent, which supports the theory of hypogonadotrophic hypogonadism as the possible cause of the decreased fertility seen in males with unilateral cryptorchidism[6, 9]. Histopathologic studies in younger cohorts of patients have provided evidence of abnormal germ cell maturation correlating with spermiograms in adulthood. Biopsy findings from children with unilateral cryptorchidism typically demonstrate reduced total germ cell counts as a result of failure of the two prepubertal steps involved in maturation and proliferation of germ cells: 1) transformation of the fetal stem cell pool (gonocytes) into adult stem cell pool (Ad spermatogonia) at 2 to 3 months of age and 2) transformation of Ad spermatogonia into primary spermatocytes (meiosis) at 4 to 5 years[10].

When specific stage of germ cell maturation was examined, transformation of gonocytes into Ad spermatogonia between 2 and 3 months of age appeared to be critical for male fertility, not the total number of germ cells. Lee [11] postulated that paternity would be a better index for verification than the sperm count because it is known that men with subnormal sperm counts can have normal paternity rates. When compared with a control group, paternity was significantly compromised in men with previous bilateral, but not unilateral cryptorchidism (53% versus 75%, respectively) [12].

It is a well established fact that children born with undescended testes are at increased risk for testicular malignancy. Approximately 10% of testicular tumors arise from an undescended testis [13]. The incidence of a testicular tumor in the general population is 1 in 100,000 , and the incidence of a germ cell tumor in men formally cryptorchid is 1 in 2550 ; therefore , the relative risk is approximately 40 times greater [13]. It is controversial whether orchiopexy affects the natural history of development of a testicular tumor, although emerging evidence supports the claim that prepubescent orchiopexy may lessen the risk. Moller and associates [14] reported on a large cohort of men in Denmark and found the relative risk for testicular cancer in men with treated or persisting cryptorchidism to be 3.6 (95% confidence interval (CI), 1.8 to 6.9) , but no increase in risk was observed in men who reported a history of undescended testes that underwent spontaneous descent . Studies provide evidence to support the contention that early orchidopexy may protect against the development of malignancy.

2. Management of cryptorchidism

Definitive treatment of an undescended testis should take place between 6 and 12 months of age. Spontaneous descent occurs by 3 months of age in most boys. Early intervention should be considered in order to theoretically prevent the complications of cryptorchidism that may be manifested before 1 year of age. Every effort should be made to preserve any testicular tissue at an early age, especially in children with unilateral or bilateral intra-abdominal testes. This recommendation is based on the poor paternity rates in men with a history of bilateral cryptorchidism. Orchiectomy is typically reserved for postpubescent males with a contralateral normally descended testis when the cryptorchid testis is either anatomically or morphologically abnormal or too far from scrotum to allow for tension free placement without compromising the vascular integrity of the testis.

Laparoscopy has achieved its greatest degree of general acceptance, both diagnostically and therapeutically, in the realm of pediatric urology for the management of a nonpalpable testis. Several thousand cases in the literature have documented the impact of laparoscopy in the management of a nonpalpable testis, over a quarter of century. Clear advantages of laparoscopy with regard to specificity and sensitivity have been shown compared to ultrasonography and magnetic resonance imaging in detecting intra-abdominal testes. The principles of surgery for a nonpalpable testis are equal to, if not enhanced by a laparoscopic approach; exposure, lighting and magnification remain critical to this pediatric procedure. The advantages of laparoscopy over conventional open surgical approach to a nonpalpable testis include accurate anatomic assessment of testicular position and viability and, when necessary, optimal accessibility to the crux of the surgical problem [15].

3. Indications for laparoscopy

- All cases of nonpalpable testes: integrated concept of diagnostic laparoscopy combined with open surgery (revision of inguinal canal, with or without orchiopexy) or combined with therapeutic laparoscopy (staged orchiopexy or orchiectomy for intra-abdominal testes).

- Suspected intersex (laparoscopy for diagnosis, eventually biopsy and/or orchiectomy).

Several limitations can be associated with laparoscopy especially in children as smaller body size implies smaller space tolerances of the abdominal wall, which makes standard trocar placement more dangerous. Looser attachments of the peritoneum to the extraperitoneal structures in children makes trocar placement more difficult. Use of a dull trocar is a potentially dangerous instrument in children. Acute infectious disease, coagulopathy and prior abdominal surgery with suspected adhesions form contraindications for a laparoscopic procedure.

Instruments for laparoscopic procedures should include a video cart with insufflators, light source, video camera, video monitor, video recorder and electrocautery unit. In smaller children it is preferable to use mini-laparoscope (1.9 mm) with 2.7 mm trocar shaft, and for older children 3.5 or 5 mm laparoscopes. 3.5 mm trocars and laparoscopic forceps/graspers/scissors are used in smaller children, whereas 5 mm trocars and instruments are used in older children. 5 mm or 10 mm clipping instruments may also be necessary.

4. Diagnostic laparoscopy for a nonpalpable testis

A nonpalpable testis accounts for approximately one fifth of children with an undescended testis. Diagnostic laparoscopy has been commonly used for the assessment of a nonpalpable testis, with the accuracy of testicular localization reported to be greater than 95%[16, 17]. Radiologic imaging studies carried out to identify a nonpalpable testis, carry unacceptable false-negative and false-positive rates [18, 19]. Elder [20] reported that inguinal ultrasound, rarely localises a true nonpalpable testis and in only 18% of cases correctly identified testes located in the inguinal canal. Magnetic resonance imaging has been shown to be an effective method of detection in 37% of cases [21]. Radiographic imaging is also not adequately sensitive enough to determine the quality of the testis when compared with direct visualization. This includes assessing whether the testis is dysmorphic or hypoplastic or whether epididymal or vassal non-union anomalies coexist that would ultimately have an impact on the type of surgical procedure performed. Whatever be the technique used , radiographic or surgical , it must be highly accurate because the fate of a missed intra-abdominal testis is potentially serious with respect to preserving testicular function and can be catastrophic because of the risk of malignancy . Diagnostic laparoscopy has also been shown to be useful in the management of a previous inconclusive open exploration for a nonpalpable testis[22, 23].

5. Technique

The technique of diagnostic laparoscopy begins with patient in supine and 10° head down position. A bladder catheter is placed and if need arises a nasogastric tube is also inserted. Access is gained either with a modified veress needle technique where the rectus fascia is identified and incised prior to needle introduction, or via the open technique. The open technique involves a semilunar supraumbilical or an infraumbilical incision carried down to the rectus fascia. The rectus fascia is opened and the preperitoneal fat is spread enough to expose the peritoneum. The peritoneum is grasped and brought up to the incision. The peritoneal layer is opened sharply and the trocar placed usually between the obliterated umbilical arteries. This open (Hasson technique) method lessens the risk of inadvertent trauma to the intra-abdominal structures, as well as extraperitoneal insufflation. Pneumoperitoneum is created with CO_2 at a flow rate between 8 and 10 L/min with a pressure limit of 8 to 10 mm Hg. A 2-0 absorbable U stitch is placed in the rectus fascia to help maintain the pneumoperitoneum and facilitate quick closure, especially if the fasciotomy has been generous. The anaesthesiologist is requested not to use NO_2 during induction or any portion of the procedure to avoid bowel distension.

The pediatric laparoscope is introduced to view the intraperitoneal pelvic anatomy. The various anatomical landmarks are identified which include the bladder and the urachal ligament, lateral umbilical ligaments, inferior epigastric vessels, internal ring, vas deferens and spermatic vessels. Examining the side opposite the pathology is useful for comparing normal anatomy, especially in the case of a vanishing testis, so that the degree of atresia can be directly measured.

There are three distinct possibilities and courses of action that can arise when diagnostic laparoscopy is used to assess a nonpalpable testis.

1. All spermatic cord structures are present and enter into the inguinal canal (viable intracanalicular testis or an intracanalicular or scrotal atrophic testis)
2. Spermatic vessels and vas deferens can be identified. They end blindly on the psoas muscle without any detectable testis (vanishing testis , anorchia)
3. Intra-abdominal testis present with or without open inguinal canal

Examination of the contralateral testis has been helpful in predicting the fate of the nonpalpable testis; however, it is not a reliable method of definitely determining testicular presence or absence. Hypertrophy of a normally descended testis may connote monorchia. A dysgenetic or hypoplastic testis will not usually result in contralateral testicular hypertrophy, defined as a testis greater than 2 ml or testicular length greater than 2 cm. A contralateral testis length of 2 .0 cm or greater predicted monorchia in over 90% of cases [24-26]. Approximately 34% to 64% of children with a nonpalpable testis will be monorchid [27]. An intra-abdominal vanishing testis will demonstrate the classic anatomy of a blind ending vas and spermatic vessels, usually within a few centimetres of the internal ring. No testicular tissue will be present. When blind ending spermatic vessels are found, no further surgical intervention is necessary, although considerations should be given to performing a trans-scrotal testicular fixation procedure on the normally descended contralateral testis because of the reported risk for abnormal testicular fixation[28].

When the spermatic vessels and the vas are seen exiting the internal ring, including those that are comparatively hypoplastic, one must consider viable testicular tissue within the caudal extent of the descent. An inguino-scrotal exploration must be performed and the cord remnant excised. Even though most testicular remnants or nubbins demonstrate histologic evidence of ischemia and necrosis, in up to 13% of cases viable residual testicular elements will be present [29, 30].

An intra-abdominal testis usually is seen within a few centimetres of the internal ring. In most of these cases, the processus vaginalis is patent and the vas deferens is seen exiting into the inguinal canal (long looping vas deferens). Occasionally an intra-abdominal testis can be much further from the internal ring and has been reported though rarely, in the perinephric, perihepatic or crossed ectopic sites. The vas deferens can demonstrate non-union with any cryptorchid testis and therefore, when blindly ending, is not confirmative of a vanishing testis[30]. The entire abdomen should be inspected at the time of diagnostic laparoscopy. Inspection of the ipsilateral internal ring during diagnostic laparoscopy is important because in 91% of boys with a patent processus vaginalis the testis will be viable whereas if the processus vaginalis is closed 97% of the testes will be vanished or absent [31] .

6. Open inguinal versus laparoscopic exploration for a nonpalpable testis

The choice of traditional open surgical exploration versus primary laparoscopy for assessment of a nonpalpable testis is a matter of debate. Open surgical exploration via an inguinal incision was the procedure most commonly used before the introduction of laparoscopy in the management of a nonpalpable testis. The arguments exist that inguinal-scrotal exploration is nonetheless necessary to evaluate the cord and gonadal structures exiting the internal ring, and thus laparoscopy may have been avoided altogether[32] . Kanemoto et al[33] combined inguinal exploration and transinguinal laparoscopy to test this strategy as an alternative. They found that an extended incision was unnecessary in the case of a blind ending vas and vessels in the peritoneum because this could be easily assessed with transinguinal laparoscopy. Laparoscopy was avoided in 73.3% of cases altogether because the testis, its remnant or testicular vessels, and the vas deferens were detected by inspecting the inguinal region. Ravasse et al[34] felt that laparoscopy was critical to a change in management in only 23% of patients. Several other reports have appeared, wherein utility was found in at-least 50% of patients when diagnostic laparoscopy was performed as the primary approach to a nonpalpable testis. Cisek et al[27] reported that in 66% of their patients benefitted from a primary laparoscopic diagnosis and treatment strategy that would have otherwise resulted in compromised exposure via an inguinal exploration. Laparoscopy, whether primary or adjunctive to an open exploration, offers a logical extension of surgical principles, especially if conversion to a therapeutic laparoscopic procedure is anticipated.

7. Laparoscopic orchidopexy

One of the first indications for laparoscopy in pediatric urology was a nonpalpable testis, reported more than 30 years ago[35]. Originally this procedure was only for diagnostic purposes. As laparoscopy became more and more feasible in pediatric patients, the procedure has progressed to complete laparoscopic orchidopexy in the intervening time. Laparoscopic orchidopexy is now standard in the management of an intra-abdominal undescended testis. A laparoscopic approach has advantages over standard open orchidopexy, in that it accurately assesses the presence, absence, viability and entire anatomy of an intra-abdominal testis. Laparoscopic orchidopexy allows accessibility to the entire course of the spermatic vessels to their origin, usually the limiting factor in tension-free mobilization of an intra-abdominal testis. Dissection close to the origin of the spermatic vessels is possible because the surgeon's range of motion with laparoscopic instrumentation extends across the entire abdominal cavity. Magnification of these delicate vessels aids in dissection and preservation of the main and collateral blood supply.

Technique : The age at which laparoscopic orchidopexy should be performed is the same as for standard open orchidopexy , usually between 6 and 8 months and certainly before 1 year of age . The surgical procedure for a boy with a nonpalpable testis begins with examination under anaesthesia. In approximately 18% of boys a previously nonpalpable testis will be palpable[27]. An 8 Fr catheter or infant feeding tube is placed per urethra to drain the bladder before and during the entire procedure. Diagnostic laparoscopy is performed initially. We prefer a modified open technique for placement of the first trocar in a child so as to reduce the inherent complications associated with blind placement of a Veress needle, such as extraperitoneal emphysema or bowel injury. A semilunar incision is made within the umbilical groove and carried down to the rectus fascia. The fascia is grasped with 2-0 absorbable sutures and then incised in the midline until the peritoneum is visualized. The Veress needle is then introduced and radially dilated to allow a 5 mm port. This modified open technique allows a tight seal and minimizes loss of insufflation during the procedure.

An intra-abdominal testes is usually found within 1 to 2 cm of the internal ring, which is usually patent (Figure 1). Once it has been decided to proceed with laparoscopic orchidopexy, two more 3 or 5 mm ports are placed under direct vision. As to where these ports should be placed, it is the surgeon's preference so as to achieve the greatest degree of instrument freedom and avoid crossing instruments during dissection (Figure 2). Attention to the distal paratesticular elements is necessary to determine whether the vas deferens exits beyond the internal ring into the inguinal canal as in a looping vas. The first element of testicular mobilization is drawing the gubernaculam attachment from the internal ring/inguinal canal, transecting it, and using it as a grasping point for safe testicular manipulation (Figure 3). The retroperitoneum is incised with a minimal 1 cm margin laterally to the testicle and medially alongside the vas deferens. The peritoneum is mobilized carefully across the spermatic vessels. All vessels around the vas deferens and the peritoneal plane between vas and vessels is left intact. Electrocautery is avoided as far as possible. The testis is carefully mobilized from the psoas fascia towards the inguinal ring.

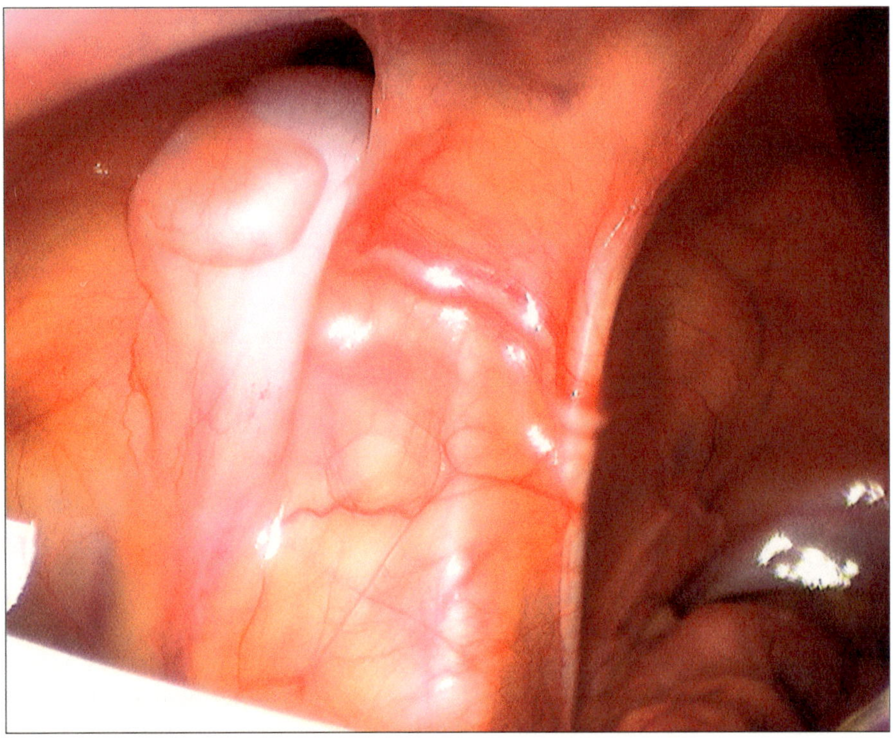

Fig. 1. A non-palpable left testis is seen at the left internal ring. The vas deferens is noted passing laterally towards the testis over the medial umbilical ligament. The spermatic vessels are seen proximal to the testis.

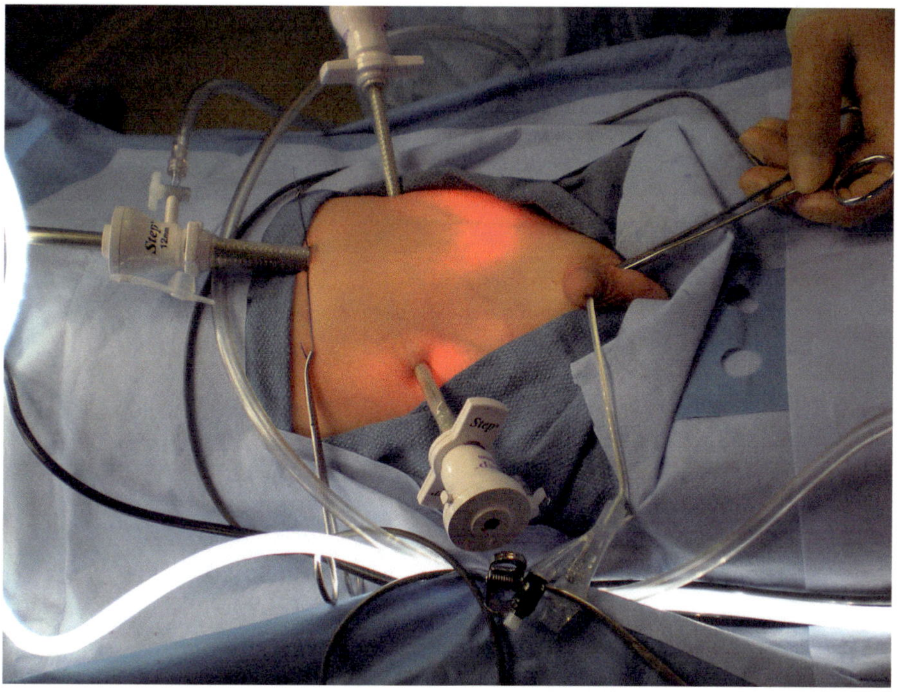

Fig. 2. A three port technique for laparoscopic orchidopexy demonstrates a single 5 mm umbilical port and 2 additional working 3 or 5 mm ports placed in the mid-clavicular line at the level of the anterior superior iliac spine. The working ports may be placed further cephalad depending on the size of the patient and length of instruments.

Care is taken to preserve the triangle of tissue medial to the spermatic vessels and lateral to the vas deferens durng mobilization (Figure 4). Adequate mobilization is complete when the testis easily reaches the contralateral internal ring without undue tension. As in the Prentis manoeuvre, a new internal ring is created medially to the epigastric vessels which shortens the overall distance to the scrotal position. An incision is made at the lower pole of the scrotum to provide a dartos pouch. A laparoscopic grasper is inserted and guided through a tunnel to the new inguinal ring and pull the mobilized testis in to the scrotum without forced tension. With an assistant maintaining the position of the testis near the scrotum, the surgeon may now incise redundant peritoneal folds laparoscopically to gain some additional length (Figure 5). It is critical for the surgeon to personally monitor tension on the spermatic cord as the testis is passed into the scrotum to avoid inadvertent avulsion of the spermatic vessels.

Before the ports are removed, bleeding should be assessed laparoscopically under low intra-abdominal pressure by releasing the pneumoperitoneum. On removing the ports , hemostasis should also be assessed at the port sites, as well as being sure that the umbilical closure does not include bowel or omentum .

Esposito et al [36] reported their experience with diagnostic laparoscopic in 85 children with nonpalpable testes, of whom 25 children had intra-abdominal testes. In 24 children laparoscopic orchidopexy was successful. Surgery lasted between 40 and 80 minutes. There was only 1 (4%) intraoperative complication namely iatrogenic rupture of the spermatic vessels. Similarly Radmayr et al [37] analyzed the success rate and long term outcome of

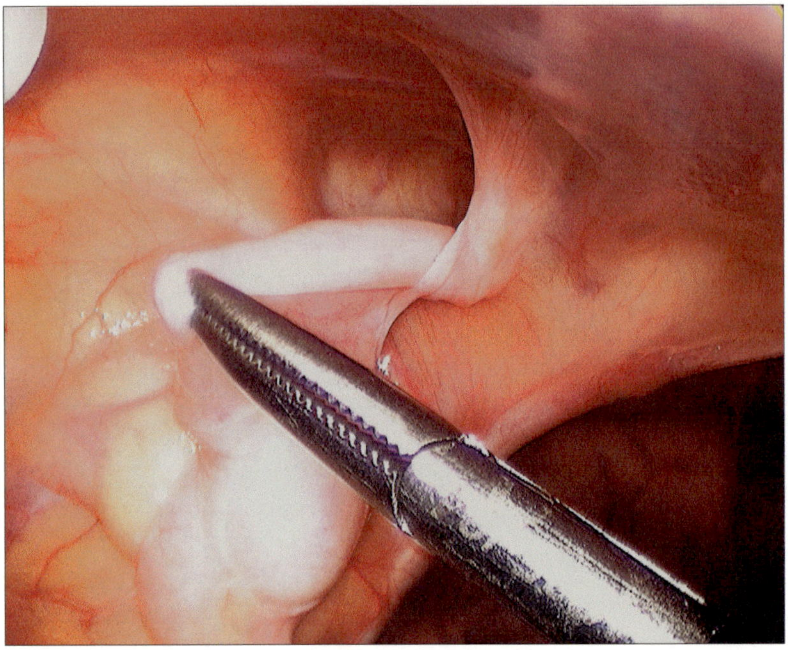

Fig. 3. The gubernaculum of the testis is mobilized. Once confirmed that a looping vas deferens is not present, the gubernaculum is divided using cautery.

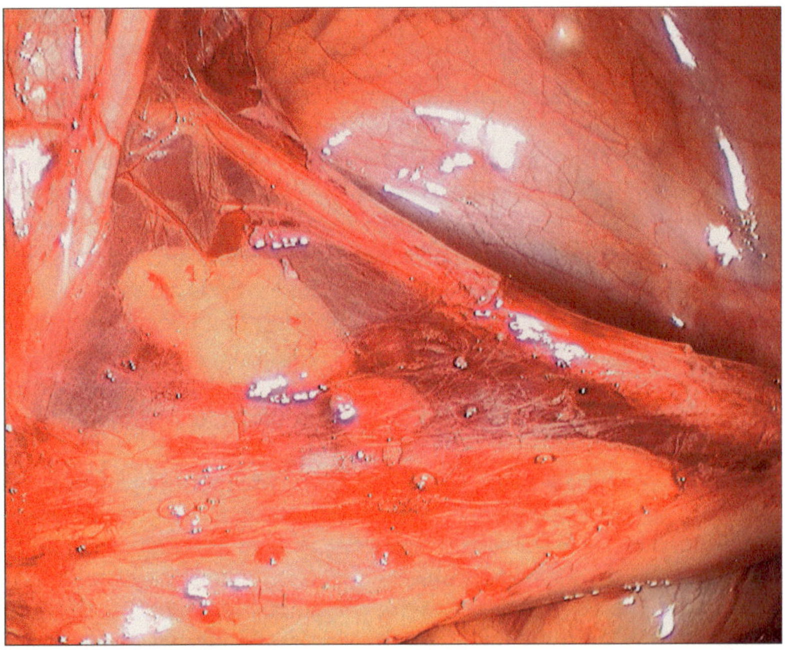

Fig. 4. The left testis is mobilized towards the contralateral right internal ring demonstrating the triangle of preserved mesentery between the vas deferens and spermatic vessels of the left testis.

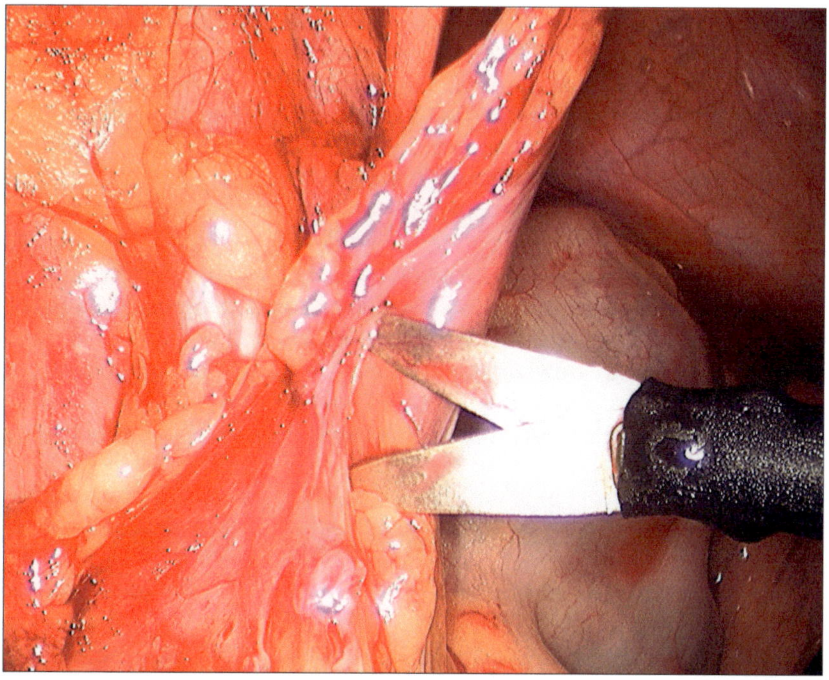

Fig. 5. With the left testis now mobilized into the left hemiscrotum via an incision medial to the medial umbilical ligament, residual peritoneal attachments may be incised laparoscopically to gain additional length to the testicle.

laparoscopic orchiopexy in 84 patients .28 were managed by direct laparoscopic orchiopexy . After a mean follow-up of 6.2 years all laparoscopically managed testicles were in a normal scrotal position with normal perfusion as revealed by colour Doppler sonography.
Riqueimo et al [38] reported on results of laparoscopic orchiopexy in children with palpable undescended testes. 28 children with 30 undescended palpable testes were treated by laparoscopic orchiopexy. The operative time was 50 minutes. On follow-up ranging 5 months to 5 years, 29 of these testes maintained good size and a correct position.

8. Laparoscopic fowler-stephens orchidopexy

If the testes is immobile and beyond 2.5 cm from the internal ring , it may be prudent to perform a staged orchidopexy consisting of clipping the internal spermatic vessels and returning 6 months later to mobilize the testis on collateral vessels and the deferential artery. Fowler-Stephens step I involves incising retroperitoneum bilaterally parallel to the spermatic vessels at-least 2 cm cranially to the upper pole of the testis. The spermatic vessels are mobilized, held with grasper and two absorbable clips applied without dividing them. Vessel ablation can also be done using the harmonic scalpel via a 5mm port.
The second stage of the orchidopexy is usually completed 6 months later. It can be performed in either open or laparoscopic fashion. The same principles apply as with an open second stage procedure if performed laparoscopically. Dissection begins in the area where the spermatic vessels were earlier clipped. The vessels are now divided. The retroperitoneum is incised with a 1 cm margin laterally to the testis and medially alongside the vas deferens. The peritoneal flap remains pedicled to the vas deferens. All the vessels

around the vas deferens and the peritoneal plane between the vas and vessels are left intact. The gubernaculum is dissected as far distally as possible. The testis is mobilized carefully from the psoas fascia towards the inguinal ring. A new internal ring is created medially to the epigastric vessels. An incision is made at the lower pole of the scrotum and a dartos pouch is created. A laparoscopic grasper is guided through a tunnel to the new internal ring and the mobilized testis is pulled into the scrotum.

Lindgren et al [39] performed 18 laparoscopic Fowler-Stephens procedure in 14 patients. Five testes were treated with a 2 stage procedure, while 11 were managed by laparoscopic mobilization followed by laparoscopic vessel clipping and orchiopexy in 1 stage. In 2 additional patients, nearly all dissection was performed laparoscopically but due to extenuating circumstances, inguinal incisions were required as well. At mean follow-up of 6 months all cases without previous surgery that were managed by laparoscopic orchiopexy were without atrophy and the testes were in scrotal position. They concluded that laparoscopic transection of the testicular vessels was safe in boys with high abdominal testes.

9. References

[1] Scorer CG, Farrington GH: *Congenital Deformities of the Testis and Epididymis,* New York, Appleton-Century-Crofts, 1971

[2] Cryptorchidism: A prospective study of 7500 consecutive male births, 1984-8. John Radcliffe Hospital Cryptorchidism Study Group. *Arch Dis Child* 1992; 67:892-899

[3] Berkowitz GS, Lapinski RH, Dolgin SE, et al: Prevalence and natural history of cryptorchidism. *Pediatrics* 1993; 92:44-49

[4] Hadziselimovic F, Herzog B, Buser M: Development of cryptorchid testes. *Eur J Pediatr* 1987; 146(Suppl 2):S8-S12.

[5] Huff DS, Hadziselimovic F, Duckett JW, et al: Germ cell counts in semithin sections of biopsies of 115 unilaterally cryptorchid testes. The experience from the Children's Hospital of Philadelphia. *Eur J Pediatr* 1987; 146(Suppl 2):S25-S27.

[6] Huff DS, Hadziselimovic F, Snyder 3rd HM, et al: Histologic maldevelopment of unilaterally cryptorchid testes and their descended partners. *Eur J Pediatr* 1993; 152(Suppl 2):S11-S14.

[7] Rune GM, Mayr J, Neugebauer H, et al: Pattern of Sertoli cell degeneration in cryptorchid prepubertal testes. *Int J Androl* 1992; 15:19-31

[8] Cendron M, Huff DS, Keating MA, et al: Anatomical, morphological and volumetric analysis: A review of 759 cases of testicular maldescent. *J Urol* 1993; 149:570-573.

[9] Huff DS, Hadziselimovic F, Snyder 3rd HM, et al: Postnatal testicular maldevelopment in unilateral cryptorchidism. *J Urol* 1989; 142:546-548.discussion 572.

[10] Huff DS, Fenig DM, Canning DA, et al: Abnormal germ cell development in cryptorchidism. *Horm Res* 2001; 55:11-17

[11] Lee PA: Fertility in cryptorchidism. Does treatment make a difference?. *Endocrinol Metab Clin North Am* 1993; 22:479-490

[12] Lee PA, O'Leary LA, Songer NJ, et al: Paternity after cryptorchidism: Lack of correlation with age at orchidopexy. *Br J Urol* 1995; 75:704-707.

[13] Farrer JH, Walker AH, Rajfer J: Management of the postpubertal cryptorchid testis: A statistical review. *J Urol* 1985; 134:1071-1076

[14] Moller H, Prener A, Skakkebaek NE: Testicular cancer, cryptorchidism, inguinal hernia, testicular atrophy, and genital malformations: Case-control studies in Denmark. *Cancer Causes Control* 1996; 7:264-274.
[15] Schnech FX and Bellinger MF ; Abnormalities of the testes and scrotum and their surgical management , in Wein AJ, Kavoussi LR, Novick AC, Partin AW and Peters CA , Ed Campbell Walsh Urology, 9th ed , Saunders Elsevier , Philadelphia, 2008 :p 3745-3798
[16] Moore RG, Peters CA, Bauer SB, et al: Laparoscopic evaluation of the nonpalpable testis: A prospective assessment of accuracy. *J Urol* 1994; 151:728-731.
[17] Tennenbaum SY, Lerner SE, McAleer IM, et al: Preoperative laparoscopic localization of the nonpalpable testis: A critical analysis of a 10-year experience. *J Urol* 1994; 151:732-734
[18] Hrebinko RL, Bellinger MF: The limited role of imaging techniques in managing children with undescended testes. *J Urol* 1993; 150:458-460.
[19] Siemer S, Humke U, Uder M, et al: Diagnosis of nonpalpable testes in childhood: Comparison of magnetic resonance imaging and laparoscopy in a prospective study. *Eur J Pediatr Surg* 2000; 10:114-118.
[20] Elder JS: Ultrasonography is unnecessary in evaluating boys with a nonpalpable testis. *Pediatrics* 2002; 110:748-751
[21] Bakr AA, Kotb M: Laparoscopic orchidopexy: The treatment of choice for the impalpable undescended testis. *J Soc Laparoendosc Surg* 1998; 2:259-262.
[22] Lakhoo K, Thomas DF, Najmaldin AS: Is inguinal exploration for the impalpable testis an outdated operation?. *Br J Urol* 1996; 77:452-454
[23] Barqawi AZ, Blyth B, Jordan GH, et al: Role of laparoscopy in patients with previous negative exploration for impalpable testis. *Urology* 2003; 61:1234-1237.discussion 1237
[24] Koff SA: Does compensatory testicular enlargement predict monorchism?. *J Urol* 1991; 146:632- 633
[25] Hurwitz RS, Kaptein JS: How well does contralateral testis hypertrophy predict the absence of the nonpalpable testis?. *J Urol* 2001; 165:588-592.
[26] Belman AB, Rushton HG: Is an empty left hemiscrotum and hypertrophied right descended testis predictive of perinatal torsion?. *J Urol* 2003; 170:1674-1675.discussion 1675-6.
[27] Cisek LJ, Peters CA, Atala A, et al: Current findings in diagnostic laparoscopic evaluation of the nonpalpable testis. *J Urol* 1998; 160:1145-1149.discussion 1150.
[28] Van Savage JG: Avoidance of inguinal incision in laparoscopically confirmed vanishing testis syndrome. *J Urol* 2001; 166:1421-1424
[29] Grady RW, Mitchell ME, Carr MC: Laparoscopic and histologic evaluation of the inguinal vanishing testis. *Urology* 1998; 52:866-869.
[30] De Luna AM, Ortenberg J, Craver RD: Exploration for testicular remnants: Implications of residual seminiferous tubules and crossed testicular ectopia. *J Urol* 2003; 169:1486-1489.
[31] Elder JS: Laparoscopy for impalpable testes: Significance of the patent processus vaginalis. *J Urol* 1994; 152:776-778.
[32] Belman AB, Rushton HG: Is the vanished testis always a scrotal event?. *BJU Int* 2001; 87:480-483.

[33] Kanemoto K, Hayashi Y, Kojima Y, et al: The management of nonpalpable testis with combined groin exploration and subsequent transinguinal laparoscopy. *J Urol* 2002; 167:674-676.
[34] Ravasse P, Petit T, Delmas P: [Impalpable testis: Complete inguinal exploration by laparoscopy.]. *Prog Urol* 2003; 13:103-105.discussion, 105-106.
[35] Cortesi N, Ferrari P, Zambarda E, Manenti A, Baldini A, Morano FP. Diagnosis of bilateral abdominal cryptorchidism by laparoscopy . Endoscopy 1976; 9: 33
[36] Esposito C, Damiano R, Gonzalez-Sabin MA, Savanelli A, Centonza A, Settimi A, Sacco R . Laparoscopic assisted orchidopexy: an ideal treatment for children with intra-abdominal testes . J Endourol 2002, 16: 659-662
[37] Radmayr C, Oswald J, Schwenter C, Neururer R , Peschel R, Bartsch G. Long term outcome of laparoscopically managed nonpalpable testes . J Urol 2003; 170: 2409-2411
[38] Riqueime M, Aranda A, Rodriguez C, Villalvazo H , Alvarez G. Laparoscopic orchiopexy for palpable undescended testes: a 5 year experience . J Lap Ad Surg Tech 2006; 16:321-324
[39] Lindgren BW, Franco I, Blick S, Levitt SB, Brock WA , Palmer LS, Friedman SC, Reda EF. Laparoscopic Fowler-Stephens orchiopexy for the high abdominal testis. J Urol 1999; 162: 990- 993

6

Absent or Non Descent of the Testis

Mohamed Amin El Gohary
Gulf medical university
UAE

1. Introduction

Cryptorchidism is a common congenital anomaly of newborns that may resolve, persist or first appear in later childhood. It affects 4% to 5% of full-term and in 9% to 30% of premature males at birth. This figure falls to around 1% to 2% after 3 months, as a significant number will descend spontaneously within the first few months of life (Barthold, & Gonzalez, 2003, Sijstermans, et al. 2008)

The testis can be found in any position along its usual line of descent; however, approximately 80% will be located in the inguinal region, just outside the inguinal canal. Approximately 20% of undescended testes are nonpalpable, and in 20% to 50% of children with nonpalpable testis, the testis is absent (Smolko& Brock, 1983)

Laparoscopy has been established as the most reliable diagnostic modality for the management of impalpable testes, It clearly demonstrates the anatomy and provides visual information upon which a definitive decision can be made. Non visualization of the testes at laparoscopy has been coined with the broad term (Absent testis), which is coined with vanishing, atrophied or agenetic testes.

In this report we will discuss the phenomena of absent testes in the light of recent discovery of a subgroup of testes that failed to descend from it is embryological subrenal position and likely to be labelled as an absent testis unless one is aware of the complexity of testicular development and descent

2. Testicular development and descent

Proper evaluation and management of cryptorchidism requires a thorough understanding of the normal testicular development and descent which depend on a complex interaction among endocrine, paracrine, growth, and mechanical factors.

Bipotential gonadal tissue begins differentiation into a testis during the 6th and 7th weeks of gestation under the effects of the testis-determining *SRY* gene. At the eighth week of gestation, Sertoli cells appear and produce Müllerian inhibitory substance (MIS) to cause regression of the Müllerian ducts. By the 10th week, Leydig cells produce androgens and insulin-like factor 3 (INSL3). Androgens are important for differentiation of various parts of the Wolffian duct and both androgens and INSL3 are required for testicular descent (Hadziselimovic & Adham, 2007; Hutson & Beasley, 1988)

Development of the male external genitalia,including the scrotum, occurs between weeks 10 and 15 of gestation and results from the conversion of testosterone to dihydrotestosterone by the enzyme 5 alpha reductase type 2 in the primordia of these tissues. The development of the scrotum allows for the ultimate descent of the testis from the abdomen.

2.1 Wolffian duct development

The Wolffian duct is originally derived from the pronephros, whose ductal derivative elongates posteriorly through the mesonephros and extends to the cloaca. The pronephros eventually degenerates but its ductal derivative remains in the mesonephros and becomes the Wolffian duct (WD). WD structure is further differented into epididymis, vas deferens, seminal vesicle and ejaculatory ducts, and is dependent on androgens from fetal Leydig cells for its development. The anterior or upper portion of the WD adjacent to the testis elongates and folds into the epididymis. Meanwhile, the mesonephric tubules differentiate into efferent ducts that eventually connect to the rete testis and the epididymis. The middle portion of the WD remains a simple tube, to form the vas deferens. The posterior or caudal portion of the WD dilates, elongates cranially and eventually forms the seminal vesicle (Hadziselimovic et al., 1987; Hutson & Beasley, 1988; Saino et al. 1997)

Androgens are crucial for the maintenance and elaboration of the WD later in development. Their action is mediated via their receptor in the androgen receptor (AR) inside target cells. Androgens enter their target cells and bind to AR to regulate the transcription of specific genes. In humans, androgen insensitivity syndrome owing to null mutations of AR resulted in the female phenotypes (Hadziselimovic & Herzog, 2001; Wensing, 1988). Furthermore, when females were exposed to excessive androgens by testis transplantation during fetal development, the WD persisted, signifying the role of androgen in WD development (Hadziselimovic & Adham, 2007; Rajfer & Walsh, 1977).

2.2 The gubernaculum development

The gubernaculum undergoes 2 phases of development. In the first phase the gubernaculum thickness, in a process known as the swelling reaction, which is mediated primarily by Insl3. This process dilates the inguinal canal and creates a pathway for testicular descent. The first phase of descent is complete by 15 weeks of gestation. During the second phase the gubernaculum undergoes cellular remodeling and becomes a fibrous structure rich in collagen and elastic fibers. At about the 25th weeks of gestation the processus vaginalis elongates within the gubernaculum creating a peritoneal diverticulum within which the testis can descend. A central column of gubernacular mesenchyme remains attached to the epididymis. Gubernaculum then bulges out of the abdominal musculature and begins to elongate towards the scrotum, eventually arriving there between 30 and 35 weeks of gestation (Shenker et al., 2006; Wensing, 1988)

Failure of the first phase of descent is rare and results in an intraabdominal undescended testis (UDT). Failure of progression of the second stage of descent is more common, and the UDT remains somewhere between the internal inguinal ring and the neck of the scrotum

It should be noted that the gubernaculums does not provide any traction on the testis to cause its descent nor is anchored to the scrotum, but mainly attached to the epididymis. Under androgen stimulation the gubernaculum pulls the epididymis and facilitates its descent, indirectly guiding the testis into the scrotum. (Hadziselimovic, 2001, 2007)

In addition, the epidermal growth factor plays an active role at the level of the placenta to enhance gonadotropin release, which stimulates the fetal testis to secrete factors involved in descent such as descendin, an androgen-independent growth factor involved in gubernacular development. (Hadziselimovic & Adham, 2007)

Other mediators of descent include calcitonin gene-related peptide (CGRP). It is excreted by the genitofemoral nerve under androgen stimulation. It causes contraction of cremasteric muscle fibers and subsequent descent of the gubernaculum, followed by the testis. (Hutson & Beasley, 1988; Shenker et al. 2006)
Both (MIF) and testosterone act locally as paracrine hormone. Failing of the testis to secrete the MIF hormone will lead to ipsilateral persistent of mullerian tissues and abnormality of the paracrine function of testosterone is responsible for epididymal anomalies and UDT (Husmann & Levy, 1995; Shenker et al., 2006)
There are animals in which the epididymis descends and the testis remains intra abdominal, but there are no animals in which the testis descends and epididymis remaines intra-abdominal a crucial information in understating laparoscopic finding of impalpable testes (Hadziselimovic &Adham, 2007)
If the testis is agenetic, one would expect that the ipsilateral mullerian structure not be suppressed. The absence of Mullerian remnants means that the there has been a testis at one stage of development that survived well above the 9th week of gestation.

2.3 Processus vaginalis

The processus vaginalis grows along and partially encircles the gubernaculum, creating a potential space in the inguinal canal and scrotum. Although the testis is stationary between the 3rd and 7th months of fetal life, the gubernaculum and the processus vaginalis together distend the inguinal canal and scrotum,thus creating a "path" for testicular descent.

2.4 Testicular agenesis

A testis may be unable to form in a 46, XY individual because the gonadal ridge fails to form or its blood supply fails to develop. Individuals with testicular agenesis may have either a male or a female phenotype. The variable phenotypic appearances, including the presence of some form of the internal genitalia, relate to the time during gestation when the testis was lost. The key clinical sign indicating testicular agenesis rather than a vanished testis is the presence of ipsilateral Müllerian structures. This entity is totally different from the vanishing testis syndrome. It is virtually impossible to have a testicular agenesis in a normal phenotype male with no remnant of mullerian structures on the affected site.

3. Management of impalpable testes

3.1 Imaging of impalpable testes

When the testis is not clinically palpable, a battery of imaging investigations are described to locate the testis. These include ultrasound scanning (USS), magnetic resonance imaging (MRI), magnetic resonance angiography (MRA) and Computed tomography (CT). Despite these many options, it is still commonly believed that none of them accurately predict either the position or morphology of the testis, with the overall accuracy of radiological investigations being estimated at only 44%. (Fritzsche et al. 1987, Kullendorff et al. 1985, Malone & Guiney, 1985; Weiss, 1979,1986)
However there are occasions in which imaging is undoubtedly beneficial especially in obese children where although a testis appears to be impalpable following clinical examination; it can be located either intracannicular or at superficial inguinal pouch position by simple US. These patients can then proceed to inguinal exploration with the option to convert to laparoscopy if no testis was found. Although some centers still advocate groin exploration in impalpable testes

(Lakhoo et al. 1996, Ferro,et al. 1999) several studies have shown that a significant proportion of testes that appear absent at the time of inguinal exploration can subsequently be identified at laparoscopy. (Boddy et al, 1985; Patil at al. 2005; Perovic; Janic 1994)

3.2 Laparoscopy for impalpable testes

Laparoscopy has been established as the most reliable diagnostic modality for the management of impalpable testes. In experienced hands, laparoscopy is capable of providing nearly 100% accuracy in the diagnosis of the intra-abdominal testis with minimal morbidity. It clearly demonstrates the anatomy and provides visual information upon which a definitive decision can be made. Both internal rings can be inspected; the location and size of the testes, their blood supply and the nature, course and termination of the vas, and epididymis can be determined. All of these anatomical landmarks individually or collectively have bearing on the operative management of the Impalpable testes. (Atlas & Stone 1992; Bianchi, 1995; Bogaert et al. 1993;Elder, 1993; EI Gohary, 2006; Froeling et al.1994;Humphrey et al. 1998; Poenaru et al.1994; Perovic& Janic 1994)

In our series of 1652 UDT seen between 1986-2009, 431 were impalpable representing 26.5%. We used both diagnostic and/or operative laparoscopy in the management of 362 testes from 1992 to 2009.Table 1 depicts our updated figures of laparoscopically managed UDT

LAPAROSCOPIC FINDING OF IMPALPABLE TESTES (362)	
Vanishing testis	72
Atrophic Abdominal	08
Atrophic Scrotal	38
No vas	03
Superf cial inguinal pouch	25
Canalicular	46
Abdominal	170

ABDOMINAL TESTES (170)	
High Abdominal	79
Above ring	74
Subrenal	12
Persistent Müllerian	04
Spleno Gonadal Fusion	01

OPERATIVE PROCEDURE FOR ABDOMINAL TESTES	
FSO	91
One Stage Lap. Orchedopexy	79

The possible findings at laparoscopy is either a normal testes at variable distance of the closed or opened internal ring atrophied or no testes. Fig 1-4. If no testes are identified, one is left with the possibility of vanishing or absent testes. Vanishing abdominal testes are readily diagnosed when a blind-ending vas meets a leach of flimsy testicular vessels, and are thought to result from a prenatal vascular accident or intrauterine testicular torsion (Stephen & Lawrence, 1986) Fig 3. Intra-abdominal testicular torsion as a cause for testicular atrophy or vanishing testes has been postulated but as far as we can ascertain never been seen. However one of our patients aged 8 had an atrophied left testis due to several twists of its blood supply leading to atrophic changes Fig 4 (El Gohary, 1997)

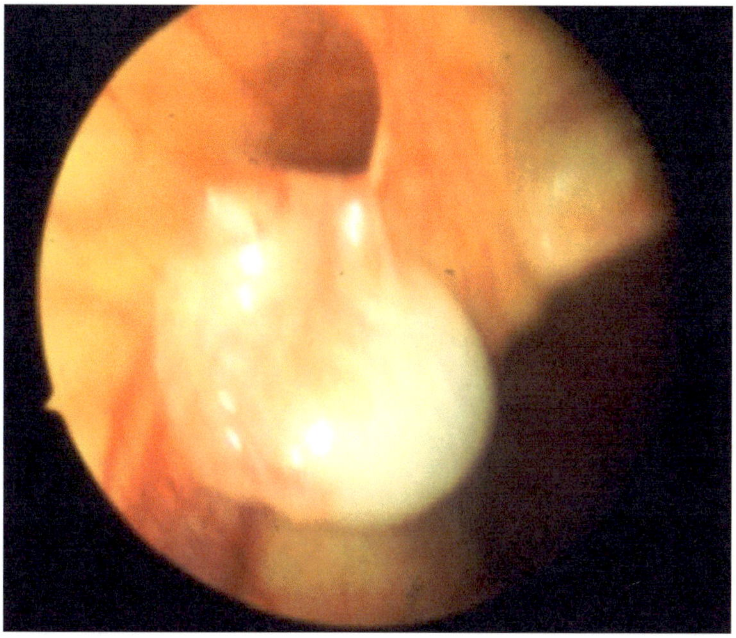

Fig. 1. Testis near opened internal ring

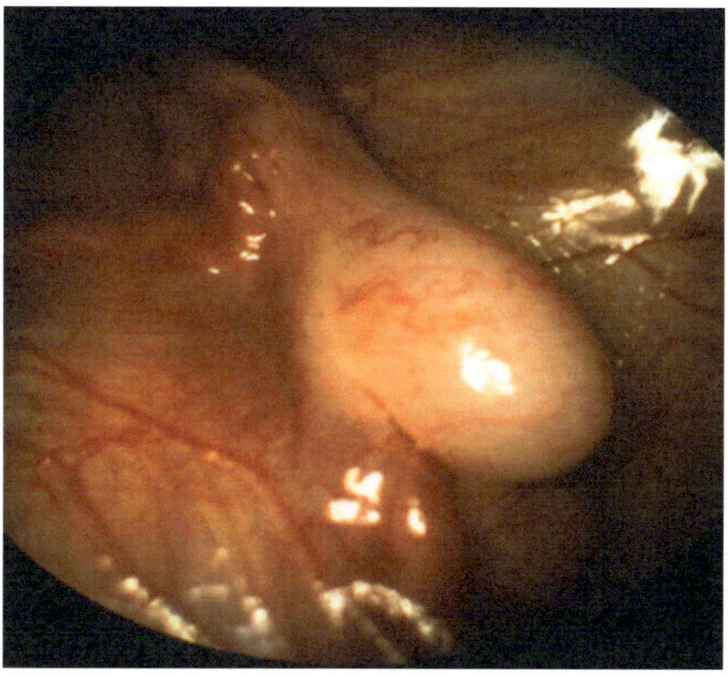

Fig. 2. Testis away from closed internal ring

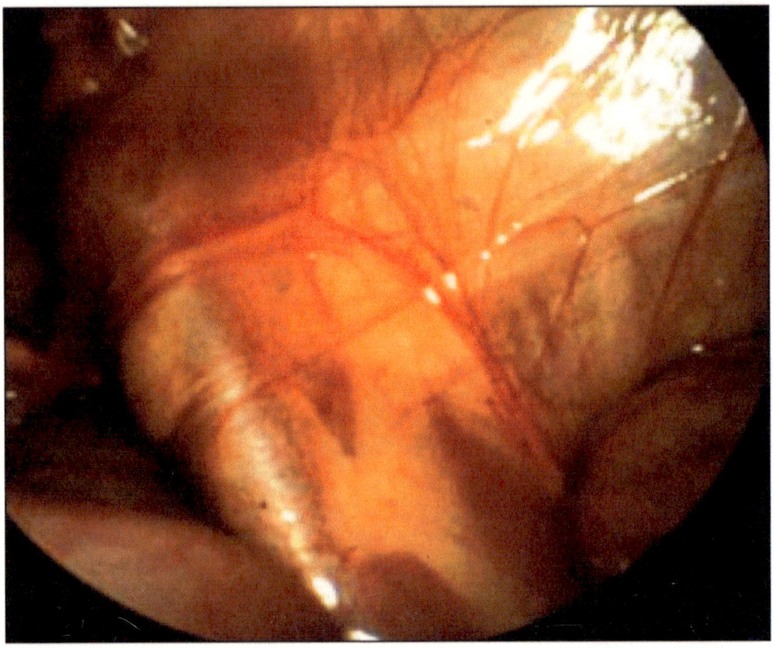

Fig. 3. Vanishing testis

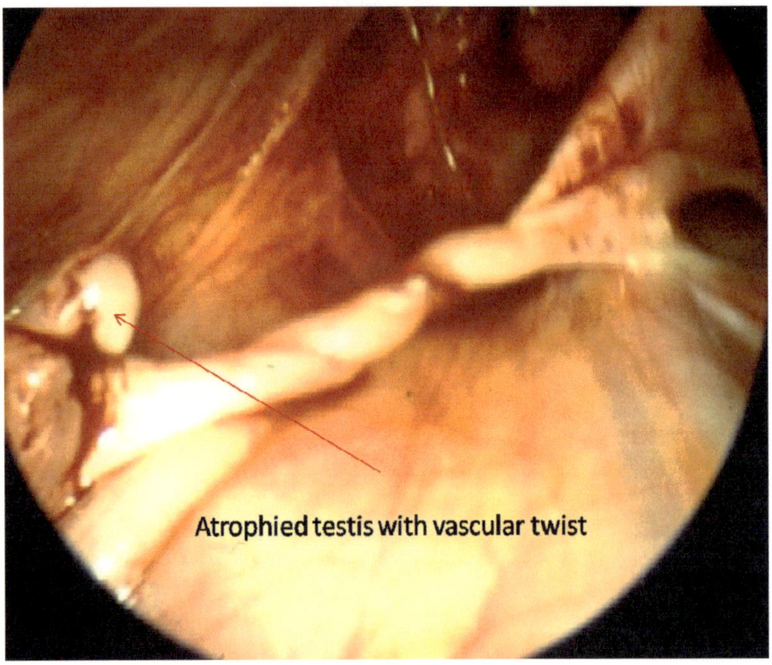

Fig. 4. Atrophied testis with vascular twist

3.2.1 Testicular epididymal separation

As the vas is embryologically derived separately from the testis (Hadziselimovic,et al.1987), finding the vas alone with no testicular vessels does not exclude an existing testis in abnormal locations or merely separated from the vas. Testicular epididymal separation allowing epididymis to elongate and descent to the scrotum without associated testicular descent is a known phenomena (Marshall& Shermeta, 1997, Shereta, 1979) Fig 5,but there are rare situation of complete urogenital nonunion in which there are no communication between the descended epididymis and the UDT. (Emanuelet, 1997; Wakeman, 2010; El *Gohary*, 2009). An extreme example of this was one of our reported cases in which the vas enters closed internal ring and a normal testis lying completely dissociated from the vas in the pelvis (El *Gohary*,2009) Fig 6. This particular case would have been labeled as an atrophied testis, but for the diagnostic accuracy of laparoscopy. The explanation to these phenomena is related to the embryological development of the wolfian system separately from the testis with the gubernacular attachment to the epididymis rather than the testis. (Hadziselimovic, 2007)

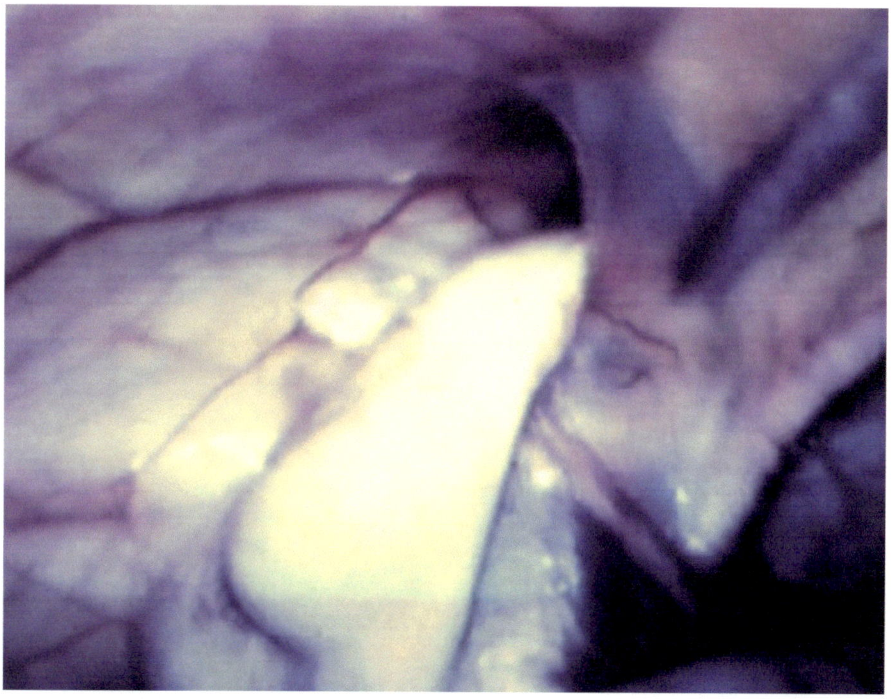

Fig. 5. Separated epididymis (vas is seen entering the canal leaving an intra- abdominal testis)

3.2.2 The testicular vessels as a landmark for testis

The testicular vessels are a good landmark for testicular localization and there is a relationship between the size of the feeding vessels and the testicular tissue. (El Gohary, 1997; Smolko 1983) Visualizing of well developed spermatic vessels predicts the presence of a good-sized testis whereas poor blood supply is invariably associated with poorly developed or atrophied testes (fig 7,8)

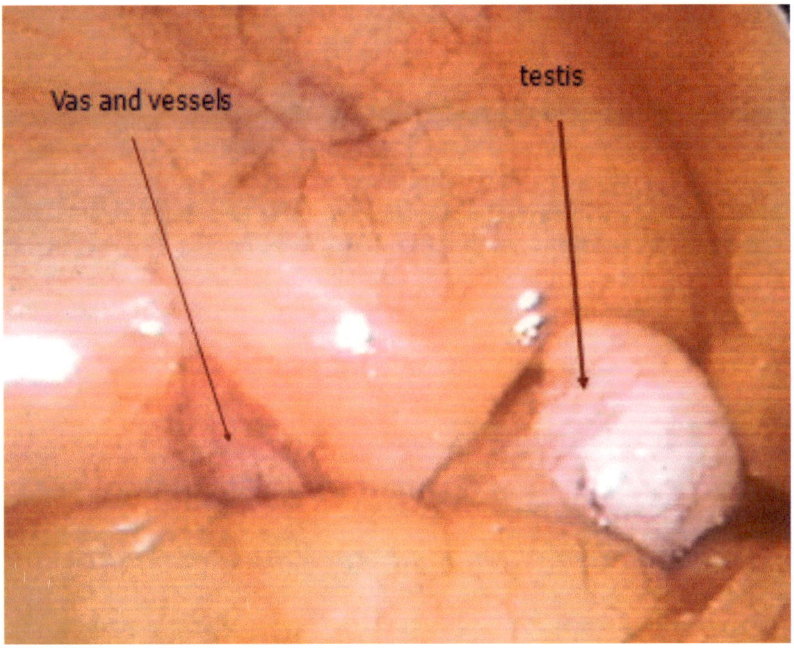

Fig. 6. Urogenital none union

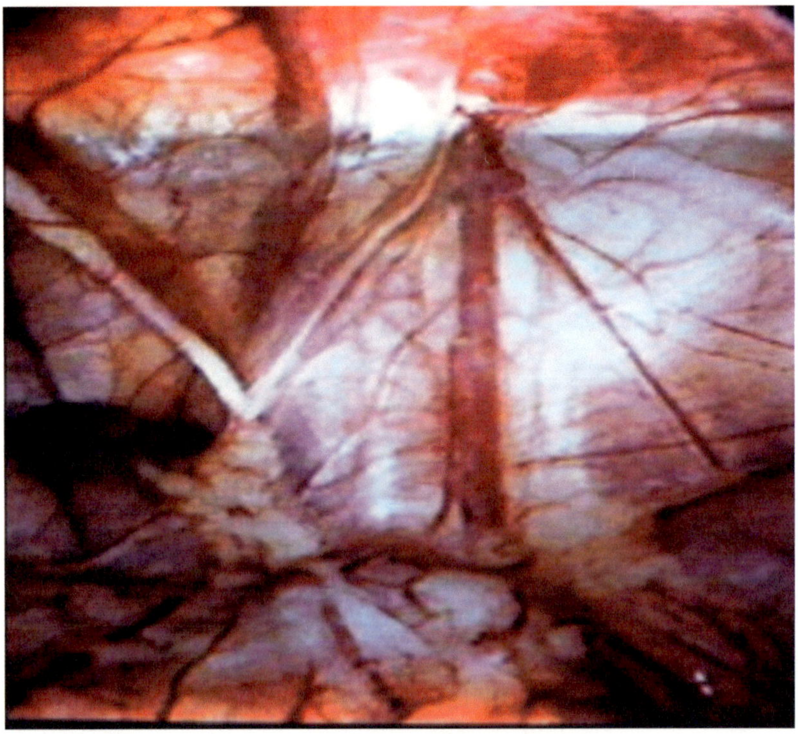

Fig. 7. Normal size testicular vessels and vas deferens entering closed ring

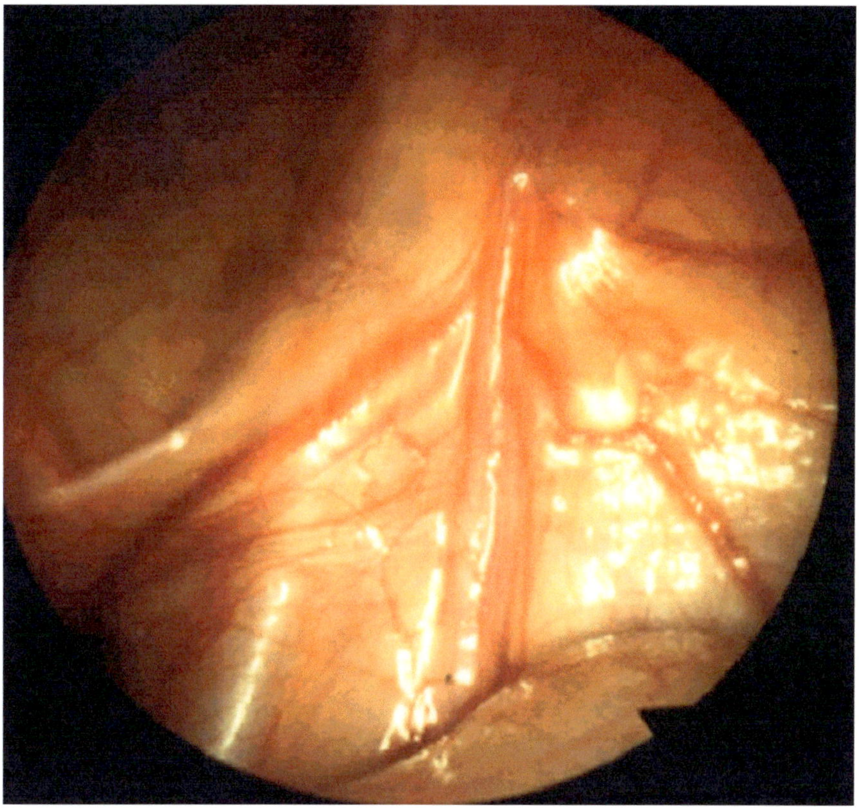

Fig. 8. Hypoplastic vessels entering closed ring

Obese boys with UDT are difficult to examine even under GA. Those group of patient may benefit from an initial ultrasonography and groin exploration before embarking upon diagnostic laparoscopy. These children represent the majority of our patient subjected to diagnostic laparoscopy with the finding of good testicular vessels leading to a good size testes outside abdominal cavity during groin exploration

3.2.3 Absent testes

The term absent testes has been used in the literature to denote vanishing, atrophied, nubbin of tissue at the end of the spermatic or agenetic testes. Agenetic testes in a 46, XY individual do occur because the gonadal ridge fails to form or its blood supply fails to develop. Individuals with testicular agenesis may have either a male or a female phenotype. The variable phenotypic appearances, including the presence of the internal genitalia, relate to the time during gestation when the testis was lost (Shenkeret al. 2006). The key clinical sign indicating testicular agenesis rather than a vanished testis is the presence of ipsilateral Müllerian structures. True congenital absence of one testis is virtually impossible in a phenotype male with no remnant of mullerian structures on the affected site.

3.2.4 Non-descent of the testes

Non-descent of the testes is a subgroup that may cause confusion about the real status of the testes. They are located at their initial embryological position below the kidneys, in contrast to the high abdominal testes which are present along the line of descent at a variable distance from the internal ring (fig 2). This entity was realized when, during routine laparoscopy for impalpable testes, a leach of flimsy vessels was encountered entering an open inguinal canal with no vas (Fig. 9). The initial impression was that of an absent testis. During further inspection a vas was found hidden under the caecum and going in an upward direction toward the right hypochondrium.

When followed the vas was seen to join the epididymis which was attached to a subrenal testis (Figs. 10 and 11). In 2008 we reported eight testes in 7 patients found at the sub-renal position after an initial finding of no testes and no vas at the pelvic inspection; seven on the right side and 1 on the left. The later belong to a patient with bilateral UDT (El Gohary, 2008). We have since found another 4, all were on the right side.

The predominance of right side for this particular cases is difficult to explain and it is rather early to generalize before we collect more cases

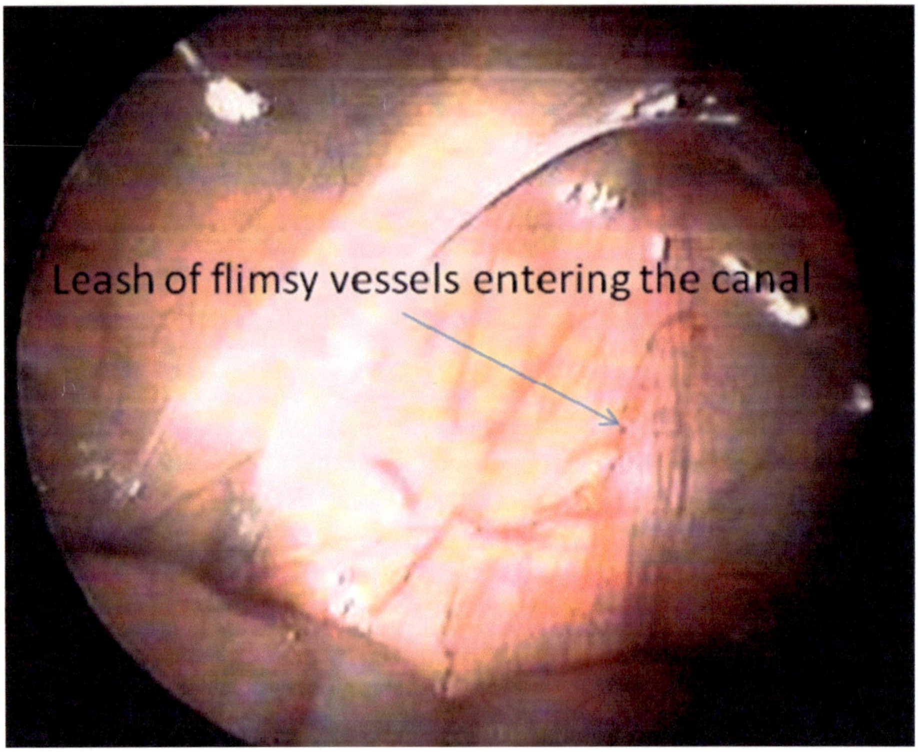

Fig. 9. Initial finding of no vas and flimsy vessels in patients with subrenal testis

The etiology might be attributed to poorly developed or absent gubernaculum. This is highlighted by the fact that the only trace of gubernacular tissues in the present cases was a leach of vessels along the course of testicular descent. Gubernaculum is attached to the epididymis and plays an integral part in testicular decent.

There are 2 reports of subrenal testes with initial finding at laparoscopy very similar to our cases, but with the difference that they had no vas or epididymis and associated with ipsilateral muticystic kidney. There is a correlation between absent vas and renal anomalies (Deane & May,1982; Ellsworth & Cheuck, 2009; Kim et al. 2005) but those cases of absent vas

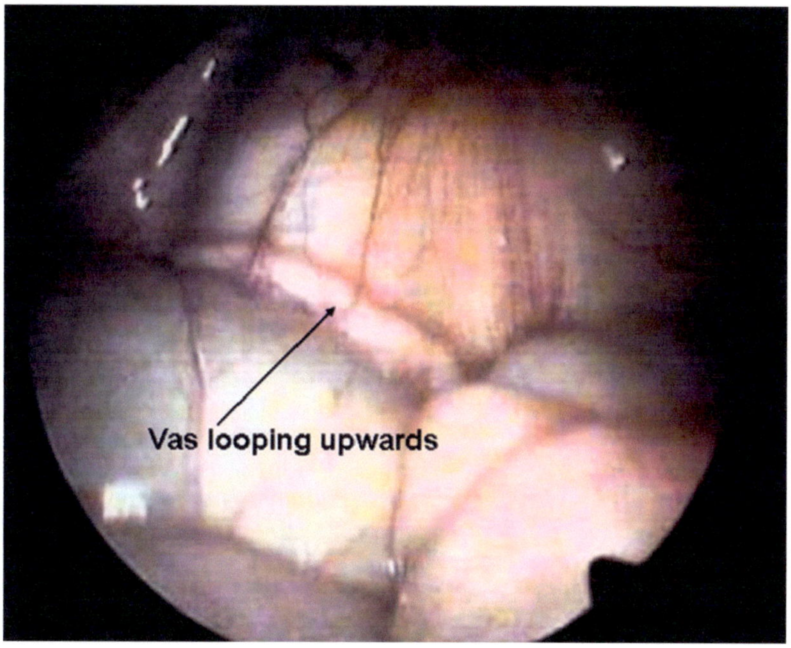

Fig. 10. Vas looping up towards subrenal testis

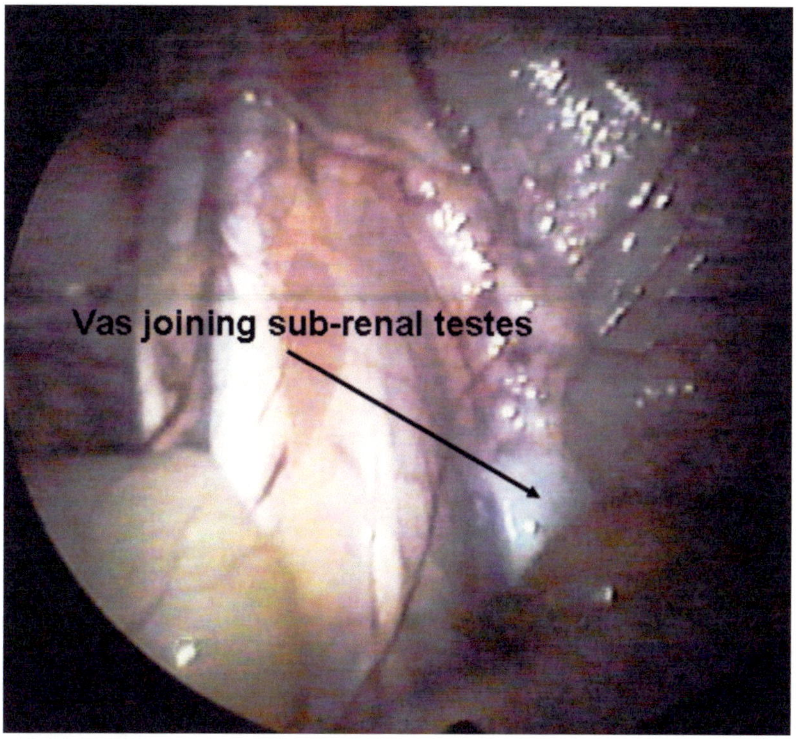

Fig. 11. Vas joining sub-renal testis

and non visualization of the testis are extremely rare. And in patients with normal male phenotypic appearance warrant through laparoscopic exploration to locate the hidden testes along the course of descent.

3.2.5 Spermatic vessel ligation

In 1903, Bevan suggested division of the spermatic vessels to allow for scrotal placement of high abdominal testes. Fowler and Stephens,1959 expanded on this approach by dividing the spermatic vessels well above the testis and carefully preserving the collateral vassal arteries by leaving a strip of peritoneum attached to the vas when dissecting it into the pelvis. Ransley et al. 1984 reported a two-stage Fowler Stephen orchedopexy (FSO); This involved preliminary ligation of the spermatic vessels and after an interval of several months to allow for compensatory dilatation of collateral blood supply. Bloom, 1991 described performing the first stage laparoscopically. Lindgren et al. 1999 reported on laparoscopic single-stage FSO. Although it has been proposed that a single-stage FSO is more favorable than 2satge procedure, as it avoids repeat anesthesia and the potentially difficult dissection associated with re-operation, (Boddy, 1991; Docimo, 1995); The majority of published series favors two-stage procedure as it allows for compensatory dilatation of collateral blood supply and have a better chance for testicular vascularization (Bloom, 1991; Boddy et al.1991; Daher et al. 2009; Dave et al. 2009).

The blood supply to subrenal testes are very short and cannot be mobilized to gain enough

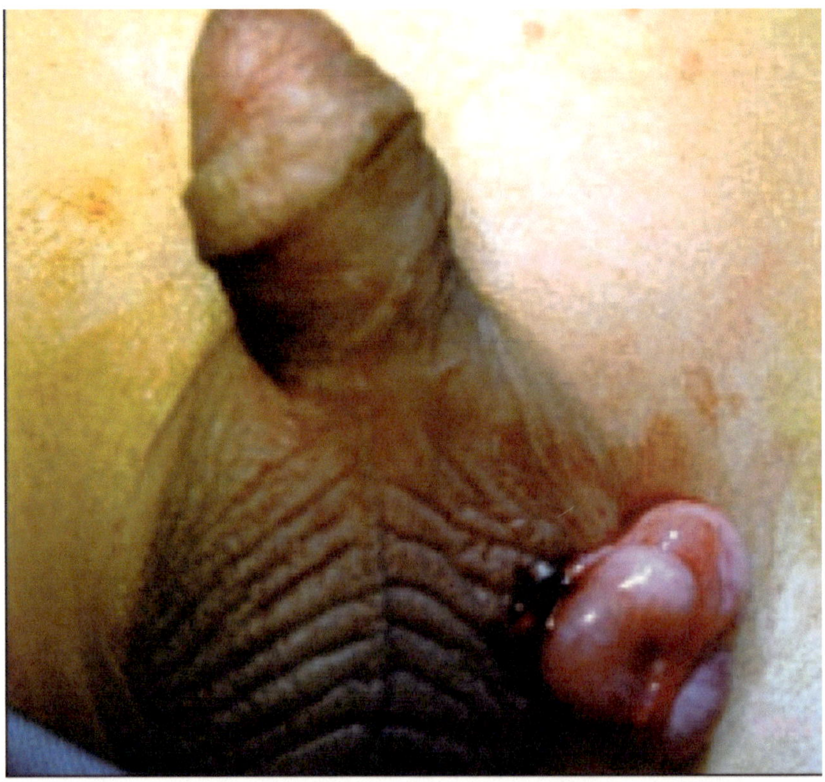

Fig. 12. 2nd stage FSO in a patient with subrenal testis showing good vasculature (clips are close to the testis as the blood supply in subrenal travels short distance)

length of the cord, but the vas runs a log course in upward direction and its blood supply can be used as a support for the mobilized testis using FSO.
We have used one stage FSO in 2 patients, one of them became atrophied and the other attained good scrotal position. Two stage Fowler Stephen were used in the management of 10 subrenal testes with good result in 7, (Fig 12) one reached to mid scrotal position and 2 atrophied. The overall success rate for all Fowler-Stephens procedures was 85%, (Daher et al. 2009; Dave et al. 2009; Hutson & Clarke, 2007)

4. Conclusion

When no testis could be identified during laparoscopy, the vas and the testicular vessels are traced as leading points for testicular localization. As the vas develops separately from the genital ridge; its absence does not exclude the presence of a testis in an unusual location. Testicular vessels proved to have high accuracy as a land mark for the developing testis and its size has a relationship with the fictional testicular tissues, however poorly developed gubernaculums can easily be mistaken for hypoplastic testicular vessels.
Subrenal none descended testes represent a variant of abdominal testes that are likely to be missed unless one is aware of its possible anatomical location. In this subset of cases there are no vas at initial laparoscopy and what looks like flimsy vessels represent poorly developed gubernaculum. Based upon embryological facts of testicular development, in a phenotypically normal male it is virtually impossible to be associated with an absent or agenetic testis. The absence of Mullerian remnants means that the there has been a testis at one stage of development that survived well above the 9th week of gestation. There are reported cases in which the testis was absent during initial laparoscopy and was subsequently found under the renal lower pole; which makes laparoscopic examination of the site of origin below the kidneys an essential step in all cases apparent absent testes. We do believe that testicular absence does not exist in normal males and that cases that were labeled as (absent testes) should be re-scoped to exclude sub-renal testes. An algorithm for management of impalpable testes is highlighted.

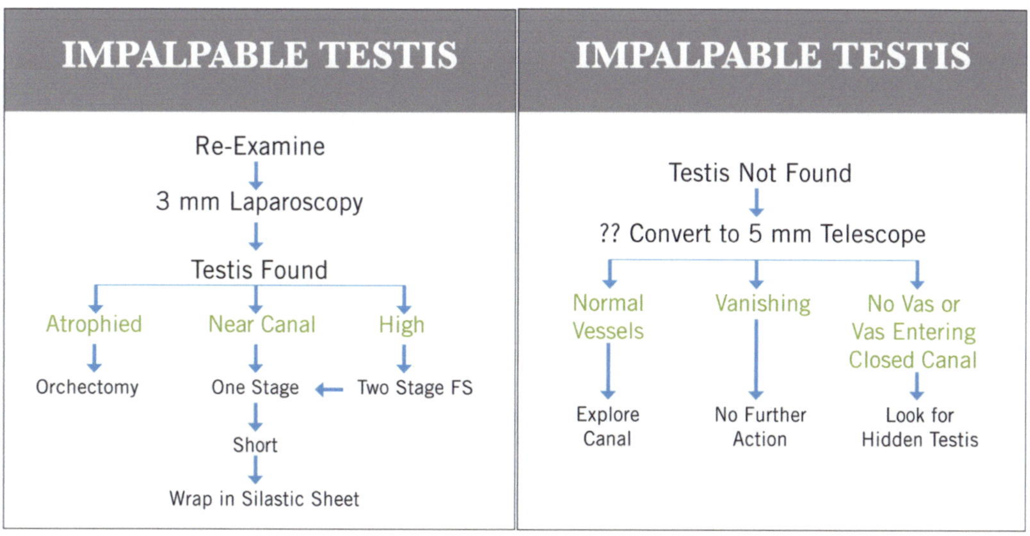

5. References

Atlas, I; & Stone, N; (1992).Laparoscopy for evaluation of cryptorchid testis. *Urology*. 40:256-8.

Baillie, C; Fearns, G; Kitteringham, L; & Turnock R;.(1998) Management of the impalpable testis: the role of laparoscopy. *Arch Dis Child*. 79:419-22.

Barthold J. & Gonzalez R. (2003) The epidemiology of congenital cryptorchidism, testicular ascent and orchiopexy. *J Uro*,170:2396-401.

Bevan, A;. (1903).The surgical treatment of undescended testis: a further contribution. . JAMA .41:718-723.

Bianchi, A;.(1995). The impalpable testis. Ann R Coll Surg Engl .77:3-6.

Bogaert, G; Kogan, B;, & Mevorach, R;.(1993).Therapeutic laparoscopy for intra-abdominal testes. *Urology* 42:182-8.

Bloom, D;. (1991). Two-step orchiopexy with pelviscopic clip ligation of the spermatic vessels. *J Urol* 145:1030-3

Boddy, S; Corkery, J; & Gornall, P;. (1985). The place of laparoscopy in the management of the impalpable testis. *Br J Surg* . 72:918-9.

Boddy, S; Gordon, A; Thomas, D; & Browning, F;. (1991). Experience with the Fowler Stephens and microvascular procedures in the management of intraabdominal testes. *Br J Urol* .68:199-202.

Daher, P; Nabbout, P; Feghali, J; & (2009). Riachy, E; Is the Fowler-Stephens procedure still indicated for the treatment of nonpalpable intraabdominal testis? *J Pediatr Surg*. 44:1999-2003.

Dave, S; Manaboriboon, N; Braga L;, et al. (2009).Open versus laparoscopic staged Fowler-Stephens orchiopexy: impact of long loop vas. *J Urol*. 182:2435-9

Deane, A; & May, R;.(1982). Absent vas deferens in association with renal abnormalities. *Br J Urol*.54:298-9.

Docimo, S;.(1995). The results of surgical therapy for cryptorchidism: a literature review and analysis. *J Urol*.154:1148-52.

Elder, J;.(1993) Laparoscopy for the nonpalpable testis. Semin Pediatr Surg.2:168-73.

El-Gohary M.(1997). The role of laparoscopy in the management of impalpable testes. Pediatr Surg Int.12:463-5.

El Gohary, M;.(2006). Role of Laparoscopy in the Management of Impalpable Testes. *JIAPS*. 11:207-210.

El Gohary, M.(2008).Non-descent of the testis: An overlooked laparoscopic finding. *J Pediatr Urol* .4:364-6.

El Gohary, M;(2009). Failure of fusion of epididymis and testis: a rare laparoscopic finding. *Eur J Pediatr Surg*19:108-9.

Ellsworth, P; & Cheuck, L;. (2009). The lost testis: Failure of physical examination and diagnostic laparoscopy to identify inguinal undescended testis. *J Pediatr Urol*. 5:321-3.

Emanuel, E; Kirsch, A; Thall, E; & Hensle, T;.(1997) Complete separation of the testis and epididymis. *J Pediatr Surg*. 32:754-5.

Fritzsche, P; Hricak, H; Kogan, B; Winkler, M; & Tanagho E.(1987) Undescended testis: value of MR imaging. *Radiology* 164:169-73.

Ferro, F; Spagnoli, A; Zaccara, A; De Vico, A, La Sala E; (1999) Is preoperative laparoscopy useful for impalpable testis? *J Urol*.; 162: 995-996.

Folwer, R;,& Stephens F. (1959).The role of testicular vascular anatomy in the salvage of high undescended testis. . Aust New Zeal J Surg .29:92-106.

Froeling, M; Sorber M; de la Rosette J, de Vries J.(1994) The nonpalpable testis and the changing role of laparoscopy. *Urology* .43:222-7.

Hadziselimovic, F; Herzog, B; & Buser M;.(1987). Development of cryptorchid testes.Eur J Pediatr. 146 Suppl 2:S8-12.

Hadziselimovic, F; & Herzog, B;(2001). Importance of early postnatal germ cell maturation for fertility of cryptorchid males. *Horm Res* .55:6-10.

Hadziselimovic, F ; &Adham I.(2007). Insulin 3-Like Hormone and its Role in Epididymo-Testicular Descent. International Braz *J Urol.* 33 (3): 407-413.

Hutson, J;& Beasley, S;.(1988).Embryological controversies in testicular descent. Semin *Urol.* 6:68.

Hutson, J; & Clarke M;.(2007) Current management of the undescended testicle. *Semin Pediatr Surg* .16:64-70.

Humphrey, G; Najmaldin A; & Thomas D;.(1998). Laparoscopy in the management of the impalpable undescended testis. Br J Surg .85:983-5.

Husmann, D;&Levy, J. (1995) Current concepts in the pathophysiology of testicular undescent. *Urol.* 46:267.

Malone, P; & Guiney, E;(1985) A comparison between ultrasonography and laparoscopy in localising the impalpable undescended testis. Br J Urol. 57:185-6.

Kim, C; Baneet, N; & Docim S.(2005) .Missed testis on laparoscopy despite blind ending vessels and closed processus vaginalis. *Uro* 65:1226.e7–1226.

Marshall, F; & Shermeta D;.(1997). Epididymal abnormalities associated with undescended testis. *J Urol.* 121:341-3.

Patil, K; Green, J; & Duffy P;. (2005). Laparoscopy for impalpable testes. *BJU Int.* 95:704-8.

Perovic, S; & Janic, N;.(1994).Laparoscopy in the diagnosis of non-palpable testes. *Br J Urol* 73:310-3.

Poenaru, D; Homsy, Y; & Peloquin, F;.(1994). Andze GO. [The value of laparoscopy in the diagnosis and treatment of non-palpable testicular cryptorchism]. *Prog Urol.* 4:206-13.

Rajfer, J; &Walsh, P. 1977; Hormonal regulation of testicular descent: experimental and clinical observations. *J Urol* 118:985.

Ransley, P; Vodermark J;Caldamone, A; & Bellinger, M;.(1984) Preliminary ligation of the gonadal vessels prior to orchidopexy for the intra-abdominal testicle: a staged Fowler-Stephens procedure. . *World J Urol.* 2:266-268.

Saino, k; Hallsted,P; Kreidberg J; Saxén, L.&, Sariola.H. (1997). Diffrential regulation of two sets of mesenephric tubules by WT-!. Development, 124: 1293-1299

Shenker, N; Huynh, J; Farmer, P; & Hutson, J. (2006). A new role for androgen in testicular descent: permitting gubernacular cell proliferation in response to the neuropeptide, calcitonin gene-related peptide. *J Pediatr Surg* 41:407-12

Sijstermans, K; Hack, W; & Meijer, R;. van der Voort-Doedens LM.(2008) The frequency of undescended testis from birth to adulthood: a review. Int J Androl 31:1-11.

Smolko, M; Brock, W; & Kaplan G.(1983).Location and fate of the nonpalpable testis in children. *J Urol.* 129: 1204–1207.

Stephen E; Lawrence, J;.(1986).The vanishing testis syndrome: Indication for conservative therpay. *J Urol.* 758-759.

Tsujihata, M;Miyake, O; &Yoshimura, K;.(2001).Laparoscopic diagnosis and treatment of nonpalpable testis. *Int J Urol*.8:692-6.

Wakeman, D; & Warner, B;.(2010) Urogenital nonunion--a rare anomaly associated with the undescended testis. Am J Surg.199: 59-60.

Wensing, C. (1988)The embryology of testicular descent. *Horm Res* . 30:144.

Weiss, R;, Glickman M.&Lytton B.(1979). Clinical implications of gonadal venography in the management of the non-palpable undescended testis. *J Uro*. 121:745 -749.

Weiss, R; Carter A; & Rosenfield, A; (1986) High resolution real-time ultrasonography in the localization of the undescended testis. *J Urol* 135:936-8.

Wolverson, M; Jagannadharao, B; Sundaram, M; Riaz, M; Nalesnik, W; & Houttuin, E. (1980).CT in localization of impalpable cryptorchid testes. *AJR Am J Roentgenol*. 134:725-9.

7

Laparoscopy for Impalpable Testes

Ahmed Khairi
Pediatric Surgery Unit, Department of Surgery,
Alexandria Faculty of Medicine, Alexandria
Egypt

1. Introduction

1.1 Embryology

Until the 7-8 weeks gestation embryo (sexual differentiation time), the testis and ovary have the same position. Afterwards, the testis remains close to the future inguinal canal and the ovary moves away from the groin.

Both gonads have upper suspensory ligament and lower gubernaculum. The cranial suspensory ligament persists in females and regresses in boys. This is believed to be due to androgenic hormonal control. The gubernaculum enlarges in boys. This is controlled by a non-androgenic hormone mostly mullerian inhibiting substance (MIS).

Condensation of mesenchyme around the gubernaculum forms the inguinal canal musculature. A diverticulum of peritoneum grows caudally through the mesenchyme of the gubernaculum to form the processus vaginalis. The caudal part of the gubernaculum remains solid and the proximal part is divided into a central part (attached to the epididymis) and a parietal part (the cremasteric muscle) (Heyns 1987). At the third trimenster, the caudal part of the gubernaculums migrates through the inguinal abdominal wall and across the pubic region to the scrotum.

The processus vaginalis grows inside the gubernaculum, with the testis leaving the abdominal cavity within it (Backhouse,1982).

Scrotal migration of the testis and gubernaculums is under androgenic control. This is believed to be through the release of calcitonin gene related peptide (CGRP) by the genitofemoral nerve that control gubenaculum migration (Grocock ,1988).

Intra-abdominal pressure, through the patent processus vaginalis, is a probable additional factor. This process is complete by the 35 weeks (Huston, 1996).

1.2 Incidence

Cryptorchidism is the most common anomaly of the male genital system. Around 4% of infants at birth have undescended testes. At 1 year old, the incidence is around 1%.

20% of undescended testes are impalpable. Blind inguinal exploration of the impalpable undescended testes is unlikely successful.

1.3 Etiology

Multifactorial and many possible causes are raised:

- Defects in the migratory mechanism itself.

- Genitofemoral nerve defects due to lack of gonadotrophin secretion by the pituitary or the placenta.
- Abnormal location of the genitofemoral nerve with subsequent wrong site migration (outline the line of descent).
- MIS or testosterone deficiency.
- Some inherited syndromes are associated with undescended testes:
  - microcephaly: possibly due to pituitary hormone or gonadotrophin deficiency.
  - Prune-belly syndrome: possibly due to mesodermal defect and possibly decreased abdominal pressure.
  - Abdominal wall defects: gastroschisis, omphalocele, bladder extrophy (Hadziselimovic, 1987).
  - Neural tube defects as myelomeningocele due to defect of the genitofemoral nerve motor nucleus and abdominal wall paralysis.

2. Laparoscopy for impalpable testis

2.1 History

- 1976: Cortesi et al published the first case managed by laparoscopy.
- 1991: Bloom performed the first stage of Fowler-Stephens by laparoscopy.
- 1992: Jordan performed single stage laparoscopic orchidopexy.
- 1994: Caldamone reported second stage Fowler-Stephens orchidopexy laparoscopically.

2.2 Differential diagnosis

Impalpable testis may be one of the following:

1. In the inguinal canal but can not be felt (excess fat, small testis)
2. Absent testis: either due to agenesis or intrauterine torsion *(vanishing testis).*
3. Intra-abdominal testis:

- Peeping: close to the deep inguinal ring and can be manipulated into the canal.
- Low abdominal testis.
- High abdominal testis.

2.3 Age of the procedure

As parenchymal damage is clear under electron microscope at 1 year old and by light microscope at 18 months, the optimum age for surgery is before 1 year of age.

2.4 Preoperative preparation

Informed consent including the possibility of converting to laparotomy, staged orchidopexy, orchiectomy, contraletral scrotal orchidopexy.

2.5 Technique

Under general endotracheal anesthesia. Re-examine the boy under anesthesia to confirm the diagnosis of non-palpable testis. Make sure that the stomach is empty. Nasogastric tube might be inserted in small infants. Make sure that the urinary bladder is empty. If full under anesthesia; apply suprapubic pressure (Crede' manuveur) or insert a small catheter. Prep and drape the abdomen and the scrotum

2.6 Position

The child is supine. The surgeon in the opposite side of the impalpable testis, the monitor is opposite to the surgeon, the assistant on the left hand side of the surgeon and the scrub nurse to the right.

The patient is rotated to the contra-lateral side with mild Trendelenberg position on starting intervention.

2.7 Port - placement

For diagnostic laparoscopy, an umbilical port, *by either the closed or open technique,* is inserted. If the decision is taken for intervention; insert 3 mm trocar at the side of the impalpable testis at the midclavicular line at the umbilical level, and 5 mm trocar at the contra-lateral midclavicular line at a slightly lower level.

2.8 Pneumoperitoneum

*I*s established at 10-12 mmHg. This can be tolerated even by small infants. Pressure is up to 15 mmHg in older boys.

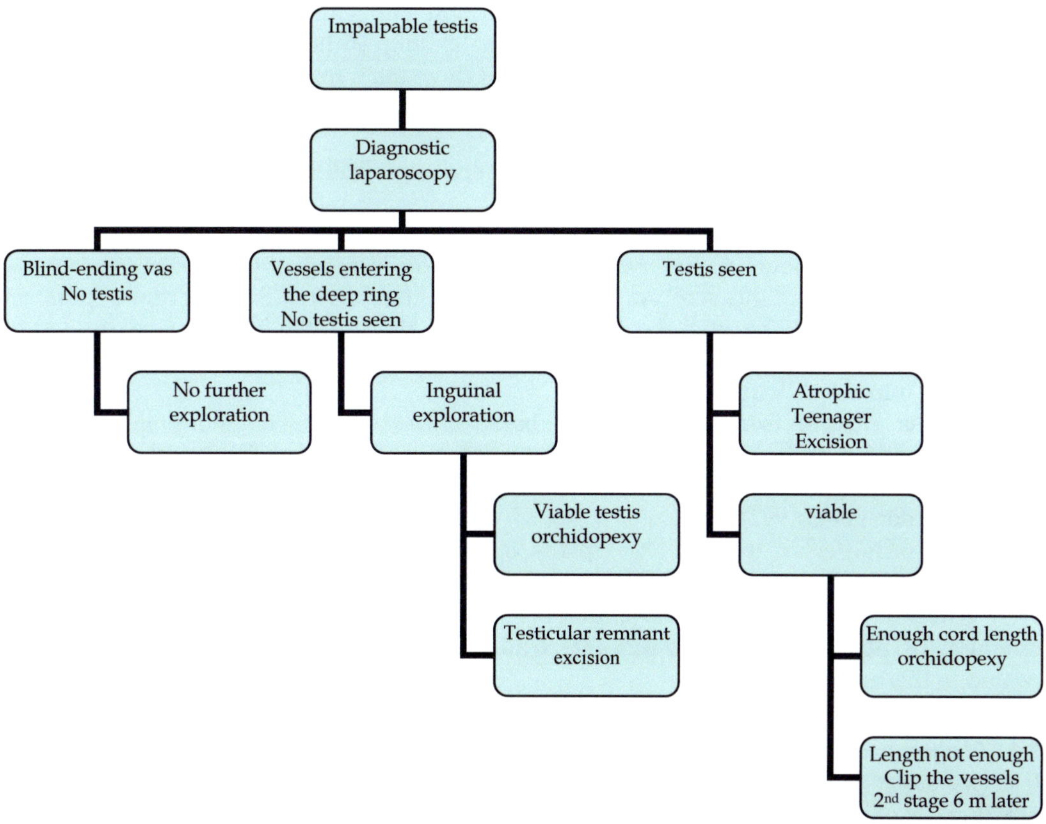

Fig. 1. Flow chart for the actions that should be taken depending on the findings on laparoscopy.

2.9 Diagnostic laparoscopy

Using O^{o} telescope, start exploration by looking for the testis at the possible sites. This could be deep to the internal inguinal ring, along its line of descent, or behind the urinary bladder. Plunging testis is detected by the presence of a patent processus vaginalis and by trying to manipulate the testis *in and out* the deep ring. Sometimes, the colon has to be retracted medially in order to detect a high testis. Further management is depending on what you find out on laparoscopy. See the flow chart for different possible scenarios and management:

2.10 Laparoscopic orchidopexy (Figures 2-15)

The colon is mobilized medially. Dissect the gubernaculum out of the internal ring and divide as distally as possible. Beware of long-loup vas around the gubernaculum.
Dissect the peritoneum around the internal ring. Proceed with the dissection around the spermatic vessels high up. Avoid dissection at the area of meeting of the vas with the vessels. The small vessels anastomoses in this area are valuable testicular supply in case in need for clipping the gonadal vessels because of short pedicle (Fowler-Stephens technique).
Dissect the bands of adhesions as needed to gain enough length. This could be as high as the origin of the gonadal vessels.
Test the gained length by pulling the testis to the contra-lateral internal ring. If this is possible, then the length is enough and it is likely to reach the scrotum without much tension.
The testis could be passed to the scrotum in one of three main routes:

1. Through the normal native internal ring through the inguinal canal if the cord length is good.
2. Medial to the inferior epigastric vessels (lateral umbilical fold): in case of short cord length *(Prentiss maneuver)*.
3. Medial to the medial umbilical fold: in case of very short cord length.

Prepare a subdartos pouch in the hemiscrotum, push an instrument (long artery forceps or 5-mm trocar) through the scrotum into the abdominal cavity. Some authors pass an instrument antegradely i,e from the abdominal cavity, through the internal ring, guided to the scrotum by palpation over the pubic area and the pass the trocar sheath over the instrument into the abdominal cavity.
The testis is grasped from the area of gubernaculums attachment and pulled into the scrotum Deflation of the pneumoperitoneum is helpful in that step. The testis is secured in the subdartos pouch with fine stitches. The pathway might need dilatation in case of large gonads (Jordan et al., 1992).
Re-inspect inside again through the laparoscope after re-inflating the peritoneum, if has been deflated, for any residual bands that need be dissected and to ensure hemostasis.
The peritoneum over the area of dissection at the internal ring might be closed with stitches or endoclips. Some authors leave this area without closure with no reported complications related to this attitude.

2.11 Staged orchidopexy

If a two-stage procedure is planned, then ligation and division of the testicular vessels proximal or cephalad to the testis is required, followed by a 6-9 month period of time to allow augmentation of the secondary collateral vasculature to the testis. This ligation and division can be performed either with endoscopic cautery, endoscopic laser (KTP) or endoscopic clips (Holcomb, 1994).

The peritoneum overlying the testicular vessels approximately 2 cm cephalad to the testicle is incised. The testicular vessels are then either coagulated with the cautery or laser or secured with the 5 mm endoscopic clip applier and divided. If the two-staged approach is used, nothing further is performed at this time.

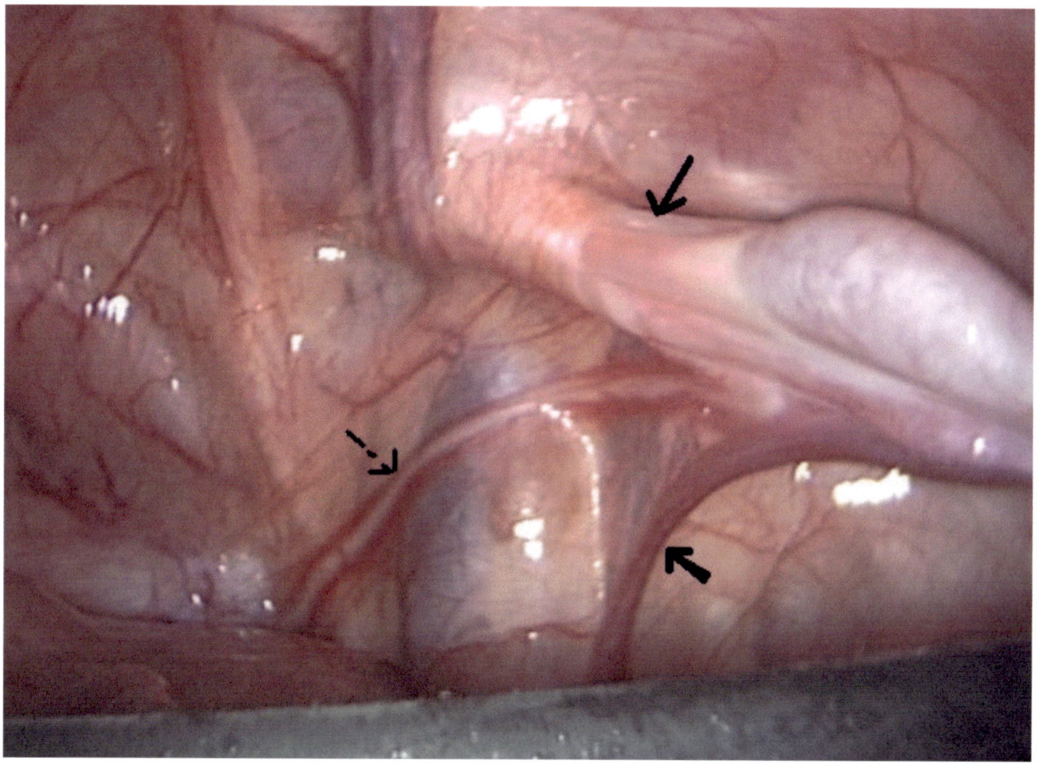

Fig. 2. Left abdominal testis. Note the vas (dotted arrow), spermatic vessels (thick arrow), gubernaculum out of the internal inguinal ring *(thin arrow)*.

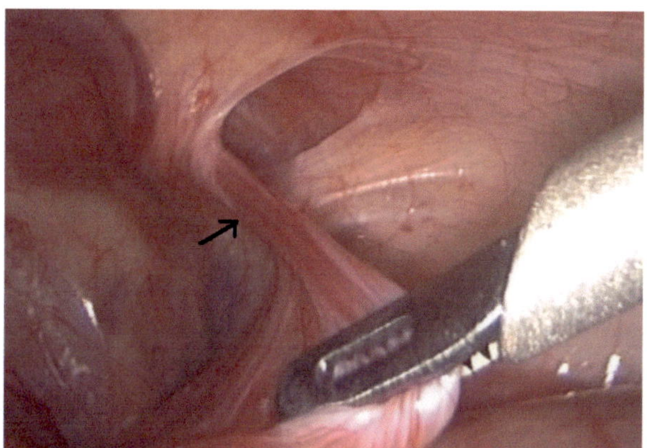

Fig. 3. Gubernaculum is pulled out of the internal ring *(arrow)*.

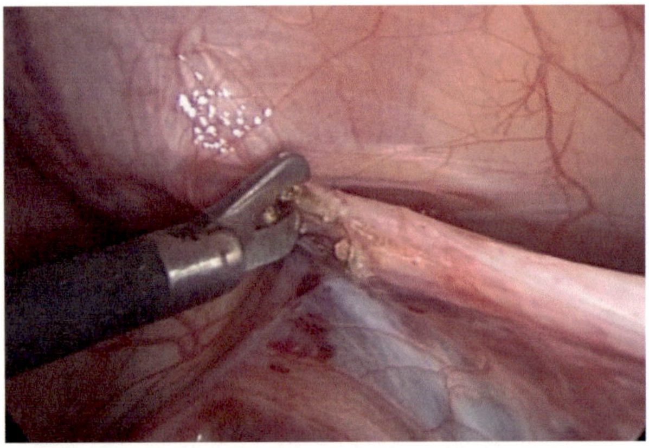

Fig. 4. The gubernaculums is dissected far from its testicular end.

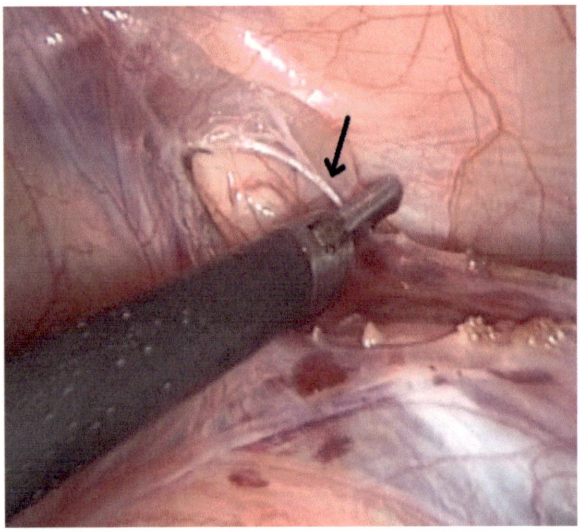

Fig. 5. The peritoneum around the internal ring is dissected.

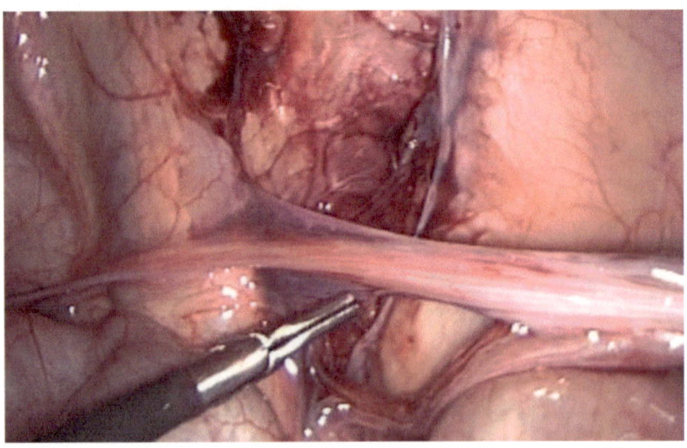

Fig. 6. The peritoneal window is dissected.

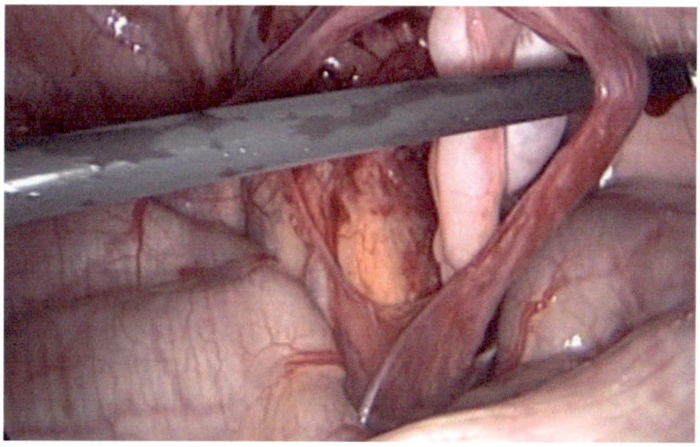

Fig. 7. The vascular pedicle after being dissected high up to its origin.

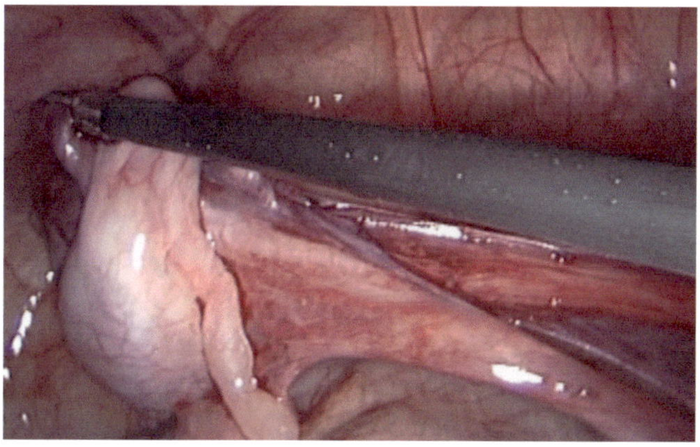

Fig. 8. Testing the cord length by pulling the testis towards the contra-lateral internal ring.

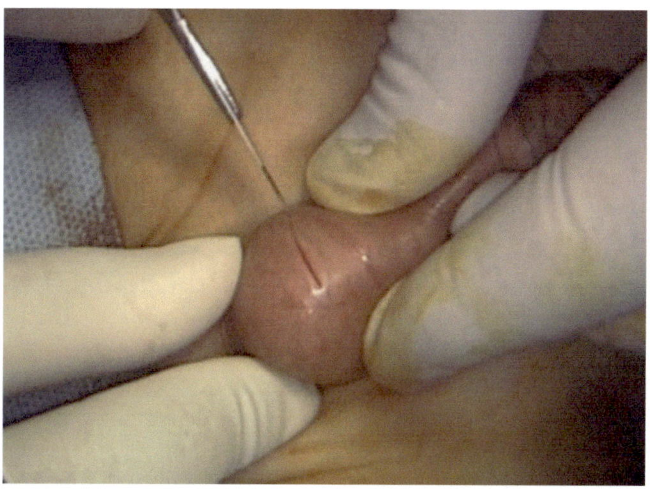

Fig. 9. The scrotal crease incision.

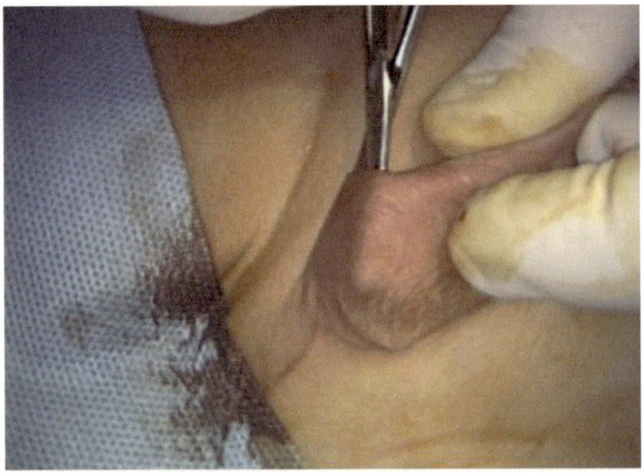

Fig. 10. The subdartos pouch is developed.

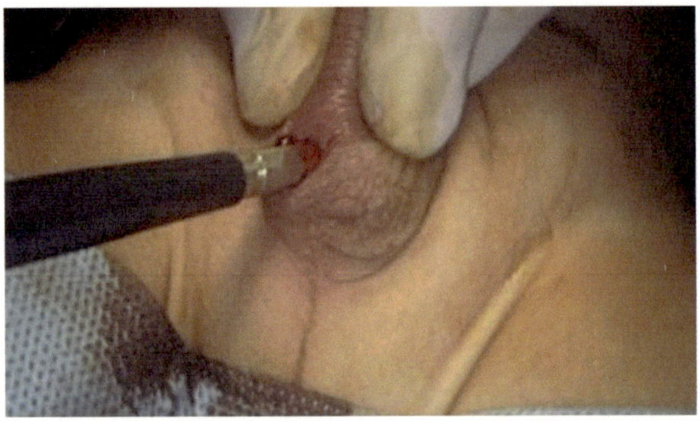

Fig. 11. 5 mm trocar is passed through the scrotal incision to inside the peritoneal cavity. This might be guided over an instrument passed from the peritoneal cavity outwards.

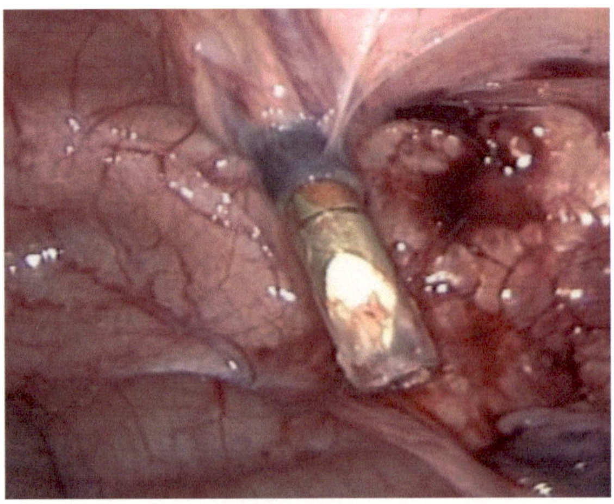

Fig. 12. The port as it is passed inside. Notice the medial relation to the inferior epigastric vessels. This rout is useful in case of relatively short cord.

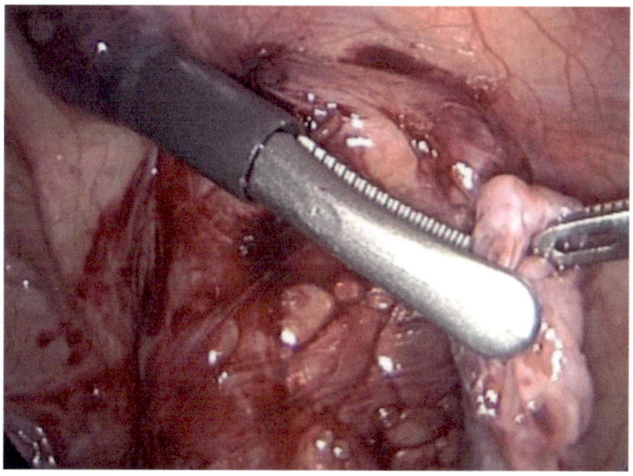

Fig. 13. The testis is grasped from the gubernaculum by an atraumatic instrument and pulled to the scrotum; *not necessarily inside the sheath but rather following its tract.*

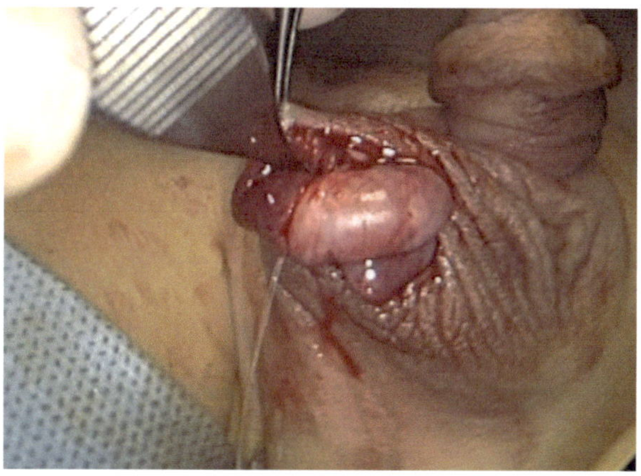

Fig. 14. The testis after being pulled and positioned in the subdartos pouch.

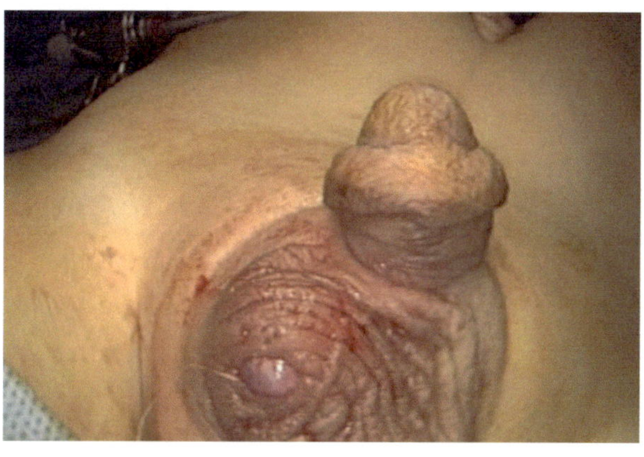

Fig. 15. The testis is secured in the scrotum without tension.

3. Conclusions

Laparoscopy is the gold standard for management of impalpable testes. Its diagnostic as well interventional potentials make it the routine technique for dealing with that problem.

4. References

Backhouse KM: Embryology of testicular descent and maldescent,Urol Clin North Am 9:315,1982.

Bloom DA .Two-step orchiopexy with pelviscopic clip ligation of spermatic vessels. J Urol 145:1030-33, 1991.

Caldamone AA & Amaral JF. Laparoscopic stage 2 FowlerStephens orchiopexy. J Urol 152:1253, 1994.

Cortesi N et al. Diagnosis of bilateral abdominal cryptorchidism by laparoscopy. Endoscopy 8:33, 1976.

Diamond DA & Caldamone AA. The value of laparoscopy for 106 impalpable testes relative to clinical presentation. J Urol 148:632-34, 1992.

Docimo SG et al. Laparoscopic orchiopexy for the high palpable undescneded testis: preliminary experience. J Urol 154: 1513-15, 1995.

Grocock CA, Charlton HM & Pike MC: Role of the fetal pituitary in cryporchidism induced by exogenous maternal oesterogen during pregnancy in mice. J Reprod Fertil 83:295,1988.

Hadziselimovic F et al. Omphalocele, cryptorchidism and brain malformations, J Pediatr Surg 22:854, 1987.

Heyns CF: The gubernaculum during testicular descent in the human fetus. J Anat 153:93, 1987

Holcomb GW III, Brock JW, Neblett WW et al. Laparoscopy for the nonpalpable testis. Am Surg 1994; 60:143-147.

Huston JM: Normal and abnormal testicular distention. In Stephens FD, Smith ED, Huston JM, editors: *Congenital anomalies of urinary and genital tracts*, Oxford, 1996, Isis Medical.

Jordan GH, Robey EL, Winslow BH. Lapendoscopic surgical management of the abdominal/transinguinal undescended testicle. J Endourolo 6:159-63, 1992.

8

Transubilical Laparoscopically Assisted Pediatric Surgery

Stjepan Visnjic
Children's hospital Zagreb, KBCSM
Medical school University of Zagreb
Croatia

1. Introduction

Endoscopic surgery has revolutionized pediatric surgery in the past twenty years. Number of operations that were previously performed through abdominal wall incisions can now be completed using endoscopic surgical techniques. The degree to which pediatric surgeons have incorporated minimally invasive surgery into their daily practice is amazing as well as the range of performed procedures. By the end of the year 2010, more than 43000 papers have been published in prereviewed medical literature with the title containing words minimally invasive or laparoscopy. Among them, more than 3500 were in the field of pediatric surgery. Around seventy procedures have been described and one quarter of them has wide acceptance as the treatment of choice.

Continuous efforts to minimize scarring from surgery led surgeons to explore new innovative and even less invasive solutions. Laparoscopic surgery using instruments in reduced sizes (mini & microlaparoscopy), two-port endoscopic surgery and less visible port laparoscopy (suprapubic and lateral -"hidden incisions") were described as initial attempts. NOTES natural orifice translumenal endoscopic surgery as a completely non visible scar procedure advocated by some general surgeons hasn't found supporters among pediatric surgeons. Idea of an endoscope passing through a natural orifice and then a internal incision in the stomach, vagina, bladder or colon, thus avoiding any external incisions or scars to perform surgery has numerous limitations. Question whether the improved cosmesis is worth the risk of visceral injury is the basic complaint about NOTES.

So for the vast majority of surgeons the most promising less invasive endoscopic surgery concept is a single incision laparoscopic surgery. This is a broad concept of single entry port surgery, applicable in abdomen, pelvis and thorax, performed by laparoscopes, scopes with working channels and endoscopes with flexible tips, and completed intraabdominaly or partly extracorporealy. Plenty of terms and acronyms exist to describe broad concept of single incision surgery. Laparoendoscopic single-site surgery consortium for assessment and research (LESCAR), a multidisciplinary group of experts of various specialties, has recently reached a consensus on nomenclature and advocate the term laparoendoscopic single-site surgery (LESS).

This concept has gained immense popularity throughout the world within the past few years. General surgeons as well as pediatric surgeons perform LESS in wide range of indications and volume of procedures inclines steadily.

In pediatric surgery, two basic concepts of single incision surgery exist and appropriate terminology for some of the procedures performed is still missing. One group of procedures is single site laparoscopic surgery using multiports and the set of LESS- adjusted instruments. Multiports (Endocone, X-cone, TriPort, UNI-X, SSL3P) are specially designed ports based on the principle of one-entry-multiple-working channel devices. Some instead of multiports use one large caliber and two adjacent trocars trough the single fascia incision. Surgery was performed using two or three specially adjusted, highly maneuverable instruments (S-shaped, bent or articulating instruments) in the manner similar or very much alike conventional laparoscopy. LESS performed by multiports provide independence of instrument movements and a steady field of vision. Traction and triangulation of tissue prior to dissection are in limited extent but still sufficient to fulfill basic requirements of laparoscopic operative technique.
Another concept is single port laparoscopic surgery with the use of a operative laparoscope. These scopes reduce the number of ports placed during minimally invasive operations by providing both visualization and a operative channel. Surgeons use laparoscopic instruments and operate trough the working channel of the operative endoscope. Procedures could be completed intraabdominaly or a part of the surgery could be done in the manner of open surgery extracorporealy. The group of procedures which combines laparoscopy and extracorporeal open surgery is the most known as transumbilical laparoscopically assisted surgery- TULA surgery. Completion of procedure extracorporeally in the manner of conventional surgery eliminates need for expensive devices; staplers cartridges, endoloops and clips, consequently TULA gained additional popularity because of low expenses. Some authors report favorable results of TULA in term of operative time comparing to open and conventional laparoscopy. The reported advantages of TULAA as a technique that reduces the cost of laparoscopy, while preserving all the benefits of laparoscopic surgery made this technique widely popular in developing countries. This is an update of the possible uses of TULA for the anomalies and conditions encountered in infants and children.

2. Basic principles of operative technique

A traditional laparoscopic procedure involves three trocars and requires three separate incisions. One port is placed for the laparoscope, and two additional ports are placed for retraction and dissection. Surgeons use instruments freely while the field of vision is steady and visualization could even be improved as the assistant rotates 30 or 45 degree scopes.
TULA is basically a single port technique. In some cases an accessory port is placed to assist in retraction. What makes this procedure specific for use is the fact that all intraabdominal dissection that needs to be done is made with an instrument which passes through the working channel of the telescope. Therefore, special equipments are necessary, including a telescope with a working channel and long shaft 420-430 mm instruments(Figure 1). Standard set of long shaft 420-ø5mm instruments include; a Maryland dissector, fine grasping forceps, a hook-cautery, curved scissors and a aspiration catheter because standard suction devices usually can not pass through the working chancel of the scope or the length of the suction device in not sufficient. The approach can sometimes be demanding because of the unsteady field of vision. Movements of the instrument change the position of the laparoscope and produce sliding of the operated substrate out of the field of vision. Another problem concerning visibility is the parallax of working instruments and the field of vision. Therefore, an adjusted operative technique using minimal and gentle movements is required.

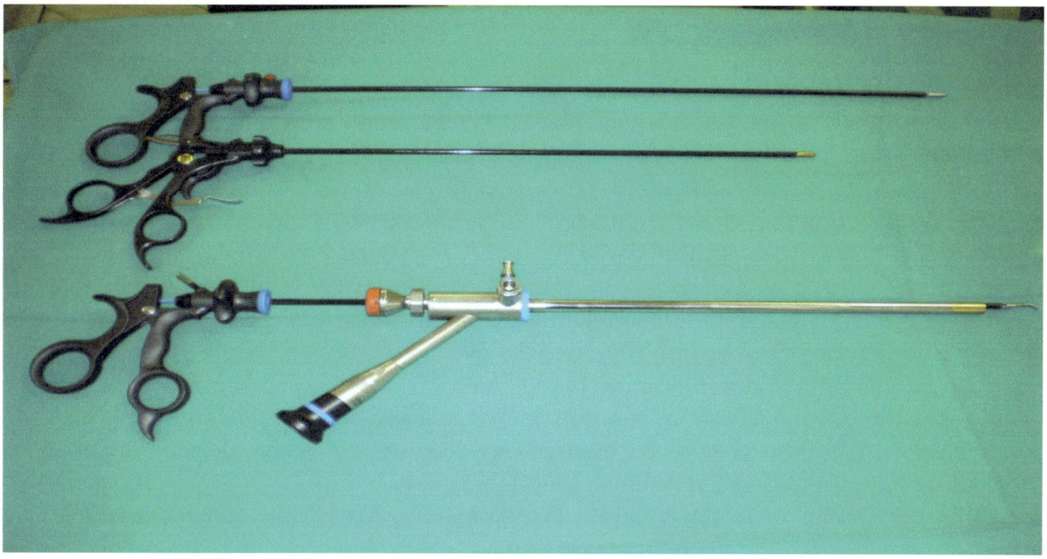

Fig. 1. Telescope with a working channel and long shaft 420-430 mm instruments

Basic preoperative considerations include thorough explanation of the procedure to the patient and parents. As with any surgical procedure, the patient will be required to sign a consent form. Proper selection of patients that are not seriously compromised would be wise choice during the learning curve. Precise procedure planning based on accurate preoperative diagnostic is necessary.

Operative room set up and instrumentation check up are mandatory. Compatibility of instruments and accessories is of utmost importance because most commercially available suction devices are too short for usage through the working channel of the scope. All suction activities need to be done by suction catheters. Procedure should be understood by all team members to reduce confusion during procedure and reduce operative time.

All procedures are performed under general anesthesia, with endotracheal intubation, assisted ventilation, muscle relaxants and proper analgesia. Nasogastric tube decompression and bladder catheterization are done routinely. Single perioperative dose of antibiotic can be administered.

Transumbilically assisted procedures usually have four main steps. Target organ is freed from intraabdominal adhesions. Exposition of the operative substrate onto the abdominal surface with precautions of slippage and spillage is the next step. Removal of substrate by open technique is the third part. Finally, the scope is reinserted to check the condition of the stump, exclude bleeding and perform final washings.

While several port reinsertions are frequently necessary to complete the operative procedure, creation of an appropriate easy-entry abdominal approach is recommendable. The 12 mm port is inserted through the umbilical incision by open technique. Some procedures could be accomplished through 5 mm ports and a small diameter scope, but these scopes provide poor visibility, mostly due to the instrument's optics and the fact that part of the screen is obstructed by the grasper. The open insertion of the first port could be sometimes time consuming, but much safer, especially in neonates with elastic abdominal wall, proximity of vital structures and potentially still patent umbilical vessels. The possibility of patent umbilical vessels in neonates is not a reason to abandon umbilical placement of the laparoscopic port as it is feasible to identify and avoid these structures by meticulous preparation. Once, the incision in the midline is done, traction sutures on the both ends will help to manipulate with the abdominal wall, help to reduce accidental air leakage by approximating incision edges and help to reinsert the port in the case of substrate slippage during extraction. Pneumoperitoneum of 8 mmHg is standard for neonatal laparoscopy and usually sufficient to enable excellent visualization of the whole abdomen and pelvis. Visualization could be further improved by a cranio-caudal slope and an additional abdominal wall lifting by traction sutures on the edges of the incision site. Adjusted intraabdominal pressures are necessary with increasing age. For preschool and school children, pressure up to 10mmHg is usually sufficient, while for adolescents, pressures could reach values for mature population.

Gentle synchronous movement of the camera and instruments provide sufficient visibility and exposure. Caution should be focused on coagulation while thermal injury is a threatening complication in a very limited working space.

After the port removal, fascia is closed by interrupted absorbable sutures and a single anchorage skin suture umbilicoplasty is performed to restore the shape of the umbilicus.

Finally, it is important to stress out three tips which enable safer and simpler procedure. Traction sutures on edges of fascia incision enable easier port reinsertion and wound closure at the end of procedure. Testing mobility of the operative substrate intraabdominally prevents substrate slippage during extraction and tears of the mesentery and adhesions, so in this way serious bleeding can be prevented. Finally, inspection of the abdominal cavity at the end of the procedure can be performed equally well in number of cases with manual abdominal wall lifting, so there is no need for CO_2 reinsufflation and time can be saved.

3. Indications

In a particular condition, several important facts will determine the indication for TULA. The clinical status and the overall patient condition, previous experience in endoscopic surgery, available technology and willingness of hospital management to afford special telescope and adjusted set of instruments, the availability of OR, support from other staff and legislative. However, for some conditions widely accepted for conventional laparoscopy, TULA is suitable. TULA is for simple appendicitis, as the most common pediatric emergency, a diagnostic and a therapeutic approach with potentially numerous advantages. At the same time, TULA is suitable for various elective pediatric surgical procedures as follows; nonpalpable testis, exploration for abdominal pain, diagnostic and staging lymph node biopsies, ovarian cysts, biopsies for Hirschsprung's disease and leveling colostomy creation, urachal remnants surgery, gastrostomy and treatment of empyema. Although feasibility has been demonstrated in some procedures such as lung wedge resection and ingiunal hernia repair, I prefer to use other than TULA approach.

3.1 Simple appendicitis

Transumbilical laparoscopically assisted appendectomy is the most common single-port operation performed in pediatric surgery. Procedure begins with universal steps; operative creation of easy-entry abdominal access, pneumoperitoneum and insertion of the working scope. The omentum should be moved away and appendix properly exposed. Sometimes, cranial retraction of the cecum helps. Rarely an additional port for traction is necessary. Once located; the appendix is freed from adhesions with a dissector, then grasped at the tip and extracted onto the abdominal surface via the umbilical port, with simultaneous release of the pneumoperitoneum. All three tools; port, scope and instrument should be brought out of abdomen together with appendix (figure 2) for this maneuver. The appendix is skeletonized off its mesenteric supply and divided at its base as in the open technique. The covering of the stump with the peritoneum is described, but it is not clear whether peritonealization has any particular benefit in reducing frequency of intra abdominal infections. Majority of surgeons advocate exposed appendicle stump as in conventional laparoscopy. The stump is dropped back into the peritoneal cavity and the umbilical port is replaced. Manual lifting of the abdominal wall usually enables sufficient working space and eliminates need for reestablishing of pneumoperitoneum. Then, the scope is reinserted to ascertain stump condition and check up for bleeding. Eventually, washout of the abdominal cavity is undertaken. Method is suitable even during infancy. According to currently published reports, TULA appendectomy technique seems to result in more complications but this difference is not statistically significant. Complications were minor port-site wound infections successfully treated with wound care and sometimes antibiotics. Complication rate may be explained by the technique of drawing the inflamed appendix through the umbilical wound. The absence of intraoperative complications and the minimal conversion

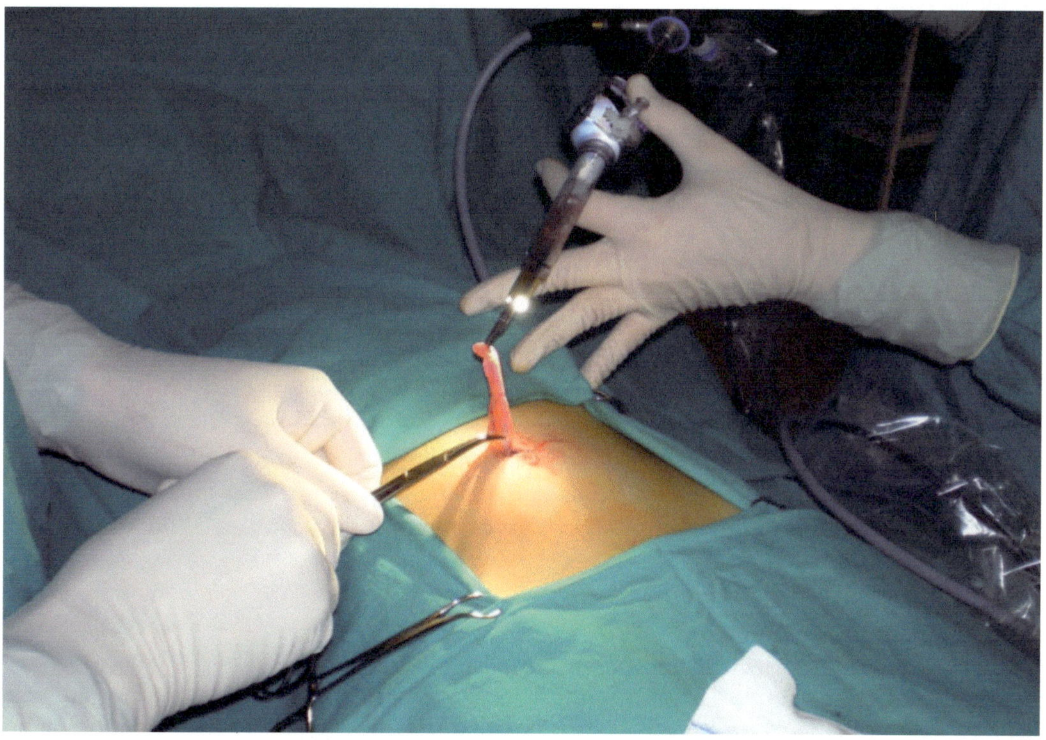

Fig. 2. Port, scope and instrument should be brought out of abdomen together with appendix

rates confirm the safety of the technique. Reduced number and length of incisions lead to better cosmesis. Reduced cost is an additional advantage of TULAA. It is shown that higher cost of conventional laparoscopy is solely attributable to the purchase price of the used supplies. In limited resources, saving achieved by TULAA could be significant.

3.2 Exploration for abdominal pain

Almost all diagnosis and conditions clinically indistinguishable from appendicitis could be verified by operative scope and a vast majority of verified conditions could be solved in very similar manner as TULAA. The same principles as for appendectomy can be applied to any operation in which the operative telescope is used for acute abdominal pain. Mesenteric adenitis and inflammatory conditions of the terminal ileum can be verified and extension of the inflamed bowel can be accurately measured. The terminal loop of inflamed bowel can be brought outside for biopsies and enlarged mesenteric lymph nodes can be taken for histology. Omental torsion can be clearly indentified, infracted omentum can be brought extracorporeally and partial or subtotal omentectomy can be done very easily, followed by peritoneal washings and control of haemostasis at the end of the operation. Meckel diverticulum could produce pain secondary to ulceration or inflammation. Other omphaloeneteric duct remnant; sinus or band can produce pain due to mechanical obstruction. In the presence of Meckel diverticula, exposure on the umbilical incision and extraabdominal resection of the diverticula is feasible. Wedge excision or total resection and end to end anastomosis is possible. If an end to end anastomosis is performed, the bowel might be congested and it may be extremely difficult to reduce bowel loop back in to the abdomen. Incision should be enlarged at the beginning of procedure to prevent vascular bowel injury during surgery. Fibrous bands or other Vitelline duct remnants can be brought outside and resected. If coagulation and dissection is performed intraabdominally, the same principles as for adhesion release after previous abdominal operations should be applied. Idiophatic intussusception can be noticed and gently reduced by traction but sometimes additional port for counter traction is necessary. Gonadal pathology and ovarian torsion can be found even in infancy and prompt reaction and detorsion could prevent infarction and rupture of the ovary and definitive lost of gonadal tissue.

3.3 Diagnostic biopsies, tumor staging and lymph node sampling

3.3.1 Diagnostic biopsies for uncertain benign conditions

Biopsies could help in differentiation in the cases of persistent hepatomegaly and splenomegaly of uncertain etiology, whether it is infective, metabolic or malignant. The hepatosplenic form of Cat scratch disease is a rare occurrence among children with intact immune system, and we previously published personal experience with laparoscopy. Liver and splenic masses of unknown origin, giant granulomas or tiny nodules could by precisely collected and analyzed.

3.3.2 Lymph node sampling

Patients who require mesenteric or pelvic lymph node sampling or lymphadenectomy are candidates for single-port laparoscopy. It is especially applicable for pediatric hematologic malignancies with primary abdominal presentation; lymph node involvement, wide dissemination and malignant ascites. In juvenile myelomonocytic leukemia abdominal symptoms could last over a period of weeks or months. The primary indication for diagnostic laparoscopy in pediatric hematological malignancies and lymphomas is a tissue diagnosis through biopsy of intraabdominal lymph nodes in the absence of peripheral lymphadenopathy, particularly when percutaneous core needle biopsy has been nondiagnostic. Procedures were performed through a single umbilical incision using an operative scope. Lymph node could be extracted or enucleated from bulking sites by meticulous preparation. For single nodules, problems could arise in the yield of adequate nodal counts. Another possibility is mesenteric nodules sampling. Exposure of a bowel loop on the umbilical incision and extracorporeal lymph node dissections could be the simplest solution.

3.3.3 Biopsies for abdominal masses

An abdominal mass in an infant or a child is a challenging diagnostic problem. It includes a spectrum of lesions of diverse origin and significance. Beyond the newborn period, there is a significant increase in malignant tumors. Therefore, all soft-tissue lumps that persist or grow should be biopsied. Biopsy is the only reliable way to determine or exclude malignancy. If needle biopsy fails to obtain sufficient or appropriate sample, tissue can be obtained via surgical biopsy. Although port site metastases are now reported less frequently, this serious complication of laparoscopic cancer surgery can still occur. Another serious complication is peritoneal seeding due to malignant spillage and tumor implantation. However, same complication can occur in open surgery. We prefer laparoscopic guidance for needle biopsies and active hemostasis in cases of persistent bleeding on biopsy site. For identification of the most appropriate puncture site operative scope could play a crucial role. Natural topography or adhered organs can make an obstacle for proper puncture so they should be gently removed by a grasper or a dissector to provide most appropriate biopsy samples.

3.3.4 Staging

Indications for staging laparoscopy in pediatric surgery are rare. Staging laparoscopy is indicated for primary staging or even restaging of Hodgkin's lymphoma when accurate staging affects decisions for appropriate treatment and prognosis. Single port laparoscopy with operative scope is a worthily attempt and additional port could be a reasonable spare solution. Gynecologists tend to expand the role of laparoscopy in the treatment of more gynecological malignancies. There are reports of single-site staging surgery for oncologic procedures. Potential benefits remain to be assessed in comparison with more conventional minimally invasive approaches. Pre-treatment laparoscopic staging in early-stage disease for therapeutic strategies planning and the laparoscopic second-look procedures in disease status assessment at the completion of adjuvant chemotherapy could be done in selected patients.

3.4 Nonpalpable testis – Fowler-Stephen procedure stage I

The length of testicular vessels is the main limiting factor in the descent of the testes in the scrotum. Since Fowler and Stephen proposed the division of testicular vessels, high and as far from the testes as possible to maintain collateral blood supply, this approach became standard in the treatment of high intra-abdominal testes, although testicular atrophy as a potential complication exists. Cortesi introduced the diagnostic laparoscopy and Jorden first completed a laparoscopic orchidopexy. Further investigations proved laparoscopic transection of the testicular vessels as safe in boys with high abdominal testes that do not reach the scrotum after laparoscopic high retroperitoneal dissection. Two-stage Fowler-

Stephens orchiopexy appears to carry a higher rate of success than the single stage approach. First step in the treatment of nonpalpable testes is abdominal exploration by an operative scope. The decision to perform a staged Fowler-Stephen orchidopexy was based on the distance of the testis from the deep inguinal ring on laparoscopy. If the distance was more than three centimeters, we proceeded to a staged Fowler-Stephen orhidopexy. In the first stage, performed completely as single port, opening in the parietal peritoneum is created by 430-ѳ5mm scissors connected to diathermy for minor coagulation. Dissector is used for vascular plexus mobilization and testicular vessels are finally cautherized by a hook cauthery. This procedure yields a fair success rate. The magnification and wide mobilization of laparoscopy probably allows better preservation of the collateral vascular supply than open exploration. Transsection of the vessels by diathermy is a very safe, cost-effective method.

3.5 Gastrostomy

Gastrostomy may be indicated in numerous situations. For all children with conductible esophagus PEG (percutaneous endoscopic gastrostomy) is the treatment of choice according to less invasiveness. The principle is endoscopic approximation of the stomach and peritoneum followed by percutaneous entrance into the stomach by cannula. Percutaneous cannula insertion is guided by transillumination. However, the morbidity of PEG placement still remains around or slightly less than 10%, due to injury to the intestine, colon or esophagus.

For those children whose esophagus is not passable for flexible endoscopy, e.g. refracter strictures, epidermolysis bullosa, (Figure 3) etc, endoscopic guidance by transstomach illumination is not possible. Then, gastrostomy made by an operative laparoscope placed trough the umbilical port could be one of the options. The stomach and abdominal wall can be visualized directly thus limiting the chance of inadvertent injuries. Stomach is fixed by a fine grasper and approximated to the abdominal wall. Two percutaneous sutures are placed and PEG cannula can be inserted into the stomach as in endoscopic PEG placement, but now

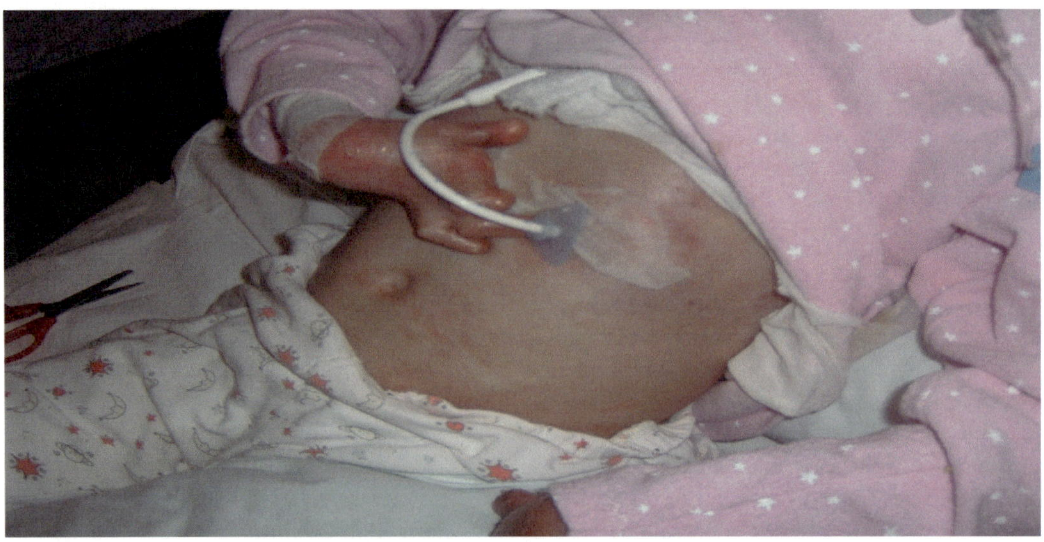

Fig. 3. Laparoscopic gastrostomy in epidermolysis bullosa

under visual control. Rest of the procedure is very much alike PEG procedure (Russell introducer technique). A guidewire is inserted through the cannula and dilation of ostomy channel is performed using dilators from PEG set. A series of dilators are used to increase the size of the gastric opening. Once sufficient width is achieved, PEG tube is inserted over the wire into the stomach under visual control and catheter balloon is insufflated with fluid. The fixation plate is then placed ensuring that sutures pass through the holes of fixation plate. Finally, knot tying anchorages fixation plate and stomach. This type of laparoscopic gastrostomy involves two skin incisions an umbilical and a stoma site incision.

Some authors prefer gastrostomy with a single incision performed on stoma site. After introduction of port and operative scope, the stomach is indentified by the instrument which passes through the scope working channel. Greater curvature is grasped at the appropriate location and brought out through the trocar site. The gastrostomy is then sutured to the fascia and a primary gastrostomy button is placed.

3.6 Urachal remnants

Urachal defects are rare with urachal cysts, being the most common anomaly occurring in approximately 1/5,000 births. Urachal cyst, embryological remnant of the allantois originally communicates with the vertex of the bladder. Symptoms could be infection or less often recurrent umbilical secretion. Excision is curative. Abdominal exploration by usage of an operative scope provides clear insight in retropubic Retzius space and as a diagnostic procedure should be advocated in all cases of umbilical secretion when routine imaging techniques fail to show pathologic substrate. Procedure provides reliable diagnosis and enables safe and efficient treatment of pathology as single port. The dissection is performed on the anterior peritoneal wall. Cyst or urachal bend can be grabbed and exposed together with the vertex of the bladder on umbilical port. Cyst should be excised and the vertex of the bladder sutured with sutures in two layers. Bladder decompression by a catheter is mandatory. Laparoscopic approach shown in the previous case made it possible to minimize a long vertical incisional scar and related complications.

3.7 Biopsies and leveling colostomy for Hirschsprung's disease

Once the diagnosis of Hirschprung disesase is established by rectal biopsy, primary pull through is the treatement of choice. The presence of associated anomalies may dictate a staged approach. Immediate operation should be undertaken if irrigations are ineffective and leveling colostomy should be performed.

By the use of the operative scope, mobile parts of the colon can be exposed on the umbilical incision and serial full thickness biopsies can be made in order to identify the most distal segment of the bowel with ganglion cells. In spite of the fact that gross appearance of the colon can suggest a transition zone it is smart to perform biopsies on at least four locations of the colon. We recommend biopsies on the rectosigmoid, the sigmodescendent flexure, the splenic flexure, and the hepatic flexure. All these segments can be easily brought to the umbilical incision and biopsies can be performed as in open surgery with full thickness sampling and closure of the biopsy sites by sutures. The transition zone should be identified with a frozen section biopsy. A colostomy above the transition zone in such cases is life protecting and should be performed in the same act. Additional trocar should be inserted at the place of the ostomy creation and the appropriate segment of the colon marked by sutures during biopsies should be brought out through the trocar site. A loop of bowel is secured by sutures to the incision in the abdominal wall. Colostomy is then finished in the traditional way. By this approach it is possible to create colostomy on all levels of colon, sigmoid, splenic or hepatic flexure (Figure4).

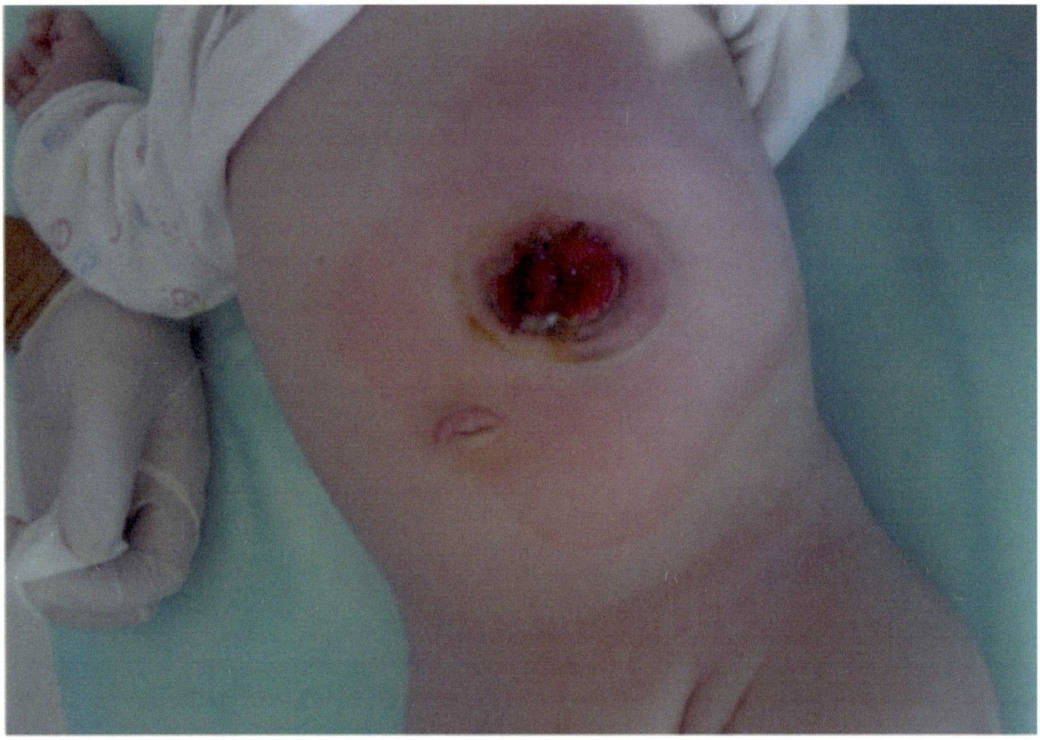

Fig. 4. Single port leveling colostomy after serial biopsies

3.8 Ovarian cyst torsion, infarction and amputation

Due to the stimulation by maternal hormones, cystic changes in fetal ovaries can be noticed in as much as one third of all female newborns. Hormonal imbalance during puberty is the reason for another peek of incidence among adolescents. The routine ultrasound scan as well as the improved US resolution have increased detection of cysts and allied gonadal pathology. Ultrasound patterns and cyst size have a prognostic value. Simple cysts greater than 5 cm in diameter have a greater chance of complications such as enlargement, rupture, bleeding and torsion. Shift from simple to a complex US pattern during follow up and verified debris, septation and solid component suggest complications. High incidence of complications is an argument in favor of surgical intervention regardless of symptoms or age of the patient.

Author prefers two basic approaches. For simple cysts larger than 5 cm, laparoscopic decompression can be done. Cyst is identified and drained percutaneously by a suction needle.

For complicated cysts, partial decompression and size reduction is done as the initial procedure by a puncture of the cyst. Second step is cyst exposure through the usage of a instrument and a operative scope on the umbilical incision. Incision enlargement is done if necessary. Rest of the cyst is removed on the abdominal wall as a open technique either by free cyst wall resection or by deflated cyst enucleation and if possible, ovary sparing surgery and tunica albuginea reconstruction.

Three major issues exist with single port laparoscopy during infancy and puberty considering dissection, elimination and puncture needle manipulation.

If the cyst wall is attached to the parietal peritoneum, dissection is necessary. By pushing cyst forward, loose adhesions are exposed. Dissection of adhesions can be done by scissors' tip (curved tip scissors) as close as possible to the peritoneal side in order to preserve the integrity of cyst wall until the whole cyst is completely freed and mobile (Figure 5).

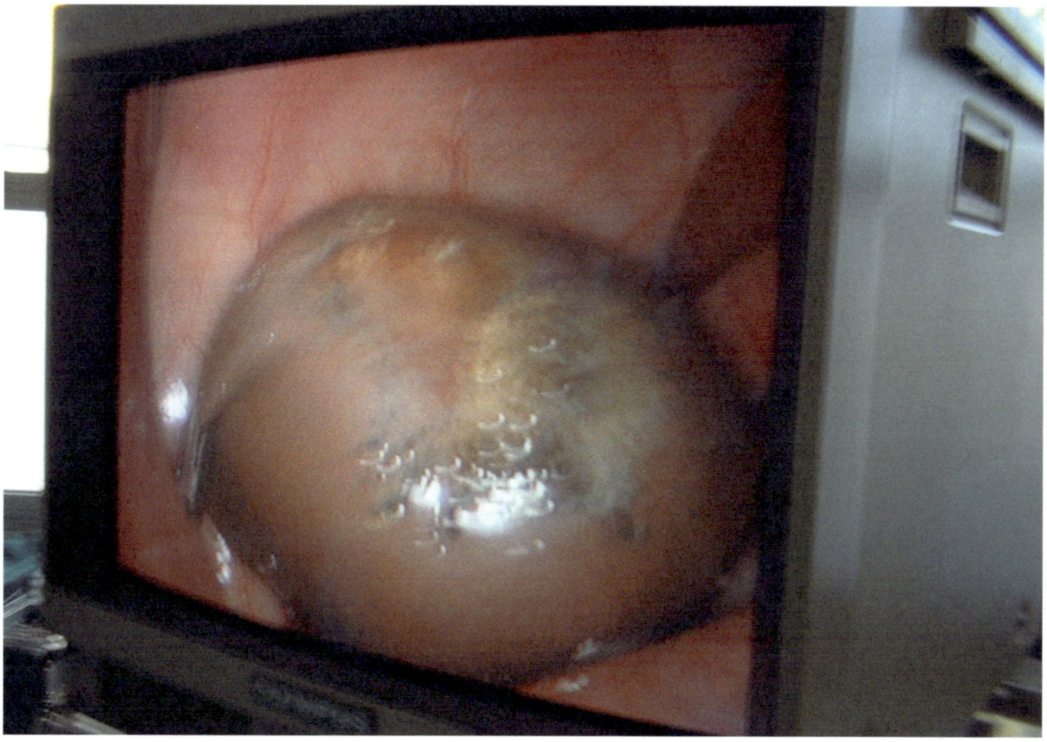

Fig. 5. Preserved integrity of the cyst after laparoscopic mobilization

If the ovary has undergone irreversible changes, elimination of bulky necrotic tissue can be a problem. Two possible solutions are available and decision should be made on case to case basis. The cyst could be suctioned to fit the size of the umbilical port and removed combined with incision enlargement, or it could be brought to the umbilical incision, capsule incised, solid component enucleated and then removed in reduced size as gall bladder removal for cholelithiasis.

Finally, some tips regarding manipulation with puncture needle. It has been previously reported that the suction needle has a tendency to slide on the cyst and to cause an injury of adjacent organs in the presence of negative pressure. Visualization of the puncture site by camera and cyst fixation during puncture by the instrument which passes through the scope working channel minimizes the risk of slippage. Once puncture is done, a grasper placed on the puncture site around puncture needle solves the problem of potential fluid leakage and needle slip-out and enables manipulation with decompression needle inside the cyst in the cases of septation.

3.9 Treatment of empyema

Inflammatory fluid and debris in the pleural space as result of ongoing infection usually resolves after therapy. Some effusions do not resolve in spite of prolonged antibiotic therapy. Inflammatory response can proceed until adhesive bands form. The infected fluid becomes loculated pus in the pleural space. No clear consensus has been reached concerning the optimal therapeutic strategy for advanced empyema. We consider thoracoscopy may be indicated only if chest tube drainage is inadequate and ineffective because of tube clogging and multiple loculations. Prior thoracoscopy, serial ultrasound examinations should be performed on daily basis in the patient in a sitting position. Ultrasonography may provide information about the size, position and the viscosity of the lesion. Ultrasonography may also reliably demonstrate septa in the pleural fluid collection but the most important sonograpy could determine trocar insertion level. Scope insertion should be planned at least two intercostals space under or above the locus of empyema collection determined by ultrasound. Intrathoracic pressure up to 5 mmHg will collapse or partially collapse the lungs and improve visualization. Decortication and fluid aspiration are procedure goals. Decortication and release of the lung is a delicate procedure and can result in serious bleeding. Therefore, it is not clear whether total decortication is necessary or only partial decortication could be sufficient, especially having in mind the high incidence of readhesions. Limited experience showed that division of adhesion is possible using a Maryland grasper through the scope. Dissection should be done as close as possible to the parietal pleura and the chest wall while preserving pulmonary tissue. We found no need for a complete excision of all adhesions but only resection of the septa and a conversion of multilocular lesion to a single volume process. Sufficient size chest tube insertion should be done on the lowest point to enable sufficient drainage.

4. Conclusion

Single-port surgery has evolved significantly in the past few years and has been shown to be valuable, safe and effective alternative to traditional laparoscopy in the performance of minimally invasive operations. Pelosi in 1992 published first appendectomy, done trough a puncture on the umbilicus incision. An idea to apply principles and strategies of both procedures, laparoscopy and open surgery and thus compile advantages, resulted in development of laparoscopically assisted techniques- TULA for various indications. This approach represents a natural progression of minimal access surgery towards less invasive approach and is now a significant portion of LESS. Elastic abdominal wall and relatively short abdominal distances to the umbilicus made transumbilical laparoscopically assisted surgery especially feasible during infancy and childhood.

Clear advantages of TULA are fewer incisions and decreasing costs. Fewer incisions minimize scars from surgery and lead to improved cosmesis. But, fewer incisions also slightly reduce operative time concerning time needed for insertion and closure of additional port sites and some authors reported statistically significant time saving for TULA-appendectomy in comparison to conventional laparoscopy. Finally, single incision eliminates most frequent complications associated with additional port insertion like hemorrhage due to injury of the inferior epigastric vessels, gastrointestinal lesion or ureter injury.

In spite of reported decline in cost of laparoscopic instruments and supplies during time, laparoscopic operative procedures are still more expensive then open surgery. Cost-effectiveness of laparoscopic surgery is based on the fact that the operative cost surplus is outnumbered by secondary savings associated with decreased hospital stay and earlier resumption to normal activities. In TULA, cost of operative procedure usually equals cost of open surgery and operative cost surplus of laparoscopy is eliminated. At the same time, TULA procedure provides clinical benefits and secondary savings associated with laparoscopy.

Some authors report improved patient outcomes like decreased pain and quicker recovery as additional advantages but controlled randomized trials to confirm that data are still missing.

However, this technique, although very popular, has certain limitations. Little or no formal guidance, training or structured protocols exist at the moment. Therefore, a significant role in maximizing patient safety is setting threshold for conversion to conventional three port laparoscopy or even open surgery appropriately low. Some argue that TULA may lead to an increase in umbilical wound infections. Further investigations and bigger series of cases are necessary to give us clear picture in the incidence of these infections. Some reported difficulties when performing TULA in larger adolescents, but with certain precaution measures, surgery is done routinely in adult population too. Finally, one instrument is not sufficient for more complex and demanding surgery, but operative scope enables creative solutions for various surgical situations even in the complex MIS procedures.

To have a complete insight into problem maybe the fact that PUBMED search for words-transumbilical single port laparoscopy gives 519 results, and if filter age is added; All Child: 0-18 years- result is 96 published papers. 72 of 96 papers were published in the last five years, and thus provide a proof how challenging and vibrant part of surgery TULA is. Simplicity of most TULA procedures and low complication rate reported so far amplified reported benefits of transumbilically assisted approach. It makes TULA potent alternative to traditional MIS.

5. References

Aziz O, Athanasiou T, Tekkis PP, Purkayastha S, Haddow J, Malinovski V, Paraskeva P, Darzi A 2006 Laparoscopic versus open appendectomy in children: a meta-analysis. Ann Surg 243:17-27

D'Alessio A, Piro E, Tadini B, Beretta F 2002. One-trocar transumbilical laparoscopic-assisted appendectomy in children: our experience. Eur J Pediatr Surg 12:24-7

Dutta S. 2009. Early experience with single incision laparoscopic surgery: eliminating the scar from abdominal operations. J Pediatr Surg. Sep;44(9):1741-5.

Jones VS, Cohen RC. 2008. Two decades of minimally invasive pediatric surgery Pediatr Surg. Sep;43(9):1653-9.

Marietti S, DeCambre M, Fairbanks T, Kling K, Chiang G. 2010. Early experience with laparoendoscopic single-site surgery in the pediatric urology patient population. J Endourol. Aug;24(8):1321-4.

Koontz CS, Smith LA, Burkholder HC, Higdon K, Aderhold R, Carr M 2006. Video- assisted transumbilical appendectomy in children. J Pediatr Surg 41:710-2

Little DC, Custer MD, May BH, Blalock SE, Cooney DR 2002. Laparoscopic appendectomy: An unnecessary and expensive procedure in children? J Pediatr Surg 37:310-7

Pelosi MA 1992. Laparoscopic appendectomy using single umbilical puncture (minilaparotomy). J Reprod Med 37:588-594

Saxena A., Hollwarth M; 2009. Essentials of Pediatric Endoscopic Surgery. Springer verlag Berlin

Visnjic S. 2008. Transumbilical laparoscopically assisted appendectomy in children: high-tech low-budget surgery.Surg Endosc. Jul;22(7):1667-71. Epub 2007 Dec 11.
Višnjić S, Popović L, Župančić B 2006. Laparoscopically assisted appendectomy. Eur Surg 38:374-375

9

Laparoscopic Varicocelectomy

Ali Shamsa
Professor of Urology and Kidney Tx
Mashhad University of Sciences
Iran

1. Introduction

Varicocele is dilatation of pampiniform plexus in the scrotum. It is one of the most common causes of male infertility. The aim of this chapter is the evaluation of the role of laparoscopy in varicocele treatment; however, because of high incidence of this disease we will discuss it in brief.

2. History

Celsus, in the first century, found that varicocele makes testicular atrophy. Abol-ghasem Khalaf Zahravi (Albucasis) mentioned this subject and added that my teacher (Celsus) suggested orchidectomy for testis atrophy due to varicocele through scrotal incision parallel to the penis (1).

Toullouch published a paper in 1952 about an infertile man with bilateral varicocele. He operated on him, and the patient became fertile. Then after two children he came in for vasectomy (2).

3. Vasculature

The main artery of the testes arises from the aorta. This artery communicates to the other arteries like cremaster and vasal arteries at the internal ring (3).

The main testicular vein has a high anastomotic condition which is called the internal spermatic vein. It has some communication with external pudendal, cremasteric and vasal veins (3).

The left internal spermatic vein drains to the left renal vein just opposite to the adrenal vein at a rectangular angle, but the right internal spermatic vein drains to the inferior vena cava, 4-5 cm below the renal vein (4).

4. Diagnosis

Physical exam is still the key to diagnosis of varicocele. However, in obese patients or during cold weather or for any other doubt, sonography, especially color Doppler sonography, is indicated. Our study showed that the standing position with and without Valsalva maneuver and looking for reflux to be the choice procedure for the diagnosis of varicocele (5).

5. Grading

Clinically, there are three grades for varicocele.
Grade I. The patient is standing and varicocele appears while the scrotum is palpated and Valsalva maneuver is done.
Grade II. Varicocele appears while the scrotum is palpated without Valsalva maneuver.
Grade III. Varicocele appears as a "bag of worms" while the patient stands, without valsalva and palpation.

6. Incidence and laterality

Left sided varicocele is more common than the right side (85% vs. 11.2-25%, 6- 7). The use of ultrasonography incidence of bilateral varicocele is more common than before. Our study on diagnosis of suspected varicocele with ultrasonography among100 patients showed bilateral varicocele was 87%, left side12%, and only right side1%(5) Incidence of varicocele among young patients is 8-20%, but in infertile cases it is up to 40% (7-8).
The reason for high incidence of varicocele in the left side may be the longer left spermatic vein and its attachment to the left renal vein with a perpendicular angle just opposite the adrenal vein established behind the descending colon.

7. Etiology

Etiology of varicocele is not really known. The most acceptable theory is absence or insufficiency of internal spermatic vein valves and resulting venous reflux with its consequent results. But Shafik (1973) suggested that varicocele is the result of cremasteric weakness and made scrotal plication for its treatment (9).
Renogonadal bypass and nutcracker phenomenon is another theory for varicocele appearance.

8. Effect of varicocele on spermatogenesis

Now, most researchers believe that varicocele has some adverse effect on spermatogenesis. It is said that retrograde venous flow increase the scrotum temperature up to 2.5 deg. C. (10), and this increased temperature change stagnation of blood and decreases blood flow from the scrotum end to decrease oxygen and finally decrease maturation of sperm at the epididymis (7).
Retrograde of adrenal metabolites through left internal spermatic vein, which have serotonin, can decrease spermatogenesis as well. It is suggested that serotonin can increase prostaglandin production and affect spermatogenesis.
Recent study by Benof et al (11) showed increased cadmium, even in unilateral varicocele, can accumulate bilaterally and induce apoptosis, decreasing sperm concentration.

9. Symptoms and siepididymisgns

The most important symptom of varicocele is infertility. From 21 March 1990 until 20 March 2003 we operated on 1,711 patients. The operation was done because of infertility in 91.7%. Dull ache and heavy sensation (48%) were another symptom. We also found two additional symptoms: early ejaculation and spouse abortion.

In one study in the city of Kerman, Iran, the incidence of spontaneous abortion was 12% (12), but it was 59% ($P<0.05$) among 117 patients with varicocelectomy (from Sept. 1997),
From September 1977 we asked about early ejaculation. 499 (58%) out of 862 varicocele patients had early ejaculation. The incidence of early ejaculation in our population was 27% ($P=0.000$) (13).
Three months postoperatively, 206 out of 499 patients that came for follow up 154 (75%) had improvement (6).
Recently we are conducting a research in our IVF Center (Montaserieh) on varicocele and DNA fragmentation on sperm of spouses with their wives' history of abortion. Varicocelectomy can decrease DNA fragmentation in most cases (not published data).
It is believed that varicocele can effect on hypothalamus - hypophyse axis (14). In this regard it decreases Sertoli cell and Leydig cell functions (15).
Sometimes we diagnosed high grade varicocele incidentally, without any symptoms and with children.

10. Treatment

10.1 Indication for treatment

Not all varicoceles need treatment. We have seen, as we mentioned earlier, that, varicoceles with no symptoms: i.e. infertility, pain, sperm abnormality and testicular atrophy, do not need intervention.
There are different treatments for a varicocele, including varicocelectomy, sclerotherapy and recently laparoscopy (16-17). Open varicocelectomy and sclerotherapy is beyond the scope of this chapter. So we will focus on laparoscopic varicocelectomy.
In 1991 Aaberge et al introduced laparoscopic varicocelectomy as the new and less invasive treatment for varicocele (18). In 1999 Piskun and Rajpal introduced laparoendoscopic single site (LEES) surgery for cholecystectomy (19). This newer technique is even less invasive than conventional laparoscopy, and it is safe and effective with a single 10 - 15mm incision. But it needs more cases and comparison with conventional laparoscopy (20). For this reason we describe the conventional laparoscopic varicocelectomy.

10.2 Technique

Patient in supine position and under general anesthesia received by nasogastric tube and urethral Foley catheter. A one-cm transverse incision is made immediately above the umbilicus, and then fascia is opened transversally. We prefer Hasson (open) rather Verese (Blind) technique. Before the insertion of a 10 mm trocar, we grasp the fascia with 0-nylon. After insertion of the trocar, the abdomen is filled with CO_2 gas (# 15 mm Hg). At this time, a 10 mm telescope is inserted into the first trocar. Now we can see abdominal organs including the internal spermatic vein.
After that two 5mm trocars are inserted through the midclavicular line at both sides of the umbilicus. Grasping with one hand and using scissors in the other hand, two perpendicular incisions are made in the peritoneum overlying the left or right internal spermatic veins. By lifting the vascular mass, arterial and lymphatic component should be separated from the vein(s) (fig.1-3). Then veins are ligated by one or two clips (fig.4).
We do not recommend cauterizing or suturing or even cutting the veins, to save time.
When a 5 mm clip- applier is not available, it is possible to change the 10 mm telescope to a 5 mm telescope and 10 mm clips applied.

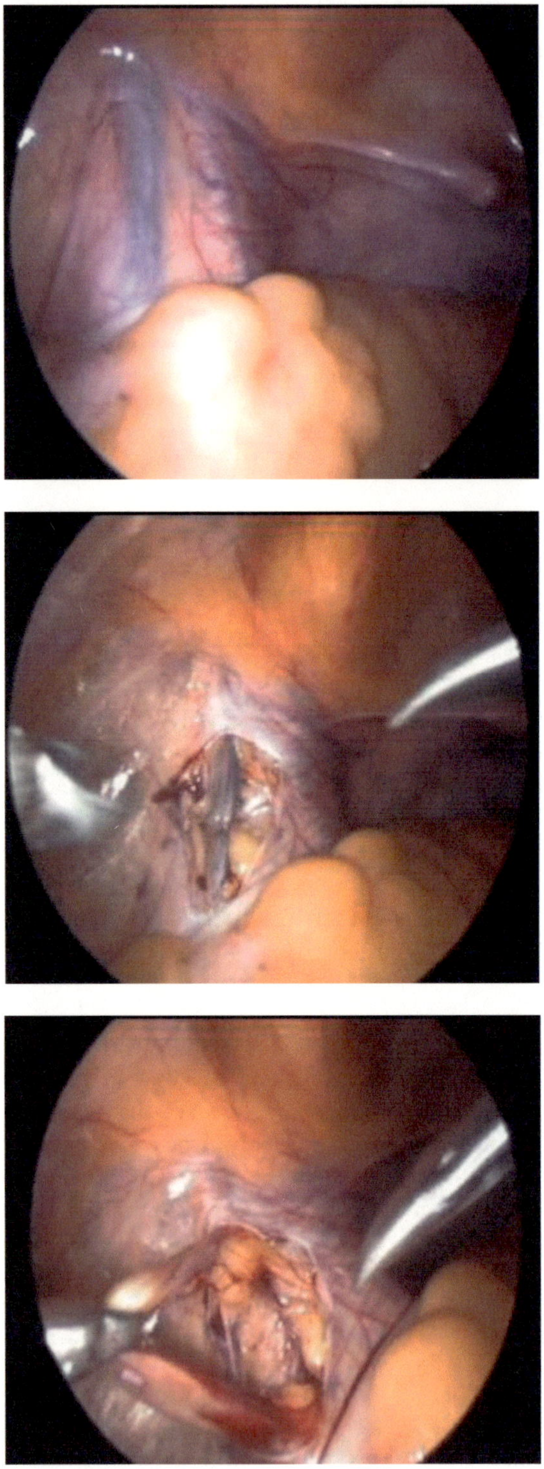

Fig. 1-3. Right int. spermatic vein

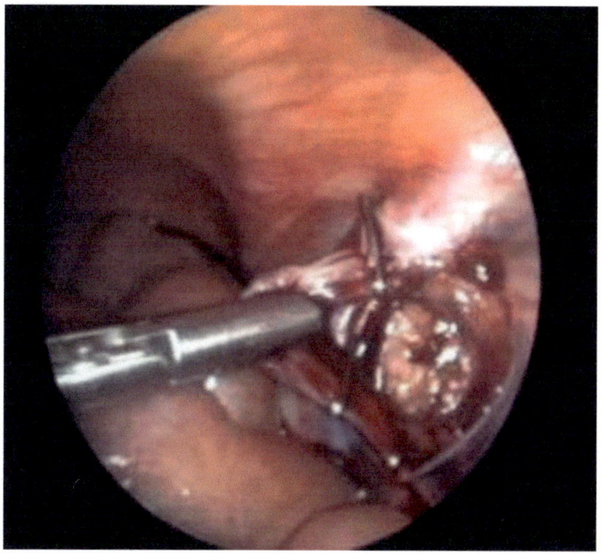

Fig. 4. Left int. spermatic vein after clipped applied

11. Our study

We conducted a randomized study comparing three different forms of varicocelectomy: Laparoscopy, open with general anesthesia and open with local anesthesia. We allocated 30 patients with bilateral varicoceles in each group. Our aim was to compare operative time, complications, and sperm analysis after surgery. SPSS Software was used for data analysis. P value <.05 considered significant (21).

12. Results

The mean operative times were 3.0 ± 5.5, 27.0 ± 3.5 and 38.0 ± 1.8 minutes respectively (P = .02).

13. Complications

Regarding complications, it occurred only in the laparoscopic group (subcutaneous emphysema (one case).
Post operative complications were summarized in table I.

Complication	Laparoscopy	Open With General Anesthesia	Open With Local Anesthesia
Hydrocele	1 (3.3)	0	0
Scrotal edema	4 (13.3)	3 (10.0)	0
Orchitis	1 (3.3)	1 (3.3)	0
Wound infection	0	3 (10.0)	0
Hematoma	0	0	1 (3.3)
Recurrence	2 (6.7)	0	0

*Values in parentheses are percents.

Table 1. Varicocelectomy Complications With Different Surgical Methods*

Sperm count after 3 months with analysis t test did not show any significant changes among the three groups, except slight improvement of sperm morphology in Group 3. It is also summarized in Table 2(21).

Varicocelectomy	Before Treatment	After Treatment	P
Laparoscopy			
Sperm count, × 10^6/mL	58 ± 42	54 ± 33	.65
Sperm motility, %	73 ± 49	92 ± 100	.26
Sperm morphology, %	69 ± 52	74 ± 41	.31
Open with general anesthesia			
Sperm count, × 10^6/mL	40 ± 25	34 ± 20	.26
Sperm motility, %	35 ± 20	35 ± 20	.91
Sperm morphology, %	31 ± 16	38 ± 18	.07
Open with local anesthesia			
Sperm count, × 10^6/mL	51 ± 23	47 ± 25	.31
Sperm motility, %	55 ± 19	58 ± 19	.18
Sperm morphology, %	51 ± 27	57 ± 22	.045

Table 2. Semen Analysis Results With Different Varicocelectomy Methods

Our results showed the Complications, cost and also operative time, laparoscopy is not superior to other methods of varicocelectomy. It is similar to other studies (22).
We recommend laparoscopic approach for obese patients, recurrent (or persistent) varicocele, history of inguinal surgery and patients who had other diseases (renal cyst, inguinal hernia, non palpable testis, etc).
One important notice: Bilateral varicocele is certainly more common than other urologic diseases that need laparoscopy surgery. So for gaining experience and increasing the learning curve, conventional laparoscopic varicocelectomy or LESS has this potential value and are good options.
We do not advocate the laparoscopic approach for unilateral varicocele except when it is concomitant with other mentioned pathology.

14. Conclusion

Laparoscopic varicocelectomy is recommended for infertile men with bilateral varicoceles. It is preferred in obese patients, history of inguinal surgery and or other diseases (renal cyst, inguinal hernia, non palpable testis, etc).
LEES varicocelectomy is promising but needs either more experience or more patients.

15. Refrences

[1] Spink MS, Lewis GL. Albucasis on surgery and instruments. Great Britain. Oxford university press, 1927.438.
[2] Tulloch WS. Varicocele in subfertility: Results of treatment. Br Med J 1955;4935(1):356-8.
[3] Brooks J.D.,Anatomy of the Lower Urinary Tract and Male Genitalia,in Wein A.J.(Eds)Campbell-Walsh Urology . Philadelphia,Saunders,2007:38-77.
[4] Redman J.F., Anatomy of the Genitourinary System,in Gillenwater J.Y.,et.al.(Eds)Adult and Pediatric Urology.St.Louis. Mosby ,1996:3-61.

[5] Oraei Abbasian F.,comparison of two methods of varicocele diagnosis(upper and supine positions) with color Doppler ultrasonography,thesis for the degree of doctorate in medicine,supervised by Shamsa A.,Nekuei C.,Shakeri M.S .2010,MUMS.
[6] Shamsa A., Nademi M., Aqaee M.,, Nouraee Fard A., Molaei M., Complications and the effect of varicocelectomy on semen analysis, fertility, early ejaculation and spontaneous abortion Saudi J Kidney Dis Transplant. 2010,21: 6; 1100-1105.
[7] Shamsa A. Varicocele in Iranian Textbook of Urology ,(eds) Simforoosh N., Nour alizadeh A.;Tehran,Behine,2007, vol 2: 1147-1153
[8] Goldstein M. Surgical management of male infertility and other scrotal disorders. In: Walsh P, Wein A, Kavoussi L, Novick A, Partin A, Peters C. (eds). Campbell's Urology. 8th ed. Philadelphia. Saunders, 2002.1532-83.
[9] Shafik A. The cremasteric Muscle: Role in varicocelogenesis and in thermoregulatory function of the testicle. Invest Urol 1973;11 (2):92-7.
[10] Marmar JL. Varicocele and male infertility: Part II the pathophysiology of varicoceles in the light of current molecular and genetic information. Hum Reprod Update 2001;7(5):461-72.
[11] Benoff SH, Millan C, Hurley IR, Napolitano B, Marmar JL. Bilateral increased apoptosis and bilateral accumulation of cadmium in infertile men with left varicocele. Hum Reprod 2004;19(3):616-27.
[12] Habibzadeh V. Incidence of spontaneous abortion in women referred to Kerman health centers. J Shahid Sadoughi Univ Med Sci Health Serv .2001;3(8);88-92.
[13] Hoseini S, Beigi D, Khoshabi K. Pervalence of early ejaculation among infertile men referred to Royan institute and society men. Articles abstract of Iran's 5th congress of Urology, Tehran. Iran university of medical sciences, p75,1381.
[14] Comhair F.,Vermeulen A.,Hormonal Testicular Function in patients with Varicocele ,in Jecht E.W., Zeitler E. (Eds):varicocele and male infertility. Berlin,Springer Verlag,1982: 110-116.
[15] Shamsa A review of 427 cases of Varicocele, Medical Journal of The Islamic Republic of Iran 1988;2(2): 115-118.
[16] Hassan JM, Adams MC, Pope JCt, Demarco RT, Brock JW, 3rd Hydrocele formation following laparoscopic varicocelectomy. J Urol. 2006;175:1076-9.
[17] Misseri R, Gershbein AB, Horowitz M, Glassberg KI. The adolescent varicocele. II: the incidence of hydrocele and delayed recurrent varicocele after varicocelectomy in a long-term follow-up. BJU Int.,2001;87:494-8.
[18] Aaberg RA, Vancaillie TG, Schuessler WW. Laparoscopic varicocele ligation: a new technique, Fertil Steril. 1991;56:776.
[19] Piskun G, Rajpal S. Transumbilical laparoscopic cholecystectomy utilizes no incisions outside the umbilicus. *J Laparoendosc Adv Surg Tech A.* 1999;9:361–364.
[20] Kawauchi A, Naitoh Y. ,Miki T. Laparoendoscopic single-site surgery for pediatric patients in urology; Current Opinion in Urology ,2011,21:303-308.
[21] Shamsa A, Mohammadi L, Abolbashari M, Shakeri MT, Shamsa S. Comparison of open and laparoscopic varicocelectomies in terms of operative time, sperm parameters, and complications. Urol J. 2009 ;6(3):170-5.

[22] Diegidio P, Jhaveri JK, Ghannam S, Pinkhasov R, Shabsigh R, Fisch H. Review of current varicocelectomy techniques and their outcomes. BJU Int. 2011 Mar 24. doi: 10.1111/j.1464-410X.2010.09959.x. [Epub ahead of print] [PubMed]

10

Radiofrequency Ablation of Renal Cell Carcinoma: A Systematic Review

Seong Kuk Yoon
Dong-A University College of Medicine
Republic of Korea

1. Introduction

The widespread use of abdominal cross-sectional imaging such as computed tomography (CT) and magnetic resonance imaging (MRI) has resulted in a significant rise in the frequency of incidentally detected renal masses (Mouraviev et al., 2006). Most tumors are small and localized renal tumors have been shown to be of a very early clinical stage. It is estimated that in 2009, 57,760 new cases of kidney caner will be diagnosed and 12,980 patients will die of the disease in the United States (American Cancer Society, 2009). Nephron-sparing surgery such as partial nephrectomy remains the gold standard in patients with small renal cell carcinomas (RCCs), with oncologic outcomes similar to the use of a radical nephrectomy (Bandi et al., 2008). However, both open and laparoscopic partial nephrectomy are associated with a significant complication rate and laparoscopic partial nephrectomy is also associated with a significant learning curve, increased warm ischemia time, and a higher morbidity rate as compared with open partial nephrectomy (Gill et al., 2003). Many cases with incidentally detected small renal tumors are found in elderly patients with significant comorbidities, and these patients may not be good surgical candidates. Therefore, several investigators have utilized a variety of energy-based tissue-ablative technologies such as radiofrequency (RF) ablation, cryoablation, high-intensity focused ultrasound, microwave thermotherapy, and interstitial photon irradiation as alternative treatment options of small renal masses (McAchran et al., 2005). Among these minimally invasive ablative techniques, RF ablation and cryoablation are the most commonly utilized methods and have been extensively studied. For short-term results, cryoablation (4.6% tumor-persistent disease and complication rate of 10.6%) is considered better than RF ablation (7.9% and 13.9%, respectively) (Weld & Landman, 2005). However, there are no prospective comparative studies to suggest that cryoablation is more effective than RF ablation for the treatment of small RCCs. RF ablation has several advantages with a superior relationship between the RF-probe diameter and the volume of ablated tissue (Mahnken et al., 2005). RF ablation also provides many potential benefits, including a low complication rate, reduced morbidity, shorter hospital stay, absence of an ischemic period, possible conscious sedation, less expensive than surgery, and the ability to avoid the higher risk of surgical resection in elderly patients (Lotan & Cadeddu, 2005; Mouraviev et al., 2006; Park et al., 2007). Furthermore, RF ablation may minimize destruction of normal renal tissue and thus minimizes removal of functional nephrons (Mylona et al., 2009). For the intermediate term, the oncologic outcomes of RF ablation appear comparable to that of partial nephrectomy for small, early stage RCCs (Stern et al., 2007). However, long-term data is still lacking.

2. Mechanism

High-frequency, alternating electric current produced by the RF generator is delivered to target tissues through an electrode. RF current returns to the generator via grounding pads and thereby completes the electrical circuit. Deposition of RF energy results in molecular friction and heat production, leading to membrane disruption, protein denaturation, vascular thrombosis, and ultimately, coagulation necrosis. Thermal damage is dependent on both the tissue temperature achieved and the duration of heating. Heating tissue to 50°C to 55°C for 4 to 6 minutes produces irreversible cell injury. At temperatures between 60°C and 100°C, near-immediate coagulation necrosis is induced. At 110°C, tissue vaporizes and carbonizes (McAchran et al., 2005; Zagoria, 2004a).

3. Patient selection: Indications and contraindications

Indications for RF ablation include significant comorbidities making the patient a high surgical risk, pre-existing renal insufficiency, advanced age, life expectancy of more than 1 year but less than 10 years, a solitary kidney, patients who refuse surgery, or multifocal RCC, such as in patients with von Hippel-Lindau disease or familial RCC (Gervais et al., 2005b; McAchran et al., 2005). The only absolute contraindications include irreversible coagulopathy or acute and severe medical instability, such as sepsis (Zagoria, 2004a).

4. Techniques

4.1 Equipment: RF systems and electrodes

RF generators are either temperature-based or impedance-based systems. A temperature-based system (RITA Medical Systems, Mountain View, CA, USA) monitors tissue temperature by the use of thermocouples at the needle tips and determines completion of treatment when the tissue adjacent to the probe has reached a target temperature for a predetermined duration of time. Impedance-based systems (Radionics, Burlington, MA, USA; RadioTherapeutics, Sunnyvale, CA, USA; CelonPOWER System, Teltow, Germany) measure the impedance of the surrounding tissue of the electrode and RF energy is delivered until the impedance exceeds a critical level (Anderson et al., 2005; Desai & Gill, 2002). To the best of our knowledge, there are no comparative clinical studies showing a clear advantage for the use of each system. All of these generators modulate the amount of electrical current delivered to the electrode. If too much RF energy is provided too quickly, charring occurs immediately surrounding the electrode. This charring highly increases the resistance of the tissue and does not allow delivery of the electric current into the tissue. Thus, ablated zones are decreased in size and results are less reproducible (Anderson et al., 2005). There is a variety of electrodes: single versus multiple tined probes versus cluster, and wet versus dry versus cooled-tip probes. However, there are no randomized comparative clinical studies for the electrode types.

4.2 Guidance and approaches

RF ablation is performed under ultrasound (US), CT, or MR guidance for exact targeting of the electrode within renal tumors. Most investigators prefer CT guidance that allows accurate placement of the electrode. Although US provides widespread availability, real-time imaging, absence of ionizing radiation, low cost capabilities, and portability, US has some limitations for guiding electrodes. (Fig. 1, US-guided radiofrequency ablation.) In some cases, it is difficult to visualize lesions due to a lack of innate tissue conspicuity or overlying bony structures or gas-containing bowel structures. During US-guided RF ablation, a tumor surrounding the electrode becomes centrifugally hyperechogenic secondary to microbubble formation in the ablated tissue. Thus, it may be difficult to appreciate the difference between tumor tissue and normal tissue. Such acoustic changes may increase the difficulty to reposition the probe for further treatment. For renal RF ablation, CT has some advantages, including superior anatomic delineation, easy visualization of small tumors, absence of obscuring artifacts after ablation, and intravenous contrast enhancement to determine the adequacy of ablation (Zagoria, 2004a). (Fig. 2, CT-guided radiofrequency ablation.)

RF ablation can be performed via open, laparoscopic, or percutaneous approach. Open RF ablation is rarely used in clinical practice. Laparoscopic RF ablation performed under general anesthesia is typically used for anterior and medial tumors or for tumors in close proximity to the ureter, renal hilum, or adjacent organs. Percutaneous RF ablation can be performed under conscious sedation or general anesthesia (Anderson, 2005; Carraway et al.,

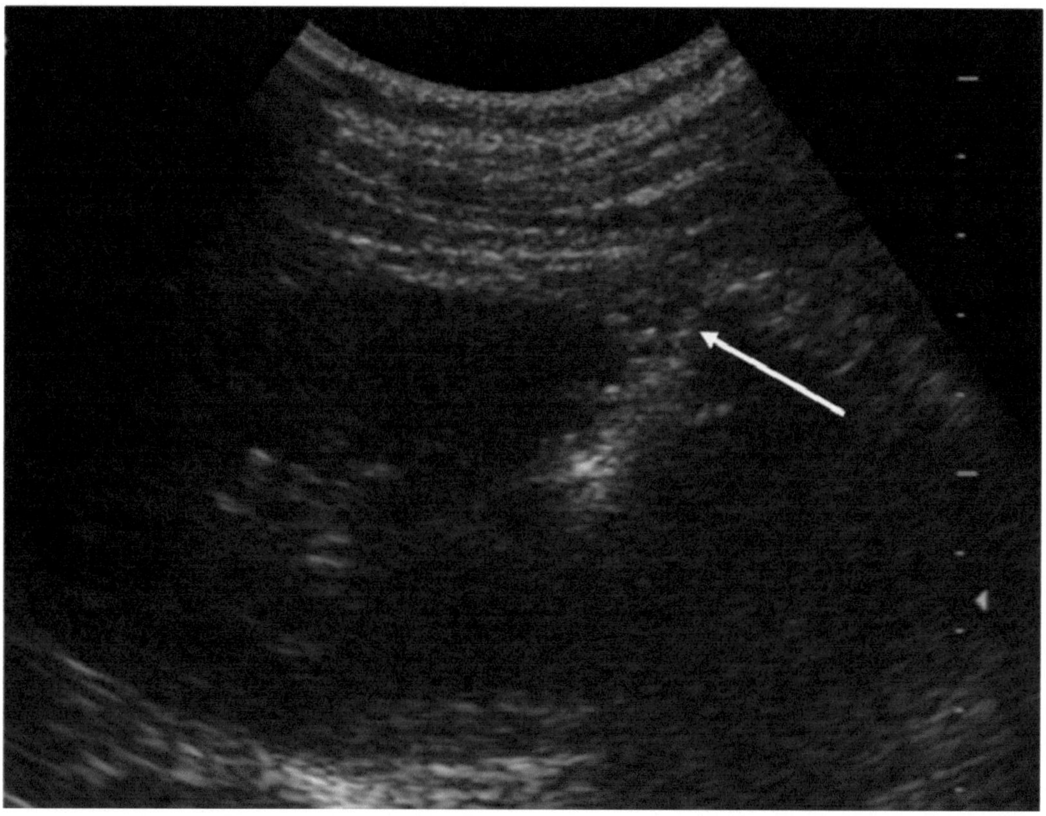

Fig. 1. US-guided radiofrequency. US image shows a echogenic electrode within the tumor (arrow).

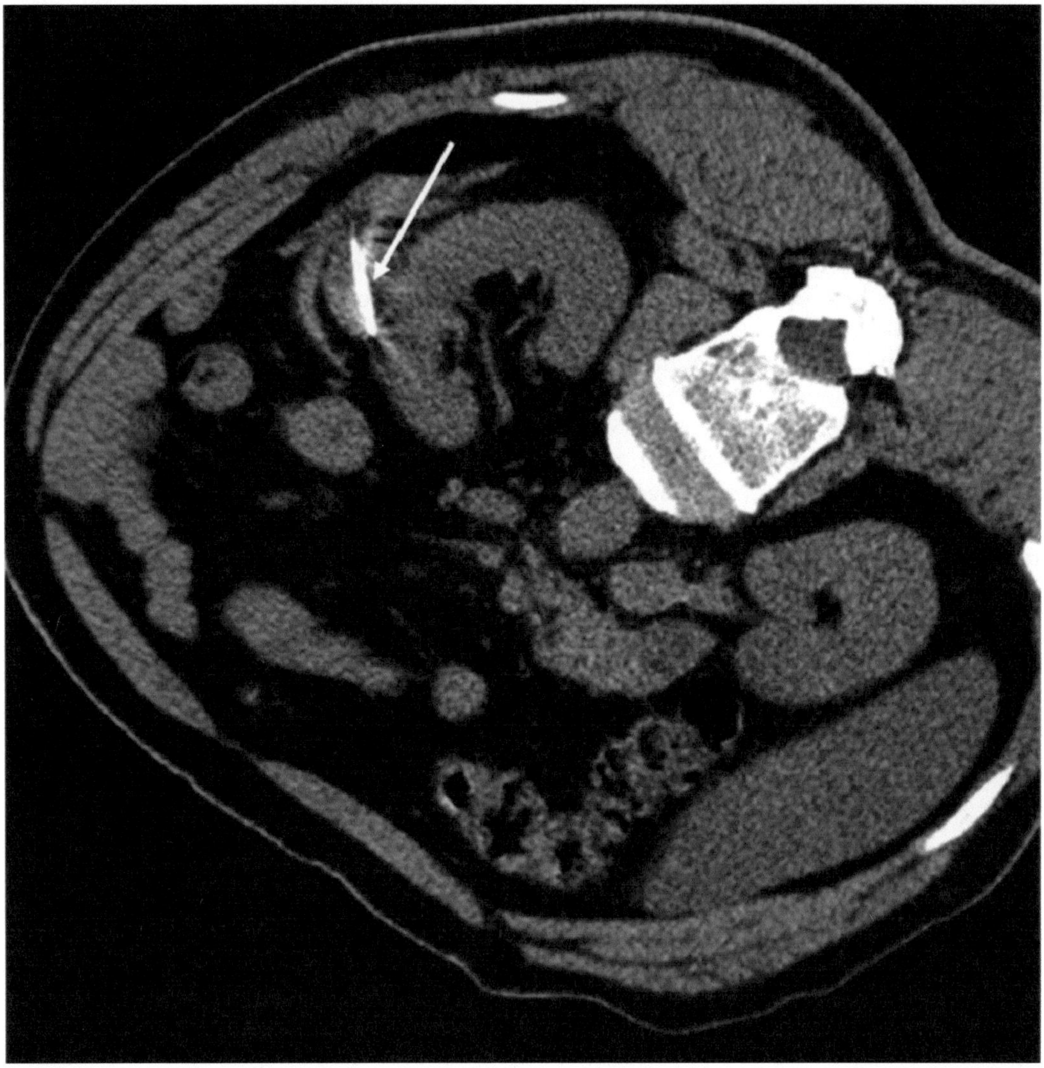

Fig. 2. CT-guided radiofrequency ablation. Unenhanced CT scan shows a targeted electrode within the tumor (arrow).

2009). Meta-analysis has shown that a percutaneous RF ablation procedure is safer and as equally effective as compared with an open or laparoscopic approach, although more than one treatment session may be needed to treat renal tumors completely (Hui et al., 2008).

4.3 Pre-RF ablation biopsy

There is no consensus on the value of performing a percutaneous biopsy prior to ablation of renal tumors. A pre-ablation biopsy is not required for treatment and a biopsy should be performed at the preference of the surgeon (Anderson et al., 2005). However, a biopsy is recommended if it is expected that the biopsy results will have an impact on patient treatment and follow-up imaging planning (Zagoria, 2004a).

4.4 Imaging follow-up

Immediate follow-up imaging on postoperative day one or two is generally unnecessary and can cause misinterpretation, as the presence of periablation enhancement suggestive of reactive hyperemia may mimic the presence of a residual viable tumor on contrast-enhanced imaging (Carraway et al., 2009). Follow-up CT examinations are performed at 1 month, 3 and 6 months, and then every 6 months thereafter in our institution. However, the timing of follow-up imaging studies varies among institutions and the optimal interval time remains to be determined (Gervais et al., 2005a).

4.5 Outcomes

4.5.1 Therapeutic efficacy

Treatment success for RF ablation is assessed by postprocedural imaging, and is typically assessed by CT imaging or MR imaging at least 1 month after treatment. Imaging immediately after the procedure can be difficult to interpret because periablation inflammation may mimic the appearance of a residual viable tumor (Hines-Peralta & Goldberg, 2004). A definition of complete coagulation necrosis and thus a completely ablated tumor after RF ablation is the absence of enhancement on CT or MR images. Enhancement (> 10 HU or > 15% with CT and MR imaging, respectively) of any portion of the tumor is considered a residual viable tumor. Recurrence is defined as new enhancement that develops after CT or MR images have been interpreted to show complete necrosis (Gervais et al., 2005b; Zagoria, 2004a). Effectiveness is defined by the proportion of tumors without residual enhancement after one treatment session (i.e., primary effectiveness) or after repeated treatments (i.e., secondary effectiveness) (Hui et al., 2008). In our series, 17 RCCs in 16 patients were subjected to RF ablation treatment. The mean tumor size was 2.2 cm (range, 1.6-5.0 cm) and all tumors were in an exophytic location. The mean follow-up period was 23.8 months (range, 17-33 months). During the radiological follow-up period, 13 tumors of 12 patients were successfully treated in one ablation session and 4 tumors of 4

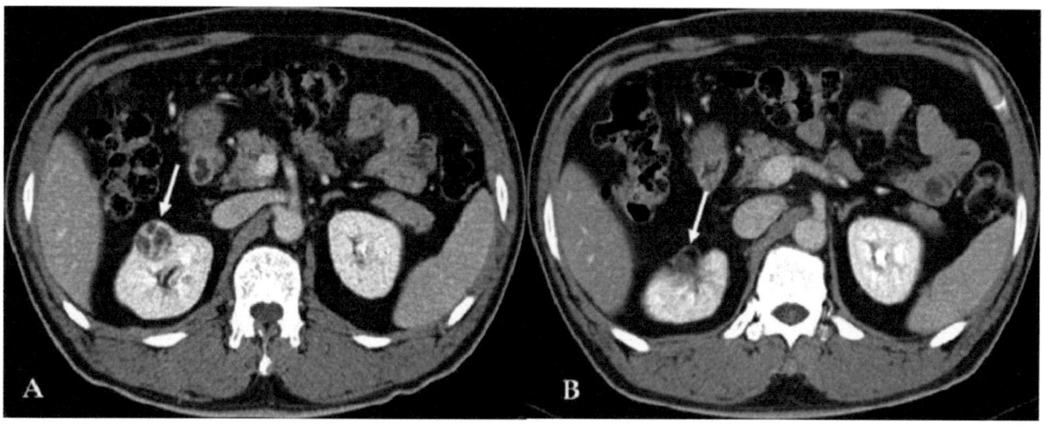

Fig. 3. Radiofrequency ablation of renal cell carcinoma. A. Contrast-enhanced CT scan shows low attenuated, exophytic tumor (arrow) with multiple, irregularly enhancing septa in the right kidney. B. Two-year follow-up contrast-enhanced CT scan after radiofrequency ablation treatment shows no intratumoral enhancement with decreased tumor size and peritumoral halo (arrow), suggesting complete ablation and no recurrence.

patients required more than one session on the basis on follow-up CT. (Fig. 3, Radiofrequency ablation of renal cell carcinoma.) One tumor required 3 sessions based on areas of persistent enhancement within the tumor. In addition, 7 tumors of 7 patients required electrode repositions, as the tumor size was too large. Technical success and technical effectiveness were achieved in all cases (100%). Local recurrence was not detected in any of the cases. On follow-up CT, all tumors showed a variable degree of size reduction (mean diameter, 0.6 cm; range, 0.2-1.7 cm) in comparison with pretreatment CT. No metastases developed in the patients during the follow-up period.

Successful rates for complete RF ablation of small renal tumors have ranged from 82% to 100% in recent series. Gervais *et al.* demonstrated that in 85 patients (100 renal tumors) who underwent percutaneous RF ablation, small (≤ 3 cm) peripheral tumors were completely ablated with 100% success; however, larger tumors (3-5 cm and > 5 cm) were ablated with 92% and 25% success rates, respectively (Gervais et al., 2005b). Zagoria *et al.* showed data on 125 RCCs in 104 patients who underwent percutaneous RF ablation. The tumor size ranged from 0.6 cm to 8.8 cm (mean size, 2.7 cm). Of 125 renal tumors, 116 (93%) tumors were completely ablated with a mean follow-up interval of 13.8 months (Zagoria et al., 2007). McDougal *et al.* presented outcomes of 16 patients with biopsy proven RCCs with greater than 4-year follow-up. These investigators showed successful outcomes in exophytic masses smaller than 5 cm. Twelve (92.3%) of the 13 tumors treated had no evidence of disease (McDougal et al., 2005). Levinson *et al.* reported data with the longest follow-up to date (61.6 months). A total of 31 patients received 34 RF ablation treatments. Tumor sizes ranged from 1.0 cm to 4.0 cm (median size, 2.0 cm). The overall recurrence-free survival rate was 90.3%. There was a 100% metastasis-free rate and disease specific survival rate in the cohort of patients. The overall patient survival was 71.0% (Levinson et al., 2008).

4.5.2 Complications

Complications are classified as major or minor based on the classification of the Society of Interventional Radiology with major complications requiring treatment or hospitalization and minor complications needing only conservative monitoring (Gervais et al., 2005a). In general, the overall complication rates of RF ablation have been reported from 2.8% to 17.6% with the majority of complications being minor complications (Carraway et al., 2009). The most common complication is hemorrhage (Gervais et al., 2005b). (Fig. 4, Perinephric hematoma.)

Major complications include superficial liver laceration, significant blood loss, congestive heart failure, conversion to open surgery, hemorrhage leading to nephrectomy, pulmonary embolism, myocardial infarction, pancreatic injury requiring surgery, ureteropelvic junction obstruction, ureteropelvic junction injury requiring nephrectomy, urine leakage, pneumonia, pelvic vein thrombosis, hematuria with significant blood clots and urinary obstruction, persistent muscle weakness, ureteric thermal injury requiring stent insertion, persistent urinoma, proximal ureteral stricture, cutaneous–urinary fistula, colon–nephric fistula, colon injury, and needle tract seeding. Minor complications include perirenal hematoma, transient hematuria, wound infection, postoperative ileus, hydronephrosis, wound separation, probe site pain or paresthesia, infection, an increased serum creatinine level, and transient neuropathy (Hui et al., 2008).

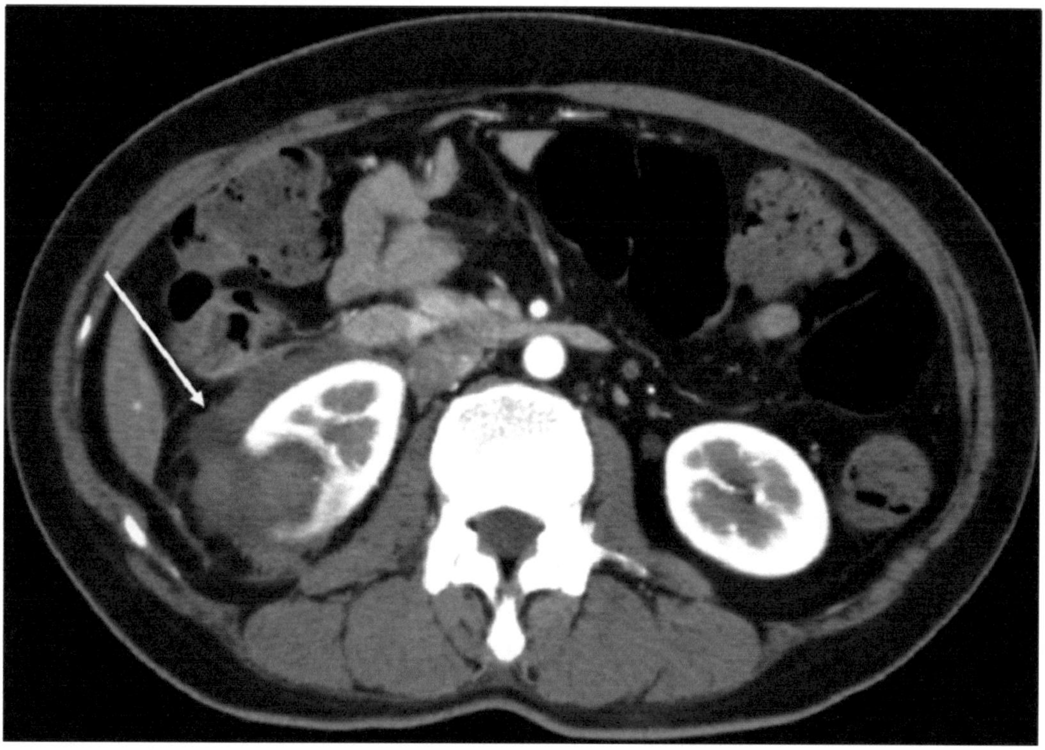

Fig. 4. Perinephric hematoma. Contrast-enhanced CT scan shows hematoma (arrow) in the right perinephric space after radiofrequency ablation treatment.

5. Factors influencing successful ablation

Tumor size and location are the two most important factors that determine whether RCCs can be treated successfully. Zagoria *et al.* found that the major determinant of successful RF ablation was tumor size. There was no correlation between the success of ablation and tumor location, histology, and the presence of renal disease (Zagoria et al., 2004b). A recent series showed that RF ablation could be reliably performed to treat RCCs smaller than 3.7 cm (Zagoria et al., 2007). However, upper size limits for consideration of renal tumors for RF ablation have not been determined. Various investigators have set this limit from 2.5 cm to 4.0 cm. (Gervais et al., 2005b). Despite advances in electrode design, successful ablation of tumors greater than 4 cm in diameter has been challenging. However, larger tumors require multiple overlapping ablations (Park et al., 2008). The location of the tumor can also influence the success of RF ablation. Even large exophytic tumors are usually treated successfully. However, central tumor ablation fails more frequently because of a heat sink effect where regional vascular flow reduces the extent of the thermally induced coagulation (Yoon et al., 2009). Gervais *et al.* found that both a small size and noncentral location are independent significant predictors of complete necrosis after a single ablation session, based on the use of multivariate analysis (Gervais et al., 2005b). The gauge and configuration of the electrode tip, intensity and length of the current, duration of energy applied, and certain characteristics of the tissue that is being ablated determine the extent of tissue ablation. Optimization of these factors is mandatory for success of RF ablation (McAchran et al., 2005).

6. Perspective

Many clinical and experimental studies have reported promising short and intermediate-term outcomes with RF ablation for the treatment of small renal tumors. However, multi-institutional, high volume, long-term follow-up data on cancer-specific survival are not as yet available and such data are required before RF ablation can be considered as a standard of management. A further prospective or a randomized trial comparing RF ablation with nephron-sparing surgery such as a partial nephrectomy is needed. Optimal techniques to perform RF ablation for renal tumors are still evolving. We are awaiting further studies on factors that influence successful ablation. Additionally, future trials should also use standard terminology. Further studies for RF ablation will likely aim to alleviate existing shortcomings by the improvement of imaging and guidance, by increasing the size of the ablation zone, and by improving performance for problematic cases.

7. Conclusion

Although nephron-sparing surgery such as laparoscopic partial nephrectomy must remain standard therapy for patients with small, localized RCCs, RF ablation for the treatment of RCC is a very promising technique that should be considered as a treatment option for patients with small renal tumors who are not good surgical candidates. For indications, RF ablation can be applied successfully for the treatment of refractory hematuria resulting from RCC, for local recurrence of RCC, and for isolated metastases from RCC (Zagoria, 2004a). RF ablation is increasingly performed and the use of RF ablation has become widespread due to comparable encouraging short and intermediate-term outcomes and a relatively low incidence of major complications. However, critical use of this procedure is emphasized until more long-term follow-up results are available. Although a number of controversies currently remain, we believe that image-guided RF ablation is a safe and effective treatment option with a very low complication rate for small exophytic renal tumors in selected patients.

8. References

American Cancer Society. (2009) Cancer Facts and Figures 2009. Available from: < www.cancer.org/downloads/STT/ 500809web.pdf>

Anderson J, Matsumoto E, & Cadeddu J. (2005) Renal radiofrequency ablation: technique and results. *Urol. Oncol.*, Vol.23, No.5, pp. 355-360

Bandi G, Hedican S, & Nakada S. (2008) Current practice patterns in the use of ablation technology for the management of small renal masses at academic centers in the United States. *Urology*, Vol. 71, No.1, pp. 113-117

Carraway W, Raman J, & Cadeddu J. (2009) Current status of renal radiofrequency ablation. *Curr. Opin. Urol.*, Vol.19, No2, pp. 143-147

Desai M, & Gill I. (2002) Current status of cryoablation and radiofrequency ablation in the management of renal tumors. *Curr. Opin, Urol.*, Vol.12, pp. 387-393

Gervais D, Arellano R, McGovern F, McDougal W, & Mueller P. (2005) Radiofrequency ablation of renal cell carcinoma: part 2, lessons learned with ablation of 100 tumors. *Am. J. Roentgenol.*, Vol.185, No.1, pp. 72-80

Gervais D, McGovern F, Arellano R, McDougal W, & Mueller P. (2005) Radiofrequency ablation of renal cell carcinoma: part 1, indications, results, and role in patient management over a 6-year period and ablation of 100 tumors. *Am. J. Roentgenol.*, Vol.185, No.1, pp. 64-71

Gill I, Matin S, Desai M, Kaouk J, Steinberg A, Mascha E, Thornton J, Sherief M, Strzempkowski B, & Novick A. (2003) Comparative analysis of laparoscopic versus open partial nephrectomy for renal tumors in 200 patients. *J. Urol.*, Vol.170, pp. 64-68

Hines-Peralta A, & Goldberg S. (2004) Review of radiofrequency ablation for renal cell carcinoma. *Clin. Cancer Res.*, Vol.15, No.10, pp. 6328s-6334s

Hui G, Tuncali K, Tatli S, Morrison P, & Silverman S. (2008) Comparison of percutaneous and surgical approaches to renal tumor ablation: metaanalysis of effectiveness and complication rates. *J. Vasc. Interv. Radiol.*, Vol.19, No.9, pp. 1311-1320

Levinson A, Su L, Agarwal D, Agarwal D, Sroka M, Jarrett T, Kavoussi L, & Solomon S. (2008) Long-term oncological and overall outcomes of percutaneous radio frequency ablation in high risk surgical patients with a solitary small renal mass. *J. Urol.*, Vol.180, No.2, pp. 499-504

Lotan Y, & Cadeddu J. (2005) A cost comparison of nephron-sparing surgical techniques for renal tumour. *BJU Int.*, Vol.95, pp. 1039-1042

Mahnken A, Rohde D, Brkovic D, Günther R, & Tacke J. (2005) Percutaneous radiofrequency ablation of renal cell carcinoma: preliminary results. *Acta Radiol.*, Vol.46, No.2, pp. 208-214

McAchran S, Lesani O, & Resnick M. (2005) Radiofrequency ablation of renal tumors: past, present, and future. *Urology*, Vol.66, No.5A, pp. 15-22

McDougal W, Gervais D, McGovern F, & Mueller P. (2005) Long-term followup of patients with renal cell carcinoma treated with radio frequency ablation with curative intent. *J. Urol.*, Vol.74, No.1, pp. 61-63

Mouraviev V, Joniau S, Van Poppel H, & Polascik T. (2006) Current status of minimally invasive ablative techniques in the treatment of small renal tumours. *Eur. Urol.*, Vol.51, No.2, pp. 328-336

Mylona S, Kokkinaki A, Pomoni M, Galani P, Ntai S, & Thanos L. (2009) Percutaneous radiofrequency ablation of renal cell carcinomas in patients with solitary kidney: 6 years experience. *Eur. J. Radiol.*, Vol.69, No.2, pp. 351-356

Park S, Cadeddu J, & Shingleton W. (2007) Oncologic outcomes for ablative therapy of kidney cancer. *Curr. Urol. Rep.*, Vol.8, No.1, pp. 31-37

Park S, Yoon S, Cho J, Oh J, Nam K, Kwon H, Kim S, Kang M, Choi S, & Sung G. (2008) Radiofrequency ablation treatment for renal cell carcinoma: early clinical experience. *Korean J. Radiol.*, Vol.9, No.4, pp. 340-347

Stern J, Svatek R, Park S, Hermann M, Lotan Y, Sagalowsky A, & Cadeddu J. (2007) Intermediate comparison of partial nephrectomy and radiofrequency ablation for clinical T1a renal tumours. *BJU Int.*, Vol.100, No.2, pp. 287-290

Weld K, & Landman J. (2005) Comparison of cryoablation, radiofrequency ablation and high-intensity focused ultrasound for treating small renal tumours. *BJU Int.*, Vol.96, pp. 1224-1229

Yoon S, Choi J, Cho J, Oh J, Nam K, Jung S, Kwon H, Kim D, & Rha S. (2009) Radiofrequency ablation of renal VX2 tumors with and without renal artery occlusion in a rabbit model: feasibility, therapeutic efficacy, and safety. *Cardiovasc. Intervent. Radiol.*, Vol.32, pp. 1241-1246

Zagoria R. (2004) Imaging-guided radiofrequency ablation of renal masses. *RadioGraphics*, Vol.24(Suppl. 1), pp. S59-S71

Zagoria R, Hawkins A, Clark P, Hall M, Matiaga B, Dyer R, & Chen M. (2004) Percutaneous CT-guided radiofrequency ablation of renal neoplasms: factors influencing success. *Am. J. Roentgenol.*, Vol.183, pp. 201-207

Zagoria R, Traver M, Werle D, Perini M, Hayasaka S, & Clark P. (2007) Oncologic efficacy of CT-guided percutaneous radiofrequency ablation of renal cell carcinomas. *Am. J. Roentgenol.*, Vol.189, No.2, pp. 429-436

11

Port-Site Metastasis Following Laparoscopic Surgery

Terence C. Chua[1], Tristan D. Yan[1],
David L. Morris[1] and Paul H. Sugarbaker[2]
[1]*Hepatobiliary and Surgical Oncology Unit, UNSW Department of Surgery, St George Hospital, Sydney*
[2]*Washington Cancer Institute, Washington*
[1]*Australia*
[2]*USA*

1. Introduction

In the 1990s, laparoscopic surgery became accepted as a standard approach for general surgical operations including cholecystectomy (Barkun et al., 1992) and appendectomy (Attwood, Hill, Murphy, Thornton, & Stephens, 1992). In these randomized studies, the laparoscopic compared to the open approach resulted in decreased length of hospital stay, fewer postoperative complications, more rapid return to normal activities with reduced analgesic requirements. This was associated with decreased cost of care and also achieved superior cosmetic results leading to increased patient satisfaction. Following this, the frontier of laparoscopic surgery was pushed further forward through experimentation of other complex intraabdominal surgery including colorectal surgery (Milsom, Lavery, Church, Stolfi, & Fazio, 1994), bariatric surgery (Cowan, 1992) and more recently hepatopancreaticobiliary surgery (Gigot et al., 2002). The growth and expanded role of laparoscopic surgery in abdominal operations meant that cancer surgery may now be performed using laparoscopy.

Despite the perioperative advantages, laparoscopic cancer surgery has been highly debated and its oncological appropriateness has been questioned. Doubts over the technique concerned compromising oncologic principles through loss of the surgeon's ability to perform tactile assessment which could otherwise have been performed in an open surgery. It was also thought that with laparoscopic approach may limit the extent of resections. For example, in the setting of laparoscopic colon resection, reduced lymph nodes harvested from insufficient mesentery may make disease staging inaccurate. Further, there are concerns regarding the development of port-site metastasis.

Port site metastasis was first described by Dobronte and colleagues (Döbrönte, Wittmann, & Karácsony, 1978) who described the case of a patient developing local tumor metastases in the abdominal wall two weeks after laparoscopy for malignancy and explained that this occurred due to infiltration of malignant ascites during needle and trocar insertion into the abdominal cavity at the port site. Since this report, there has been extensive publication of case reports in the literature, describing this phenomenon in gastrointestinal (Cook & Dehn, 1996), urological (Chueh, Tsai, & Lai, 2004) and gynaecological malignancies (Sanjuán et al.,

2005). This chapter identifies through a literature search the risk of port-site metastasis in laparoscopic surgery for cancer and discusses the current understanding to guide practice and management.

2. Incidence of port site metastasis

It was initially thought that port-site metastasis was associated with advanced malignancy. Cook and Dehn reported a rate of five of 46 patients (11%) developing port-site metastasis after undergoing laparoscopy and identified that advanced disease with serosal involvement of the tumor was associated with the occurrence of this phenomenon (Cook & Dehn, 1996). However, port-site metastasis has also been reported in patients undergoing colectomy for Duke A tumors (Prasad, Avery, & Foley, 1994). This may have been a result of soilage of tumor into the peritoneal cavity during surgery, implantation of circulating tumor cells present in the lymphatics and haematogenous system that are transacted as part of surgery or trauma during the process of specimen retrieval.

To ascertain the incidence of port-site metastasis, we undertook a literature review of large clinical trials that reported results after an adequate follow-up time to determine the risks of its occurrence. As shown in table 1, from the 17 studies reviewed that included 11,027 cancer patients undergoing laparoscopic surgery or diagnostic laparoscopy, it appears that the port-site metastasis is a rare phenomenon, occurring in less than 2% of patients (COLOR, 2009; Fleshman et al., 2007; Jayne et al., 2010; Kaiser, Kang, Chan, Vukasin, & Beart, 2004; Kim, Park, Joh, & Hahn, 2006; Koffron, Auffenberg, Kung, & Abecassis, 2007; Lacy et al., 2008; Liang, Huang, Lai, Lee, & Jeng, 2007; Lujan et al., 2009; Martinez, Querleu, Leblanc, Narducci, & Ferron, 2010; Miyajima et al., 2009; K. H. Ng et al., 2009; S. M. Ng et al., 2008; Rassweiler et al., 2003; Shoup et al., 2002; Song et al., 2010; Zivanovic et al., 2008). In eight randomized clinical trials comparing laparoscopic surgery to open surgery for cancer, there was no statistical difference in the development of port-site metastasis or wound metastasis (COLOR, 2009; Fleshman et al., 2007; Jayne et al., 2010; Kaiser et al., 2004; Lacy et al., 2008; Liang et al., 2007; Lujan et al., 2009; S. M. Ng et al., 2008).

In an international survey of port-site metastasis involving members of the German Society of Surgery, Swiss Association for Laparoscopic and Thoracoscopic Surgery and Austrian Society of Minimal Invasive Surgery, participants reported 70 of 409 cases (17.1%) of port-site metastasis in patients undergoing laparoscopic cholecystectomy for gallbladder cancer and 19 of 412 cases (4.6%) of port-site metastasis in patients undergoing laparoscopic surgery for colorectal cancer (Paolucci, Schaeff, Schneider, & Gutt, 1999). These authors further alluded to the association of port-site metastasis and the propensity for intraperitoneal spread of cancer. The incidence data reported in this study appears to be high when compared to the tabulated studies. It is likely that the high incidence may be an effect of the learning curve of laparoscopic cancer surgery during the 1990s era as modern data seems to suggest otherwise.

In summary, it appears from current data that port-site metastasis is a rare occurrence and its incidence is unlikely to be more common than wound metastasis when oncologic principles are adhered to in the technical performance of laparoscopic surgery.

3. Hypotheses for port-site metastasis

There are several mechanisms that have been proposed and studied in an experimental setting to investigate the development of port-site metastasis in animal models. Although these in-vivo experiments has provided some mechanisms to explain its occurrence, the limitations in the homology of animal models where human cancer cell lines are used due to the lack of available native tumor cells and the immunodeficient state of these animal models (de Jong & Maina, 2010). Nevertheless, animal models remain a unique opportunity to provide in vivo information in translation research. The most commonly discussed hypotheses include hematogenous dissemination, wound contamination, effects of pneumoperitoneum that including the type of insufflating gas, chimney effect, aerosolization, surgical technique and the local immune response. Experiments investigating these hypotheses have yielded both positive and negative results and it is likely the occurrence of port-site metastasis is multifactorial stemming from a combination of these various hypotheses.

3.1 Hematogenous dissemination

The concept of hematogenous dissemination goes against the concept of direct spread of cancer cells to explain port-site metastasis. The establishment of port-sites for access results in tissue trauma and during the healing process, its hyperaemic state, provide a nutrient rich environment for tumor growth and may become a sanctuary site of tumor metastasis in patients with free circulating tumor cells within the systemic circulation. It has been previously shown that tumor cells establish themselves in sites with increased blood supply at a greater rate than normal tissues (Murphy et al., 1988). Two studies specifically compared the rates of port-site metastasis in a group undergoing intravenous cancer cell injection versus intraperitoneal injection in a mice model. Iwanaka et al reported an incidence of 0% compared to 63% of port-site metastasis in immature A/J mice undergoing intravenous compared to intraperitoneal injection of TBJ-neuroblastoma cells (Iwanaka, Arya, & Ziegler, 1998). Brundell et al used male Dark Agouti rats and injected a suspension of 10^5 Dark Agouti mammary adenocarcinoma cells into the internal jugular vein and stimulated laparoscopic conditions by a 15 minute period of insufflations and compared the port-site metastasis rate in rats who had routine closure of port-sites or in another group whom they performed a mid-line laparotomy prior to closure. These authors reported one case of port-site metastasis in the laparoscopic group and no wound metastasis in the laparotomy group (Brundell, Ellis, Dodd, Watson, & Hewett, 2002). Both these studies demonstrate that port-site metastasis occurring through hematogenous dissemination is rare, even in the presence of a hyperaemic wound state induced by the mid-line laparotomy as performed in the second study.

3.2 Wound contamination

The effect of direct wound contamination stems from a variety of reasons. The extraction of tumor through a small port-site together with the leakage of CO2 that occurs may induce movement of free tumor cells that have an increased propensity to implant in the traumatised tissue of the wound (Tseng et al., 1998). During the surgical procedure, ongoing passage and extrication of instruments that are contaminated by tumor material due to the dissection process, may also explain its occurrence. Bundell et al studied the mechanism of wound contamination through detecting an increased deposition of radiolabeled human colon cancer cells that were injected intraperitoneally in trocar site due to contamination, demonstrated increased movement of tumor cells with increase in volumes of gas insufflations and decreased insufflations pressures leading to an increased contamination of trocar and port-sites (S. M. Brundell et al., 2002).

3.3 Pneumoperitoneum

Carbon dioxide is the most commonly used gas for insufflations during laparoscopic surgery. It is non-flammable, inexpensive, colourless, readily available and readily absorbed (Menes & Spivak, 2000). The effect of insufflating gas to distend the abdomen creates a high pneumperitoneal pressure and consequentially stimulate movement of free peritoneal tumor cells or may result in sloughing or shedding of tumor cells from viscera into the peritoneal cavity (Moreira et al., 2001). Hirabayashi et al further elucidated the effect of pneumoperitoneum by using a scanning electron microscope to study the effects of how tumor cells disseminate to form port-site metastases after pneumoperitoneum in a nude mice model injected with human gastric cancer cells. They found that pneumoperitoneum immediately results in peeling and destruction of the muscular layer of the abdominal peritoneum, increasing the propensity of tumor cell adhesion at port-sites and subsequently healing process occurs leading to scar formation with presence of entrapped tumor cells (Hirabayashi et al., 2002). A "chimney effect" that occurs when gas leaks out along the trocar has been thought to be implicated in the development of port-site metastases. In an experiment to examine this hypothesis, tumor cells at trocar sites were found to be higher compared to the control when leakage of carbon dioxide gas along the trocar was permitted during a rat animal model injected with CC-531 tumor cells intraperitoneally (Tseng et al., 1998). However, this may be related to the concentration of the amount of injected intraperitoneal tumor cells in the animal model as some other authors have not yielded similar results in their experiments to support this theory. Brundell et al demonstrated that increasing the tumor cell inoculums resulted in increased deposition of tumor cells on both ports and port-sites in a swine model, and further showed that displacement of the ports (removing and reinserting) increased the number of tumors cells deposited at port-sites (Brundell et al., 2003). Whelan et al failed to show that aerosolization of viable tumor cells in either in vivo or in vitro experiments with pressures up to 30 mmHg (Whelan et al., 1996). Pneumoperitoneum increases intraabdominal pressure and results in an increased in blood flow in the anterior abdominal wall. This has also been thought to increase the risk of port-site metastasis as the increased circulation provides a favourable medium for growth of tumor cells (Yavuz, Rønning, Lyng, Grønbech, & Mårvik, 2003). In addition, the type of gas has also been shown to influence the rates of port-site metastasis with helium insufflations being the least likely compared to argon and nitrogen that were more likely to be associated with port-site metastasis (Gupta, Watson, Ellis, & Jamieson, 2002).

3.4 Immune response

Carbon dioxide has been thought to be toxic to lymphocytes in vitro and hence its insufflations into the peritoneal cavity may potentially affect the peritoneal cell-mediated immunity. Mathew et al demonstrate this in an experiment where adenocarcinoma cells were injected in the left upper quadrant of the peritoneal cavity in syngeneic tumor-bearing rats and subjected to laparotomy, laparoscopy with carbon dioxide or gasless laparoscopy. The authors obtained peritoneal macrophage levels and showed that tumor-bearing rats produced significantly less TNG-alpha in vitro during laparoscopy with carbon dioxide compared to gasless laparoscopy or laparotomy (Mathew, Watson, Ellis, Jamieson, & Rofe, 1999). The results of this experiment was replicated by Ost et al who measured TNF-alpha levels from peritoneal macrophage in mice subjected to either carbon dioxide pneumoperitoneum or laparotomy and showed that peritoneal macrophage TNF-alpha secretion was significantly inhibited in mice subjected to carbon dioxide pneumoperitoneum

(Ost et al., 2008). In a human experiment, Evard et al sampled blood and peritoneal fluid before and after pneumoperitoneum from 16 patients undergoing laparoscopic cholecystectomy and measured cytokine levels, lymphocyte vitality and showed that there were significant decrease in absolute lymphocyte and cytokine counts during the early postoperatively before returning to normal levels (Evrard et al., 1997). This transient immunosuppression may facilitate implantation of tumor cells during laparoscopic surgery.

3.5 Surgical technique

Arguably, the strongest risk for port-site metastasis would be the surgical technique. Anecdotal case series reporting port-site metastasis after laparoscopic surgery have shown a decrease in rates of port-site metastasis with experience. In a large animal study of mice established with splenic tumors (n=128) who underwent either an open splenectomy or laparoscopic -assisted splenectomy, it was shown that the incidence of port-site tumor recurrence in the laparoscopic-assisted group decreased significantly with time (Lee, Gleason, Bessler, & Whelan, 2000). This was likely the experience in human laparoscopic surgery. During the 1990s, there were a large number of case reports describing the occurrence of port-site metastasis after laparoscopic surgery. This occurred during the initial learning curve of surgeons. However, in contemporary series such as the rates of port-site metastasis reported in the trials shown in table 1, port-site metastasis is a rare occurrence due to improved handling of tumor laparoscopically, meticulous resection, rinsing of instruments and the application of protective measures. Other factors that include suture closing of the peritoneum (Agostini et al., 2002) and the type of instruments have also been investigated (Nduka, Poland, Kennedy, Dye, & Darzi, 1998).

4. Clinical significance of port-site metastasis

The clinical significance of port-site metastasis should be regarded as a sign of locoregional recurrence. Although this could manifest as a "drop metastasis" during specimen retrieval, it is more compatible that the entry into the peritoneal cavity during laparoscopic surgery with insufflations of gas, repeated instrument cannulation of port-sites and tumor dissection process that leads to spillage of lymph and blood containing circulating tumor cells makes port-site metastasis a condition with high risk for peritoneal carcinomatosis. Z'graggen et al in a series of 37 patients undergoing laparoscopic cholecystectomy for unsuspected gallbladder cancer reported that all patients developed port -site metastasis as recurrence that was associated with peritoneal metastases (Z'graggen et al., 1998). The rate at which port-site metastasis develop is likely a factor of the tumor biology. Zivanovic et al reported 20 of 1694 patients developing port-site metastasis after laparoscopic procedures for gynaecologic malignancies and showed that in patients who developed port-site metastasis 7 months from the laparoscopic procedure had a median survival of 12 months compared to 37 months for patients who develop port-site metastasis after 7 months (P=0.004) (Zivanovic et al., 2008). Therefore, port-site metastasis should be regarded a strong risk factor for peritoneal dissemination in addition to other previously described factors that include full thickness penetration of tumor through the bowel wall, spillage of tumor from lymphatic channels by surgical trauma or free perforation of the tumor (Sugarbaker, 1988).

Peritoneal dissemination of cancer cells in the peritoneal cavity circulate with peritoneal fluid as a transport vector along with gravitational forces and fluid hydrodynamics driving the peritoneal circulation resulting in the pelvis and subphrenic spaces being a

First Author	Year Published	Type of Study	Number of Patients		Tumor Origin	Duration of Follow-up (Months)	Risk of Recurrence [Lap / Open] (%)	Disease-Free Survival [Lap / Open] (% at X-Years)	Incidence of Port-Site Metastasis [Lap / Open] (%)
			Laparoscopic	Open					
Jayne (Jayne et al., 2010)	2010	Randomized	526	268	Colorectal	56	NR	55 / 58 (P=0.48) at 5-years	1.7 / 0.4 (P=NR)
Lujan (Lujan et al., 2009)	2009	Randomized	97	96	Rectal	34	NR	85 / 81 (P=0.895) at 5-years	0 / 0 (P=NR)
COLOR (COLOR, 2009)	2009	Randomized	534	542	Colon	53	31 / 29 (P=0.24)	74 / 76 (P=0.70) at 3-years	1.3 / 0.4 (P=0.09)
Lacy (Lacy et al., 2008)	2008	Randomized	111	108	Colon	95	18 / 29 (P=0.07)	84 / 61 (P=0.0015) at 5-years	1 / 0 (P=0.65)
Ng (S. M. Ng et al., 2008)	2008	Randomized	51	48	Rectal	90	NR	78 / 74 (P=0.55) at 5-years	0 / 2 (P=NR)
Fleshman (Fleshman et al., 2007)	2007	Randomized	435	428	Colon	60	19 / 22 (P=0.25)	69 / 68 (P=0.94) at 5-years	0.9 / 0.5 (P=0.43)
Liang (Liang et al., 2007)	2007	Randomized	135	134	Colon	40	NR	72 / 68 (P=0.362) at 5-years	0.7 / 0.7 (P=NR)
Kaiser (Kaiser et al., 2004)	2004	Randomized	15	20	Colon	35	0 / 5 (P=NR)	NR	0 / 0 (P=NR)
Martinez (Martinez et al., 2010)	2010	Retrospective	1216	-	Uterine / Cervical	49	NR	NR	0.4 / -
Song (Song et al., 2010)	2010	Retrospective	1417	-	Gastric	41	3.5 / -	94 / -	0 / -
Ng (K. H. Ng et al., 2009)	2009	Retrospective	579	-	Rectal	56	23 / -	76 / -	0.7 / -
Miyajima (Miyajima et al., 2009)	2009	Retrospective	1057	-	Rectal	30	7 / -	NR	0 / -
Zivanovic (Zivanovic et al., 2008)	2008	Retrospective	1694	-	Gynaeco-logical	NR	NR	NR	1.2 / -
Koffron (Koffron et al., 2007)	2007	Retrospective Matched Analysis	300	100	Liver	69	2 / 3 (P>0.05)	NR	0 / NR
Kim (Kim et al., 2006)	2006	Retrospective	312	-	Rectal	30	NR	NR	0 / -
Rassweiler (Rassweiler et al., 2003)	2003	Retrospective	1000	-	Urological	58	NR	NR	0.2 / -
Shoup (Shoup et al., 2002)	2002	Retrospective	1548	-	Diagnostic Upper GI Cancers	8	NR	NR	0.8 / -

Table 1. Literature review of major clinical trials reporting the risk of port-site metastasis

common site for cancer cell implantation (Carmignani, Sugarbaker, Bromley, & Sugarbaker, 2003). Peritoneal carcinomatosis when managed with chemotherapy alone is a rapidly progressive disease state characterised by a symptomatic clinical course that occurs as a result of the peritoneal tumor masses that leads to abdominal pain and sub-acute bowel obstruction. In a single centre experience of 349 patients with peritoneal carcinomatosis from colorectal cancer, the median survival was 7 months (Jayne, Fook, Loi, & Seow-Choen, 2002). A combined modality approach of cytoreductive surgery and perioperative intraperitoneal chemotherapy introduced by Dr. Paul Sugarbaker from the Washington Cancer Centre has been shown to be effective in managing this locoregional recurrence and alter the fulminant natural history of this disease (Sugarbaker, Schellinx, Chang, Koslowe, & von Meyerfeldt, 1996). Current results of cytoreductive surgery with perioperative intraperitoneal chemotherapy for non-gynaecologic malignancies showed a potential for a median survival of 34 months with a corresponding 5-year survival rate of 37% (Olivier Glehen et al., 2010).

5. Diagnostic laparoscopy in patients at high risk for port-site metastasis

Data cited in this manuscript strongly suggests that the benefits of laparoscopic oncologic surgery outweigh the risk of port-site metastasis. However, there is a subgroup of patients who may profit greatly from diagnostic laparoscopy but who are at increased risk for cancer implantation at the trochar site. These are patients with ascites in whom there is a high index of suspicion for peritoneal carcinomatosis or peritoneal mesothelioma. Patients to be included in this group are those who may have mucinous ascites from a colorectal or appendiceal adenocarcinoma, ascites from ovarian cancer, ascites associated with a diagnosis of gastric cancer, or ascites from peritoneal mesothelioma. In these high risk patients a modification of the diagnostic laparascopic technique should be considered. The port-sites should be limited to the midline or limited to sites that can be included as part of the abdominal incision. Lateral ports should be avoided except under unusual circumstances and are rarely mandatory in this clinical setting - diagnostic laparascopy in patients with suspect carcinomatosis.

6. Management of port-site metastasis

A simple subcutaneous wide excision of port-site metastasis would constitute a failure of the understanding of the mechanism that underlies its occurrence. Owing to the high risk for peritoneal carcinomatosis, an extensive clinical work-up comprising of positron emission tomography scans and contrast enhanced computed tomography scan should be performed to identify for other sites of metastasis. In the absence of distant metastasis, a wide excision of the port site together with a laparotomy to survey the peritoneal cavity should be performed. If there are evidence of peritoneal seeding, a cytoreductive surgery combined with perioperative intraperitoneal chemotherapy should be performed in patients whose demographic and disease factors fulfil the selection criteria for treatment. For pseudomyxoma peritonei, a complete cytoreduction may achieve 5- and 10-year survival of 87% and 74% respectively (Youssef et al., 2011), a median survival of 53 months and 5-year survival of 47%may be achieved in patients with diffuse malignant peritoneal mesothelioma (Yan et al., 2009), a median survival of 30 months and 5-year survival of 27% for colorectal carcinomatosis (Elias et al., 2010), a median survival of 30 months and 5-year survival of 25% for ovarian carcinomatosis (Helm et al., 2010) and a median survival of 15 months and 5-year survival of 23% in the setting of a complete cytoreduction for gastric carcinomatosis (O. Glehen et al., 2010).

7. Conclusion

Previous reports of an increased clinical incidence of port-site metastasis needs to be re-evaluated. It appears from current data that the incidence of port-site metastasis is rare and is unlikely difference from that of wound metastasis, hence does not negate the benefits of laparoscopic cancer surgery. The reduction in incidence may in part be due to adherence to oncologic principles during laparoscopic surgery and prevention strategies that include port-site protective applications (Seow-Choen, Wan, & Tan, 2009). There may be a preponderance for the occurrence of port-site metastasis in malignancies that have a propensity for peritoneal dissemination, for example, ovarian cancer, colorectal cancer, pancreatic cancer, gastric cancer and appendiceal cancer. Port-site metastasis is a strong risk factor for peritoneal dissemination. An accurate diagnostic work-up should include imaging and exploration of the peritoneal cavity to identify peritoneal metastases. In the setting of peritoneal disease, referral to specialized peritoneal surface malignancy centres for treatment should be mandatory.

8. References

Agostini, A., Robin, F., Jais, J. P., Aggerbeck, M., Vildé, F., Blanc, B., et al. (2002). Peritoneal closure reduces port site metastases: results of an experiment in a rat ovarian cancer model. *Surg Endosc, 16*(2), 289-291.

Attwood, S. E., Hill, A. D., Murphy, P. G., Thornton, J., & Stephens, R. B. (1992). A prospective randomized trial of laparoscopic versus open appendectomy. *Surgery, 112*(3), 497-501.

Barkun, J. S., Barkun, A. N., Sampalis, J. S., Fried, G., Taylor, B., Wexler, M. J., et al. (1992). Randomised controlled trial of laparoscopi versus mini cholecystectomy. The McGill Gallstone Treatment Group. *Lancet, 340*(8828), 1116-1119.

Brundell, S., Ellis, T., Dodd, T., Watson, D. I., & Hewett, P. J. (2002). Hematogenous spread as a mechanism for the generation of abdominal wound metastases following laparoscopy. *Surg Endosc, 16*, 292-295.

Brundell, S., Tsopelas, C., Chatterton, B., Touloumtzoglou, J., Blefari, C., & Hewett, P. J. (2003). Effect of port composition on tumor cell adherence: an in vivo model. *Dis Colon Rectum, 46*(5), 637-642.

Brundell, S. M., Tucker, K., Texler, M., Brown, B., Chatterton, B., & Hewett, P. J. (2002). Variables in the spread of tumor cells to trocars and port sites during operative laparoscopy. *Surg Endosc, 16*(10), 1413-1419.

Carmignani, C. P., Sugarbaker, T. A., Bromley, C. M., & Sugarbaker, P. H. (2003). Intraperitoneal cancer dissemination: mechanisms of the patterns of spread. *Cancer Metastasis Rev, 22*(4), 465-472.

Chueh, S. C. J., Tsai, I. D., & Lai, M. K. (2004). Solitary port-site metastasis after laparoscopic bilateral nephroureterctomy for transitional cell carcinoma in a renal transplant recipient. *Transplantation Proceedings, 36*(9), 2697-2698.

COLOR. (2009). Survival after laparoscopic surgery versus open surgery for colon cancer: long-term outcome of a randomised clinical trial. *The Lancet Oncology, 10*(1), 44-52.

Cook, T. A., & Dehn, T. C. (1996). Port-site metastases in patients undergoing laparoscopy for gastrointestinal malignancy. *Br J Surg, 83*(10), 1419-1420.

Cowan, G. S. (1992). The Future of Bariatric Surgery. *Obes Surg 2*(2), 169-176.

de Jong, M., & Maina, T. (2010). Of Mice and Humans: Are They the Same?--Implications in Cancer Translational Research. *J Nucl Med, 51*(4), 501-504.

Döbrönte, Z., Wittmann, T., & Karácsony, G. (1978). Rapid development of malignant metastases in the abdominal wall after laparoscopy. *Endoscopy, 10*(2), 127-130.

Elias, D., Gilly, F. o., Boutitie, F., Quenet, F. o., Bereder, J.-M., Mansvelt, B., et al. (2010). Peritoneal Colorectal Carcinomatosis Treated With Surgery and Perioperative Intraperitoneal Chemotherapy: Retrospective Analysis of 523 Patients From a Multicentric French Study. *Journal of Clinical Oncology, 28*(1), 63-68.

Evrard, S., Falkenrodt, A., Park, A., Tassetti, V., Mutter, D., & Marescaux, J. (1997). Influence of CO2 pneumoperitoneum on systemic and peritoneal cell-mediated immunity. *World J Surg, 21*(4), 353-356.

Fleshman, J., Sargent, D. J., Green, E., Anvari, M., Stryker, S. J., Beart, R. W., et al. (2007). Laparoscopic Colectomy for Cancer is not inferior to Open Surgery Based on 5-Year Data from the COST Study Group Trial. *Ann Surg, 246*, 655-664.

Gigot, J. F., Glineur, D., Santiago Azagra, J., Goergen, M., Ceuterick, M., Morino, M., et al. (2002). Laparoscopic liver resection for malignant liver tumors: preliminary results of a multicenter European study. *Ann Surg, 236*(1), 90-97.

Glehen, O., Gilly, F. N., Arvieux, C., Cotte, E., Boutitie, F., Mansvelt, B., et al. (2010). Peritoneal carcinomatosis from gastric cancer: a multi-institutional study of 159 patients treated by cytoreductive surgery combined with perioperative intraperitoneal chemotherapy. *Ann Surg Oncol, 17*(9), 2370-2377.

Glehen, O., Gilly, F. N., Boutitie, F., Bereder, J. M., Quenet, F., Sideris, L., et al. (2010). Toward curative treatment of peritoneal carcinomatosis from nonovarian origin by cytoreductive surgery combined with perioperative intraperitoneal chemotherapy. *Cancer, 116*(24), 5608-5618.

Gupta, A., Watson, D. I., Ellis, T., & Jamieson, G. G. (2002). Tumour implantation following laparoscopy using different insufflation gases. *ANZ Journal of Surgery, 72*(4), 254-257.

Helm, C. W., Richard, S. D., Pan, J., Bartlett, D., Goodman, M. D., Hoefer, R., et al. (2010). Hyperthermic intraperitoneal chemotherapy in ovarian cancer: first report of the HYPER-O registry. *Int J Gynecol Cancer, 20*(1), 61-69.

Hirabayashi, Y., Yamaguchi, K., Shiraishi, N., Adachi, Y., Kitamura, H., & Kitano, S. (2002). Development of port-site metastasis after pneumoperitoneum. *Surg Endosc, 16*(5), 864-868.

Iwanaka, T., Arya, G., & Ziegler, M. M. (1998). Mechanism and Prevention of Port-Site Tumor Recurrence After Laparoscopy in a Murine Model. *J Pediatr Surg, 33*, 457-461.

Jayne, D. G., Fook, S., Loi, C., & Seow-Choen, F. (2002). Peritoneal carcinomatosis from colorectal cancer. *British Journal of Surgery, 89*(12), 1545-1550.

Jayne, D. G., Thorpe, H. C., Copeland, J., Quirke, P., Brown, J. M., & Guillou, P. J. (2010). Five-year follow-up of the Medical Research Council CLASICC trial of laparoscopically assisted versus open surgery for colorectal cancer. *British Journal of Surgery, 97*(11), 1638-1645.

Kaiser, A. M., Kang, J. C., Chan, L. S., Vukasin, P., & Beart, R. W. (2004). Laparoscopic-Assisted vs. Open Colectomy for Colon Cancer: A Prospective Randomized Trial. *Journal of Laparoendoscopic & Advanced Surgical Techniques, 14*(6), 329-334.

Kim, S. H., Park, I. J., Joh, Y. G., & Hahn, K. Y. (2006). Laparoscopic resection for rectal cancer: a prospective analysis of thirty-month follow-up outcomes in 312 patients. *Surg Endosc, 20*(8), 1197-1202.

Koffron, A. J., Auffenberg, G., Kung, R., & Abecassis, M. (2007). Evaluation of 300 Minimally Invasive Liver Resections at a single institution. *Ann Surg, 246*(3), 385-394.

Lacy, A. M., Delgado, S., Castells, A., Prins, H. A., Arroyo, V., Ibarzabal, A., et al. (2008). The long-term results of a randomized clinical trial of laparoscopy-assisted versus open surgery for colon cancer. *Ann Surg, 248*(1-7).

Lee, S. W., Gleason, N. R., Bessler, M., & Whelan, R. L. (2000). Port site tumor recurrence rates in a murine model of laparoscopic splenectomy decreased with increased experience. *Surg Endosc, 14*(9), 805-811.

Liang, J. T., Huang, K. C., Lai, H. S., Lee, P. H., & Jeng, Y. M. (2007). Oncologic Results of Laparoscopic Versus Conventional Open Surgery for Stage II or III Left-Sided Colon Cancers: A Randomized Controlled Trial. *Ann Surg Oncol, 14*(1), 109-117.

Lujan, J., Valero, H., Hernandex, Q., Sanchez, A., Frutos, M. D., & Parrilla, P. (2009). Randomized clinical trial comparing laparoscopic and open surgery in patients with rectal cancer. *Br J Surg, 96*(9), 982-989.

Martinez, A., Querleu, D., Leblanc, E., Narducci, F., & Ferron, G. (2010). Low incidence of port-site metastases after laparoscopic staging of uterine cancer. *Gynecologic Oncology, 118*, 145-150.

Mathew, G., Watson, D. I., Ellis, T. S., Jamieson, G. G., & Rofe, A. M. (1999). The role of peritoneal immunity and the tumour-bearing state on the development of wound and peritoneal metastases after laparoscopy. *Aust N Z J Surg, 69*(1), 14-18.

Menes, T., & Spivak, H. (2000). Laparoscopy: searching for the proper insufflation gas. *Surg Endosc, 14*(11), 1050-1056.

Milsom, J. W., Lavery, I. C., Church, J. M., Stolfi, V. M., & Fazio, V. W. (1994). Use of laparoscopic techniques in colorectal surgery. Preliminary study. *Dis Colon Rectum, 37*(3), 215-218.

Miyajima, N., Fukunaga, M., Hasegawa, H., Tanaka, J., Okuda, J., & Watanabe, M. (2009). Results of a multicenter study of 1,057 cases of rectal cancer treated by laparoscopic surgery. *Surg Endosc, 23*, 113-118.

Moreira, H. J., Yamaguchi, T., Wexner, S., Singer, L., Zhao, R., Baig, M. K., et al. (2001). Effect of pneumoperitoneal pressure on tumor dissemination and tumor recurrence at port-site and midline incisions. *Am Surg, 67*(4), 369-373.

Murphy, P., Alexander, P., Senior, P. V., Fleming, J., Kirkham, N., & Taylor, I. (1988). Mechanisms of organ selective tumour growth by bloodbourne cancer cells.. *Br J Cancer, 57*, 19-31.

Nduka, C. C., Poland, N., Kennedy, M., Dye, J., & Darzi, A. (1998). Does the ultrasonically activated scalpel release viable airborne cancer cells? *Surg Endosc, 12*(8), 1031-1034.

Ng, K. H., Ng, D. C., Cheung, H. Y., Wong, J. C., Yau, K. K., Chung, C. C., et al. (2009). Laparoscopic Resection for Rectal Cancers Lessons Learned From 579 Cases. *Ann Surg, 249*, 82-86.

Ng, S. M., Leung, K. L., Lee, J. F., Yiu, R. Y., Li, J. C., Teoh, A. Y., et al. (2008). Laparoscopic-Assisted Versus Open Abdominoperineal Resection for Low Rectal Cancer: A Prospective Randomized Trial. *Ann Surg Oncol, 15*(9), 2418-2425.

Ost, M. C., Patel, K. P., Rastinehad, A. R., Chu, P. Y., Anderson, A. E., Smith, A. D., et al. (2008). Pneumoperitoneum with carbon dioxide inhibits macrophage tumor necrosis factor-alpha secretion: source of transitional-cell carcinoma port-site metastasis, with prophylactic irrigation strategies to decrease laparoscopic oncologic risks. *J Endourol, 22*(1), 105-112.

Paolucci, V., Schaeff, B., Schneider, M., & Gutt, C. (1999). Tumor Seeding following Laparoscopy: International Survey. *World J Surg, 23*(10), 989-995.

Prasad, A., Avery, C., & Foley, R. J. E. (1994). Abdominal wall metastases following laparoscopy.. *Br J Surg 1994; 81: 1697, 81*(1697).

Rassweiler, J., Tsivian, A., Kumar, A. V. R., Lymberakis, C., Schulze, M., Seeman, O., et al. (2003). Oncological Safety of Laparoscopic Surgery for Urological Malignancy: Experience With More Than 1,000 Operations. *The Journal of Urology, 169*(6), 2072-2075.

Sanjuán, A., Hernández, S., Pahisa, J., Ayuso, J. R., Torné, A., Martínez Román, S., et al. (2005). Port-site metastasis after laparoscopic surgery for endometrial carcinoma: two case reports. *Gynecologic Oncology, 96*(2), 539-542.

Seow-Choen, F., Wan, W. H., & Tan, K. Y. (2009). The use of a wound protector to prevent port site recurrence may not be totally logical. *Colorectal Dis, 11*(2), 123-125.

Shoup, M., Brennan, M. F., Karpeh, M. S., S.M., G., McMahon, R. L., & Conlon, K. C. (2002). Port Site Metastasis after Diagnostic Laparoscopy for Upper Gastrointestinal Tract Malignancies: An Uncommon Entity. *Ann Surg Oncol, 9*(7), 632-636.

Song, J., Lee, H. J., Cho, G. S., Han, S. U., Kim, M. C., Ryu, S. W., et al. (2010). Recurrence following laparoscopy-assisted gastrectomy for gastric cancer: A Multicenter retrospective analysis of 1,417 patients. *Ann Surg Oncol, 17*, 1777-1786.

Sugarbaker, P. H. (1988). Surgical management of peritoneal carcinosis: diagnosis, prevention and treatment. *Langenbecks Arch Chir, 373*(3), 189-196.

Sugarbaker, P. H., Schellinx, M. E., Chang, D., Koslowe, P., & von Meyerfeldt, M. (1996). Peritoneal carcinomatosis from adenocarcinoma of the colon. *World J Surg, 20*(5), 585-591.

Tseng, L. N., Berends, F. J., Wittich, P. H., Bouvy, N. D., Marquet, R. L., Kazemier, G., et al. (1998). Port-site metastases: impact of local tissue trauma and gas leakage. *Surg Endosc, 12*, 1377-1380.

Whelan, R. L., Sellers, G. J., Allendorf, J. D., Laird, D., Bessler, M. D., Nowygrod, R., et al. (1996). Trocar site recurrence is unlikely to result from aerosolization of tumor cells. *Dis Colon Rectum, 39*(10 Suppl), S7-13.

Yan, T. D., Deraco, M., Baratti, D., Kusamura, S., Elias, D., Glehen, O., et al. (2009). Cytoreductive Surgery and Hyperthermic Intraperitoneal Chemotherapy for Malignant Peritoneal Mesothelioma: Multi-Institutional Experience. *Journal of Clinical Oncology, 27*(36), 6237-6242.

Yavuz, Y., Rønning, K., Lyng, O., Grønbech, J. E., & Mårvik, R. (2003). Effect of carbon dioxide pneumoperitoneum on tissue blood flow in the peritoneum, rectus abdominis, and diaphragm muscles. *Surg Endosc, 17*(10), 1632-1635.

Youssef, H., Newman, C., Chandrakumaran, K., Mohamed, F., Cecil, T. D., & Moran, B. J. (2011). Operative findings, early complications, and long-term survival in 456 patients with pseudomyxoma peritonei syndrome of appendiceal origin. *Dis Colon Rectum, 54*(3), 293-299.

Z'graggen, K., Birrer, S., Maurer, C. A., Wehrli, H., Klaiber, C., & Baer, H. U. (1998). Incidence of port site recurrence after laparoscopic cholecystectomy for preoperatively unsuspected gallbladder carcinoma. *Surgery, 124*(5), 831-838.

Zivanovic, O., Sonoda, Y., Diaz, J. P., Levine, D. A., Brown, C. L., Chi, D. S., et al. (2008). The rate of port-site metastases after 2251 laparoscopic procedures in women with underlying malignant disease. *Gynecologic Oncology, 111*(3), 431-437.

12

Transarterial Chemoembolization Prior to Early Hepatocellular Carcinoma Laparoscopic Resection in Patients with Child A Cirrhosis

Ricardo Robles, Caridad Marín and Pascual Parrilla
University of Murcia, Virgen de la Arrixaca University Hospital
Liver Surgery and Liver Transplantation Unit
Spain

1. Introduction

Hepatocellular carcinoma (HCC) is the most frequent primary neoplasia of the liver and its incidence has risen and mainly affects subjects with cirrhosis. Globally, the main risk factor for HCC is hepatitis B virus linked or not to aflatoxin (1). Nevertheless, in industrialised countries, the most frequent risk factors associated with HCC are chronic infection caused by hepatitis C virus and ethanol ingestion (2).
In the treatment of HCC, besides the size and number of nodules, also involved the patient's clinical status assessed by different methods (Child-Pough classification, MELD, ECOG performans status, indocyanine green levels, etc). Recently, the Barcelona Clinic group (3) provides a staging classification using the Child-Pough classification, performans status, Okuda classification, and evaluate the presence of portal hypertension and bilirubin levels.In the initial stages, the treatment options include: resection, liver transplant and ablation. In subjects with compensated cirrhosis, candidates for resection must be selected carefully and the liver function reserve must be tested (4). The best candidates for surgery are those with single tumours, those who present normal bilirubin and no clinically significant portal hypertension (5). HCC vascularisation is predominantly arterial and this establishes a specific vascular pattern characterised by intense contrast uptake in the arterial phase, followed by rapid wash out in the portal phase (6). Nevertheless, given that tumour spread via the veins originates in the area immediately surrounding the tumour, from an oncological point of view, it is worth performing a resection with a margin of 1 cm.
Despite the strict selection process, the recurrence rate for this disease is very high and can reach 70 % after 5 years (4), recurrences of which, 70 % correspond to intrahepatic metastasis, that were not detected when the resection was carried out, and 30% are de novo HCC (7,8). On the basis of this, it was established that when liver transplants are limited to those subjects with single tumours that measure 5 cm or less or with a maximum of 3 nodules which measure less than 3 cm and that do not present vascular invasion or extrahepatic dissemination, a 4-year survival rate of 75 % and a recurrence rate of 8 % is obtained (9).
In subjects with decompensated cirrhosis of the liver, resection is formally contraindicated and a liver transplant must be considered. In subjects with intermediate stage HCC (stage B according to HCC classification), the only treatment that has proven to be beneficial in terms

of survival outcome is transarterial chemoembolization (TACE) (10-13). However, despite the radiological treatment response obtained, in over half the cases, the main disadvantage was that most of the subjects experienced development of the disease despite the initial response. This treatment focuses on the predominantly arterial vascularisation of the HCC. It involves the selective catheterization of the hepatic artery, injecting a chemotherapy agent that is embedded inside a transport medium (usually lipiodol) and occluding the arterial flow afterwards with different embolizing substances.
Moreover, laparoscopic liver resection (LLR) of hepatocellular carcinoma (HCC) on cirrhosis is generally indicated in Child A patients with tumours minor than 5 cm located in the peripheral segments (14) and more rarely in the right posterior segments. Given the special nature of the liver and the cirrhotic patient, LLR involves a high risk of bleeding and could require the use of the Pringle maneuver. Both events (hemorrhage and use of the Pringle maneuver) could cause postoperative liver failure, the main cause of death after liver resection (LR) in child A patients.
Preoperative transarterial chemoembolization (TACE) has until now been used in large HCC with two objectives: (a) to increase resectability or liver transplantation, by achieving understaging, and (b) to increase survival, by decreasing recurrence rates. However, given that HCC is a tumour that is mainly irrigated through the artery, preoperative TACE could decrease vascularization in the segments to be resected, and therefore reduce the risk of hemorrhage during liver resection. Consequently, the use of preoperative TACE could be recommended in early onset tumours, especially when they are going to be resected laparoscopically.

2. Laparoscopic surgical technique

2.1 Pure laparoscopic hepatectomy (PLP)

The patient is placed in the decubitus supine position, independent of the location of the lesion, with the legs apart and slight bent over the pelvis. The surgeon stands between the patient's legs and the first assistant to the left, with the second assistant to the patient's right using a second monitor. Five trocars are used (four 10-mm and one 12-mm), 4 of them following a concave line to the lesion. After creation of the pneumoperitoneum (12 mmHg of CO_2), either with a verres needle or with optiview®, a 10-mm trocar is placed at the umbilicus for insertion of the straight telescope, and the 4 remaining trocars are placed under direct visual guidance.
The first and second (10-mm) to the left and the right of the umbilical trocar; the next (10-mm) in the left flank, on the mid axillary line, to insert the clamp for the Pringle manoeuvre; and the remaining in the subxiphoid areas to insert the liver separation forceps or for a better view of the suprahepatic veins and posterior hepatic ligaments. An intraoperative laparoscopic ultrasonography is performed using a probe inserted through the 10-mm trocar.
After necessary mobilisation of the liver the lesser omentum is dissected for control of the hepatic pedicle. Dissection of the hepatic parenchyma is done with 10-mm Ligasure® Atlas (Tyco©) or harmonic scalpel (Ethicon©). When the hepatectomy is finished, the haemostasis is completed with Tissuelink® (Primm©). Following, any possible bile leaks are sutured, a haemostatic substance is applied to the surgical bed and an aspiration drain is placed on the surgical bed. The tumour specimen is extracted via a Pfannestiel incisión, without fragmenting so that the resection margins can be checked (15,16).

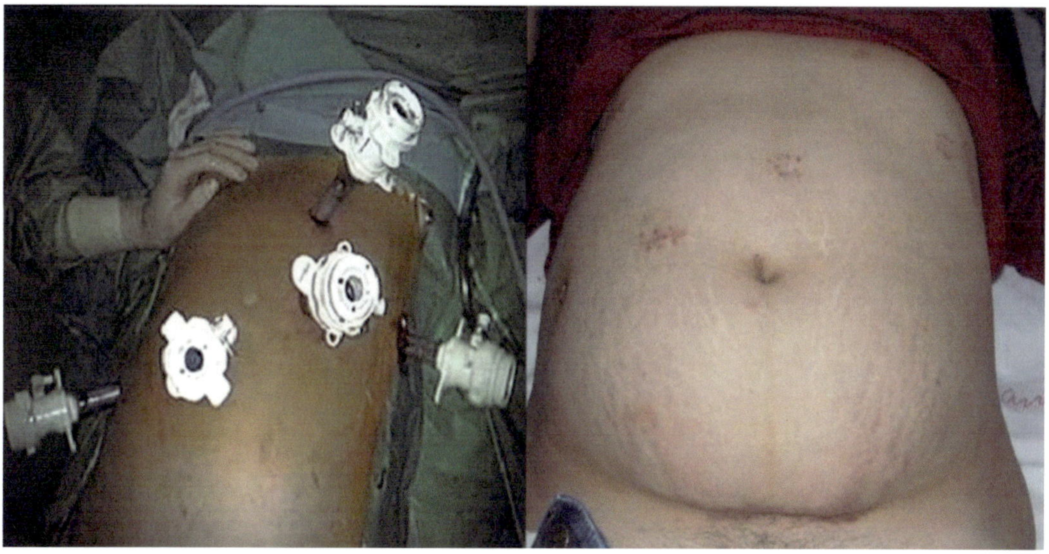

a) b)

Fig. 1. a) Pure laparoscopic surgery; b) Aesthetic results

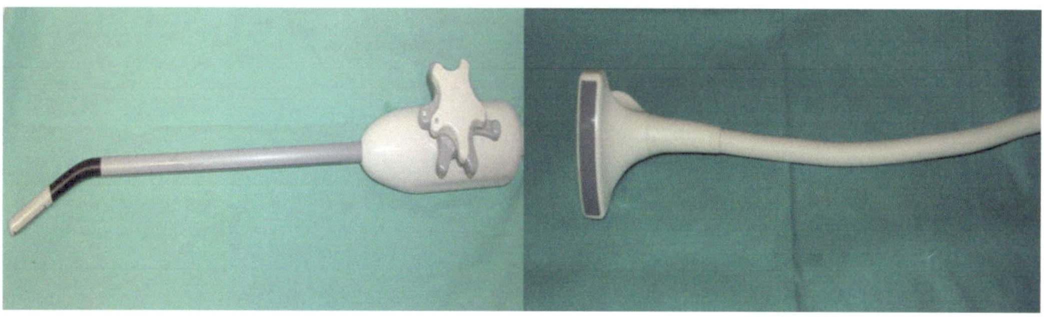

a) b)

Fig. 2. Echography probe a) Laparoscopic probe; b) Hand-assisted probe

2.2 Hand Assisted Laparoscopic Surgery (HALLS)

In cases of conversion to a (15,16), the position of the patient and the assistants is the same as with PLP. The operation is begun with a transverse incision in the right flank, 3-5 fingerwidths from the right costal edge (from the mid axillary line to the anterior axillary line).

Abdominal muscles are dissected to reach the anterior sheath of the rectus, which is generally opened in few centimetres, and the hand-port is inserted. With the surgeon's left hand inside the abdomen a 10-mm trocar is inserted into an adhesion-free area, the pneumoperitoneum is created (12 mmHg CO_2) and the 4 remaining trocars are then placed in the same location and with the same function as in PLP. Subsequently a sonography is performed with an abdominal probe inserted via the hand-port. The surgical specimen is extracted through the hand-port incision in the right flank.

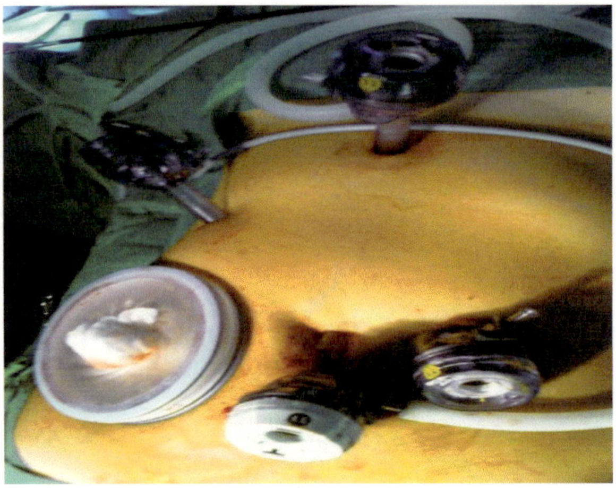

Fig. 3.1 Hand-assisted laparoscopic liver surgery

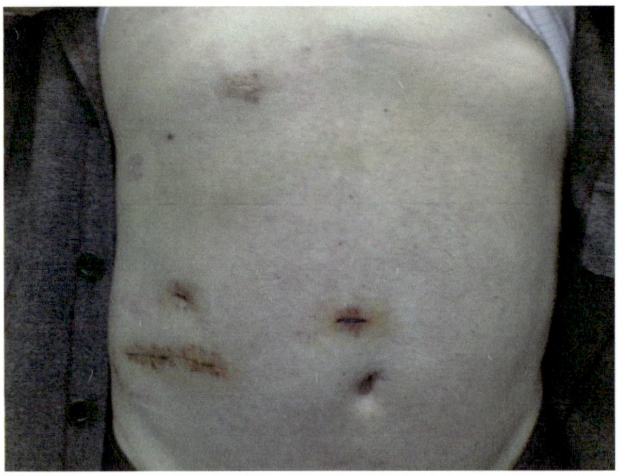

Fig. 3.2 Aesthetic results

3. Preoperative TACE technique

In 2 cases the procedure involved selective catheterization of the hepatic artery followed by an injection of adriamycin embedded in lipiodol and arterial flow occlusion using spongostan. In the other 8 cases, we used polivinyl alcohol spheres loaded with adriamycin (17).

4. Our experience

We have shown the immediate intra and postoperative results of 10 cirrhotic Child A patients with HCC stages 0 and A according to the *Barcelona Liver Cancer Classification* (3). These patients were given TACE prior to LLR.

Between January 1996 and December 2010 we performed 720 LR on solid liver tumours, of which 100 were by laparoscopy. LLR was carried out on 10 patients with HCC on cirrhosis using a preoperative TACE, which was applied in order to decrease intraoperative bleeding (Table 1). All patients were Child A cirrhosis, without portal hypertension (normal platelets, gastroscopy without varices and no splenomegaly) and a normal total bilirubin. After 3 weeks of TACE, a routine CT-scan showed tumour response to the treatment and scarce vascularization of embolized segments.

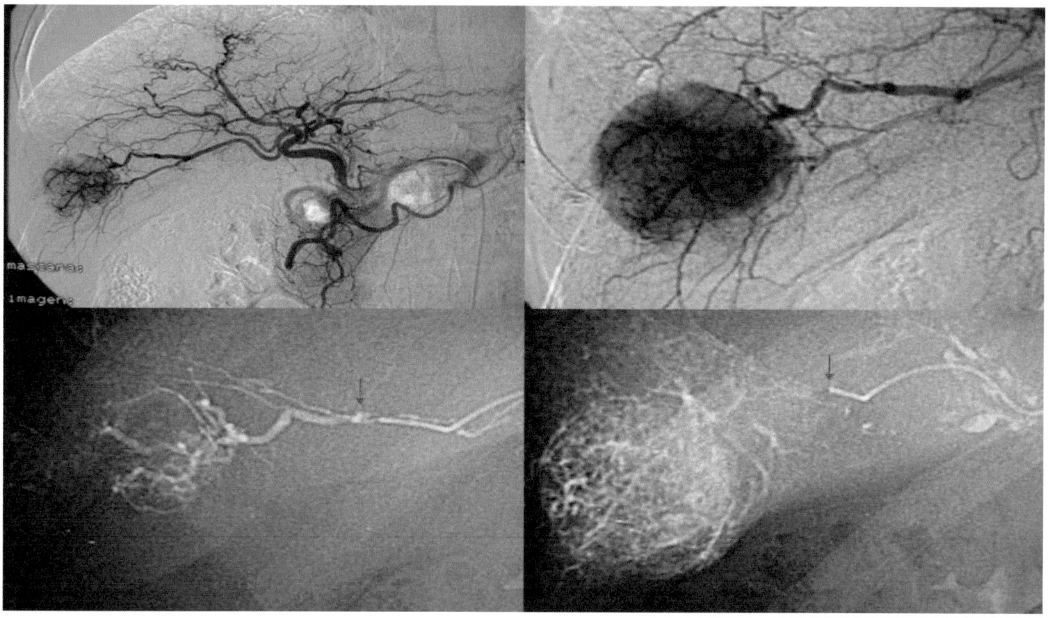

Fig. 4. TACE: we can see the tumor and where arterial occlusion is performed

Sex , years	Etiology	Nodules	Size (cm)	Location	Technique	Conversion to HALLS	Surgical time/ minutes	Blood loss	Morbidity
Male, 75	C Virus	1	4	VI-VII	VI-VII	No	210	150	No
Male, 66	Alcohol	1	3	III	III	No	240	100	No
Male, 60	Alcohol	2	3 and 2	VI + VII	VI + RF VII	Yes, for RF S. VIII	240	200	No
Female, 53	C Virus	1	5	V	V	Yes, for adherencial block	150	150	No
Male, 60	Alcohol	1	3	Left lobe	LLS	No	180	300	Ascitis
Male, 82	Alcohol	1	5	VI	VI	No	150	500	Ascitis
Female, 60	B Virus	1	4	VI-VII	VI-VII	No	120	100	No
Male, 71	Alcohol	1	3	III	III	No	180	70	No
Male, 72	Alcohol	1	3	III	III	No	150	100	No
Male, 74	Alcohol	1	2	VI	VI	No	120	50	No

Table 1. Characteristics of the 10 patients with the TACE protocol prior to laparoscopic resection until December 2010

RF. Radiofrequency

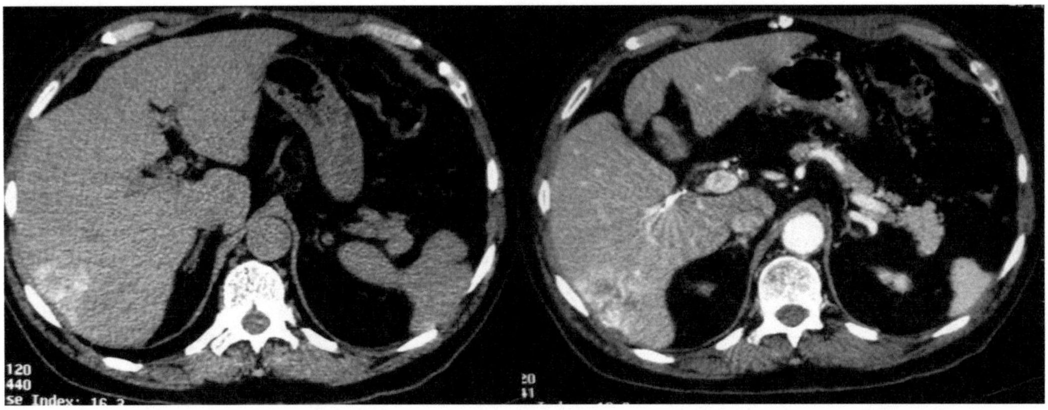

Fig. 5. The CT scan shows tumor necrosis and ischemia of the right lateral sector

The surgical technique performed was: bisegmentectomy VI-VII in 2 cases, segmentectomy VI in 3 cases (in 1 case we associated radiofrequency of a tumour located in segment VII, near to right hepatic vein), segmentectomy III in 3 cases, in 1 case segmentectomy V and left lateral sectionectomy in 1 case. No Pringle maneuver was used. No patients were transfused. There was no postoperative mortality. Two patients presented postoperative ascites that was resolved with medical treatment. The mean hospital stay was 3.7 days (range 2-12 days).

5. Comments

For most authors, HCC involves several surgical difficulties for laparoscopic approach (14-16, 18-27), especially in the cirrhotic liver (14,18,19, 24.25) due to the increased hardness of the liver, portal hypertension and alterations in blood clotting. These difficulties make conversion to laparotomy, mainly because of hemorrhages. In 27 patients with HCC resected by laparoscopy [Cherqui et al. (14)], there was a 26% conversion rate (7 patients, 5 of which were due to hemorrhage); 6 patients had blood losses greater than 1000 ml and 3 of these were given a blood transfusion (15%). Given the risk from bleeding, the authors systematically carry out the intermittent Pringle maneuver (taking a mean time of 55 min) and this could explain why they report a longer mean surgical time (240 min) (14). The technical difficulties were greater in the resection of tumours located in right lobe (even when patients were in the left lateral decubitus position) compared to tumours located in the left lateral segments (II and III segments).

Due to the greater risk of bleeding during LLR for HCC, we propose the use of TACE. As the tumour is mainly irrigated through the artery, selective TACE of the segments to be resected could lead to less vascularization, and therefore, less bleeding during LR. Consequently, there might be less need to occlude the hepatic hilum (this would prevent secondary hepatic ischemia, and therefore there could be less risk of postoperative liver failure), less surgical time and less transfusion. This seems to have been confirmed in the 10 patients in our series. In spite of several tumours being located in a position that makes tumour resection technically more difficult, when LLR was used, mean surgical time was low (174 min, range 120-240 min), mean blood loss was scarce (220 ml, range 50-500 ml) and the Pringle maneuver was not needed.

In our series, unlike other authors (14-16), the patient was placed in supine position even when the lesions were in the right lobe. In two cases we had to convert to HALLS but this was not due to bleeding, which is a factor that commonly leads to conversion in other series (24,25,28). In the first case the patient was converted in order to mobilize the right hepatic lobe enabling radiofrequency of a 2 cm nodule located posterior to the right hepatic vein (resection of segment VI had been carried out previously); and, in the second case, conversion to HALLS was necessary because of complete blockage of adhesions of the subhepatic space due to a cholecystectomy 20 years earlier.

In other series, intraoperative bleeding is lower than the levels published by Cherqui et al. (14). Belli et al. (19) carried out a retrospective study comparing 23 patients with HCC on cirrhosis treated using LLR compared to another 23 treated using open surgery (OS). Blood loss (260 ml vs. 376 ml by OS), transfusion (0% vs. 17% by OS) and the Pringle maneuver (0% vs. 21% by OS) were lower in the LLR group, although surgical time was higher (148 min vs. 125 min with OS). Furthermore, only 1 patient out of 23 was converted (4.3%), the tumour was located in S VI and there were difficulties in finding the tumour for resection, in spite of the patient being in lateral decubitus position. Perhaps these good results are related to the location of the tumour (50% in the left lobe) and due to greater patient selection given that all the tumours were subcapsular and exophitic. In this kind of tumour that is so peripheral, it would probably be inadvisable to carry out TACE.

There have been many retrospective studies of open surgery (30-32) comparing patients operated on by LR for HCC on cirrhosis with and without TACE. For Choi et al. (31) there are no differences in the 5 year survival rates between both groups and for Chen et al. (32) survival at 5 years was greater in the group with TACE. What is more, Choi et al. (31) compared the operative results of both groups, revealing slightly higher blood loss rates in the group with TACE, without statistical differences. These results are in contrast to our results and we believe that this is because the groups are not comparable because the TACE was carried out on central tumours > 5 cm and a greater % of major LR was carried out.

To conclude, selective TACE of the tumour and of the segments to be resected by laparoscopy, in patients in the early stages of HCC on Child A cirrhosis without portal hypertension, seems to reduce blood losses and the need for occluding the hilum, and any consequent complications of occlusion. Prospective randomized studies are needed with a greater number of patients comparing laparoscopic resection with and without TACE in selected cases of HCC on cirrhosis, in order to analyze the advantages in the immediate postoperative period and the possible effects on long term survival.

6. References

[1] Fattovich, G.; Stroffolini, T.; Zagni, I.; Donato, F. (2004). Hepatocellular carcinoma in cirrhosis: Incidence and risk factors. *Gastroenterology*. 127(5 Suppl 1):S35-50.

[2] Morgan, TR.; Mandayam, S.; Jamal MM. (2004). Alcohol and hepatocellular carcinoma. *Gastroenterology*. 127(5 Suppl 1):S87-96.

[3] Llovet, JM.; Fuster, J.; Bruix, J. (2004). Barcelona-Clinic Liver Cancer Group: diagnosis, staging, and treatment of hepatocellular carcinoma. *Liver Tranpl.* 10 (suppl 1): S115-20.

[4] Llovet, JM. ; Schwartz, M. ; Mazzaferro, V. (2005). Resection and liver transplantation for hepatocellular carcinoma. *Semin Liver Dis.* 25:181-200.

[5] Ishizawa, T. ; Hasegawa, K. ; Aoki, T. ; Takahashi, M. ; Inoue, Y. ; Sano, K., et al. (2008). Neither multiple tumours nor portal hypertension are operative contraindications for hepatocellular carcinoma. *Gastroenterology.*14:872-80.

[6] Kojiro, M.; Roskams, T. (2005). Early hepatocellular carcinoma and dysplastic nodules. *Semin Liver Dis.* 25:133-42.

[7] Ng, IO.; Guan, XY.; Poon, RT.; Fan, ST.; Lee, JM. (2003). Determination of the molecular relationship between multiple tumour nodules in hepatocellular carcinoma differentiates multicentric origin from intrahepatic metastasis. *J Pathol.* 199:345-53.

[8] Llovet, JM.; Fuster, J.; Bruix, J. (1999). Intention-to-treat analysis of surgical treatment for early hepatocellular carcinoma: Resection versus transplantation. *Hepatology.* 30:1434-40.

[9] Mazzaferro, V.; Regalia, E.; Doci, R.; Andreola, S.; Pulvirenti, A.; Bozzetti, F.; et al. (1996). Liver transplantation for the treatment of small hepatocellular carcinomas in patients with cirrhosis. *N Engl J Med.* 334:693-9.

[10] Lo, CM.; Ngan, H.; Tso, WK. ; Liu, CL.; Lam, CM., Poon, RT.; et al. (2002). Randomized controlled trial 1284 of transarterial lipiodol chemoembolization for unresectable hepatocellular carcinoma. *Hepatology.* 35(5):1164-71.

[11] Bruix, J., Sala, M., Llovet, JM. (2004). Chemoembolization for hepatocellular carcinoma. *Gastroenterology.* 127(5 Suppl 1):S179-88.

[12] Llovet, JM.; Real, MI.; Montana, X.; Planas, R.; Coll, S.; Aponte, J.; et al. (2002) Arterial embolization orchemoembolisation versus symptomatic treatment in patients with unresectable hepatocellular carcinoma: A randomised controlled trial. *Lancet.* 359:1734-9.

[13] Llovet, JM.; Bruix, J. (2003). Systematic review of randomized trials for unresectable hepatocellular carcinoma: Chemoembolization improves survival. *Hepatology.* 37:429-42.

[14] Cherqui, D.; Laurent, A.; Tayar, C.; Chang, S.; Van Nhieu, JT.; Loriau, J.; et al. (2006). Laparoscopic liver resection for peripheral hepatocellular carcinoma in patients with chronic liver disease: midterm results and perspectives. *Ann Surg.* 243: 499-506.

[15] Robles, R. ; Abellán, B. ; Marín, C. ; Fernández, JA.; Ramírez, P.; Morales, D.; et al. (2005). Resección de tumores hepáticos sólidos por laparoscopia. Presentación de nuestra experiencia. *Cir Esp.* 78: 238-245.

[16] Robles, R.; Marin, C.; Abellán, B.; López Conesa, A.; Pastor, P.; Parrilla, P. (2008). A New Approach to Hand-Assisted Laparoscopic Liver Surgery. *Surgical Endoscopy.* 33 (11): 2357-2364.

[17] Kirchhoff, TD. ; Bleck, JS. ; Dettmer, A. ; Chavan, A.; Rosenthal, H.; Merkesdal, S.; et al. (2007). Transarterial chemoembolization using degradable starch microspheres and iodized oil in the treatment of advanced hepatocellular carcinoma : evaluation of tumor response, toxicity, and survival. *Hepatobiliary Pancreat Dis Int.* 6 : 259-266.

[18] Belli, G.; Fantini, C.; D´Agostino, A.; Belli, A.; Rusolillo, N.; Cioffi L. (2005). Laparoscopic liver resection without a Pringle manoeuvre for HCC in cirrothic patients. *Chir Ital.* 57(1): 15-25.

[19] Belli, G.; Fantini, C.; D´Agostino, A.; Cioffi, L.; Langella, S.; Russolillo, N.; et al. (2007). Laparoscopic vs open liver resection for hepatocellular carcinoma in patients with histologically proven cirrosis: short- and middle-term results. *Surg Endosc.* 21: 2004-2011.

[20] Dulucq, JL.; Wintringer, P.; Stabilini, C.; Berticelli, J.; Mahajna, A. (2005). Laparoscopic liver resections: a single center experience. *Surg Endosc.* 19: 886-891.

[21] Gayet, B. ; Cavalière, D. ; Vibert, E. ; Perniceni, T.; Levard, H.; Denet, C.; et al. (2007). Totally laparoscopic right hepatectomy. *Am J Surg.* 194; 685-689.

[22] Dagher, I. ; Proske, JM. ; Carloni, A. ; Richa, H. ; Tranchart, H. ; Franco D. (2007). Laparoscopic liver resection: results for 70 patients. *Surg Endosc.* 21: 619-624.

[23] Vibert, E. ; Perniceni, T. ; Levard, H. ; Denet, C. ; Shahri, NK. ; Gayet, B. (2006).Laparoscopic liver resection. *Ann Surg.* 93: 67-72.

[24] Kaneko, H. ; Takagi, S. ; Otsuka, Y. ; Tsuchiya, M. ; Tamura, A. ; Katagiri, T. ; et al. (2005). Laparoscopic liver resetion of hepatocellular carcinoma. *Am J Surg.* 189: 190-194.

[25] Teramoto, K.; Kawamura, T.; Takamatsu, S.; Nakaumura, N.; Kudo, A.; Noguchi, N.(2005). Laparoscopic and thoracoscopic approaches for the treatment of hepatocellular carcinoma. *Am J Surg.* 189: 474-478.

[26] Nguyen, KT.; Gamblin, TC.; Geller DA. (2009). World Review of Laparoscopic Liver Resection—2,804 Patients. *Annals of Surgery.* 250 (5): 831-841.

[27] Buell, JF.; Cherqui, D.; Geller, DA.; O'Rourke, N.; Lannitti; D., Dagher, I.; et al. (2009). The International Position on Laparoscopic Liver Surgery. The Louisville Statement. *Ann Surg.* 250: 825–830.

[28] Koffron, AJ.; Auffenberg, G.; Kung, R.; Abecassis, M. (2007). Evaluation of 300 minimally invasive liver resections at a single institution. Less is more. *Ann Surg.* 246: 385-394.

[29] Buell, JF.; Thomas, MT.; Rudich, S.; Marvin, M.; Nagubandi, R.; Ravindra, KV.; et al. (2008). Experience with more than 500 minimally invasive hepatic procedures. *Ann Surg.* 248: 475-486.

[30] Lu, CD. ; Peng, SY. ; Jiang, XC. ; Lu, CD.; Peng, SY.; Jiang, XC.; et al. (1999). Preoperative transcatheter arterial chemoembolization and prognosis of patients with hepatocellular carcinomas : retrospective analysis of 120 cases. *World J Surg.* 23 : 293-300.

[31] Choi, GH. ; Kim, DH. ; Kang, CM. ; Kim, KS. ; Choi, JS. ; Lee, WJ. ; et al. (2007). Is preoperative transarterial chemoembolization needed for a resectable hepatocellular carcinoma?. *Worl J Surg.* 31:2370-2377.

[32] Chen, XP.; Hu, DY.; Zhang, YF.; Zhang, WG.; Qiu, FZ. (2007). Role of mesohepatectomy with or without transcatheter arterial chemoembolization for large centrally hepatocellular carcinoma. *Dig Surg* . 24: 208-213.

13

The Impact of Visceral Fat Accumulation on Laparoscopy-Assisted Distal Gastrectomy for Early Gastric Cancer

Junji Ueda, Hitoshi Ichimiya and Masao Tanaka
Department of Surgery and Oncology, Kyushu University, Fukuoka
Department of Surgery, Hamanomachi Hospital, Fukuoka
Japan

1. Introduction

Gastric cancer is one of the most common malignancies in Japan. Laparoscopic techniques have been used for the treatment of cancer in several organs, and laparoscopy-assisted distal gastrectomy (LADG) has recently been widely accepted for the treatment of early gastric cancer in Japan (Shimizu et al., 2003; Noshiro et al., 2005; Kitano et al., 2007). The potential benefits of LADG include less pain, less operative blood loss, earlier resumption of oral intake and shorter hospital stay compared to conventional open surgery (Adachi et al.,2000; Shimizu et al., 2000; Kitano et al., 2002).

Obesity is a rapidly growing epidemic, and has been considered a risk factor for postoperative complications (Dhar et al., 2000; Inagawa et al., 2000). Special caution may be required when performing laparoscopic surgery on obese patients. Although several studies have reported that obesity adversely affects the technical difficulty and postoperative outcome of laparoscopic surgery (Noshiro et al., 2003; Senagore et al., 2003; Yasuda et al., 2004), some recent studies have reported that obesity does not adversely affect these factors (Leroy et al.; 2005; Kim et al., 2006). The impact of obesity on the technical feasibility and outcome of laparoscopic surgery remains controversial.

Obesity is characterized by an excess of visceral fat (VF) and subcutaneous fat (SF) accumulation. In Japan, the prevalence of obesity, defined by the World Health Organization as body mass index (BMI) ≥ 30 kg/m^2, is only 2-3 %, in contrast to 30-35 % in the United States (Yoshiike et al., 2002; Kanazawa et al., 2005; Ogden et al., 2006). However, recent papers have shown that Japanese have more VF tissue than Caucasians (Tanaka et al., 2003; Kadowaki et al., 2006). The accumulation of VF is thought to be one of the important factors affecting operative difficulty in laparoscopic gastric surgery. Although many surgeons feel that excess VF accumulation increases operative difficulty, the relationship between fat accumulation and operative difficulty has not been fully studied (Tsukada et al., 2004; Seki et al., 2007).

It is well known that excess VF accumulation is associated with cardiovascular disease, diabetes and hypertension (Fujioka et al., 1987; Kanai et al., 1990; Despres & Lemieux, 2006). We hypothesized that VF accumulation is also associated with technical difficulty and postoperative outcome of LADG. In this study, we evaluated the impact of VF accumulation on the technical difficulty and postoperative outcome of LADG (Ueda et al., 2009).

2. Patients and methods

2.1 Patients

The medical charts of 34 consecutive patients who had a preoperative diagnosis of early gastric cancer and underwent LADG in our hospital (Hamanomachi Hospital, Fukuoka, Japan) between November 2000 and November 2006 were analyzed. Three patients who underwent simultaneous LADG and cholecystectomy and one patient whose preoperative computed tomography (CT) was not performed in our hospital were excluded from the study. LADG was performed for lesions located in the antrum or body of the stomach. As the ability to perform extended lymphadenectomy is limited in LADG, the procedure was performed only for lesions thought preoperatively not to be infiltrating beyond the submucosal layer. The depth of infiltration of the lesion was assessed preoperatively using radiography, endoscopy and endoscopic ultrasonography.

2.2 Measurement of visceral and subcutaneous fat accumulation

VF and SF accumulation were quantified on preoperative abdominal CT images. The area of VF and SF tissue on cross-sectional CT at the level of the umbilicus was measured using FatScan software (N2 system corporation, Kobe, Japan) (Fig. 1A and 1B) (Yoshizumi et al., 1999). Patients were divided into high and low VF accumulation groups based on the area of VF tissue, according to the criteria for VF accumulation recommended by the Japan Society of the Study of Obesity. Patients in the high VF accumulation group had an area of VF tissue ≥ 100 cm^2, and patients in the low VF accumulation group had an area of VF tissue < 100 cm^2.

2.3 Surgical procedures

All LADGs were performed with 4 or 5 trocars under a pneumoperitoneum of 8 - 12 mmHg. Operative techniques consisted of the following procedures as described in other papers (Noshiro et al., 2005; Kitano et al., 2007): 1) laparoscopic dissection of the lesser and greater omentum, and ligation and division of the vessels to mobilize the stomach, 2) resection of the distal two-thirds of the stomach with D1+α, D1+β, or D2 lymph node dissection based on the Guidelines of the Japan Gastric Cancer Association, and 3) Billroth I reconstruction through a 5-8cm minilaparotomy incision.

2.4 Statistical analysis

We obtained the following clinical data from medical charts: age, sex, concurrent illnesses, tumor characteristics, operation time, operative blood loss, number of dissected lymph nodes, time to first flatus, time to resumed food intake, length of fever, white blood cell count, serum C-reactive protein (CRP) level and postoperative complications. Values were expressed as mean ± SD. Correlation between the area of fat accumulation and operative difficulties was analyzed by Pearson's correlation test. Differences between the two groups of patients were analyzed by either Student t-test or X^2 test. All statistical analyses were performed with StatView 5.0 software (SAS Institute, Cray, CA). A P value of < 0.05 was considered statistically significant.

3. Results

3.1 Correlation between fat accumulation and operative difficulty

To investigate the effect of fat accumulation on the technical difficulty of performing LADG, the correlation between fat accumulation and operation time was analyzed. The area of VF

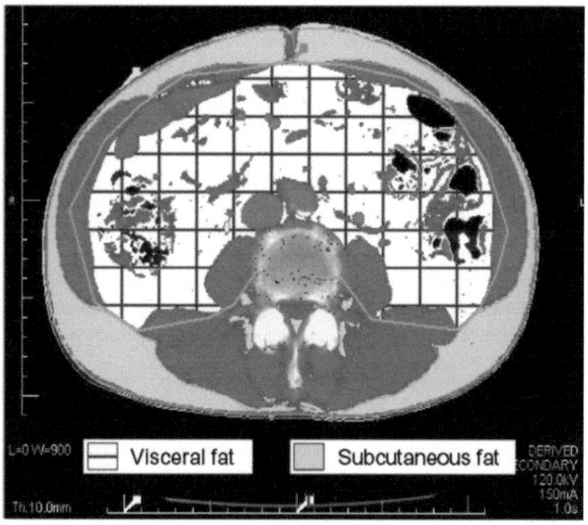

Fig. 1a.

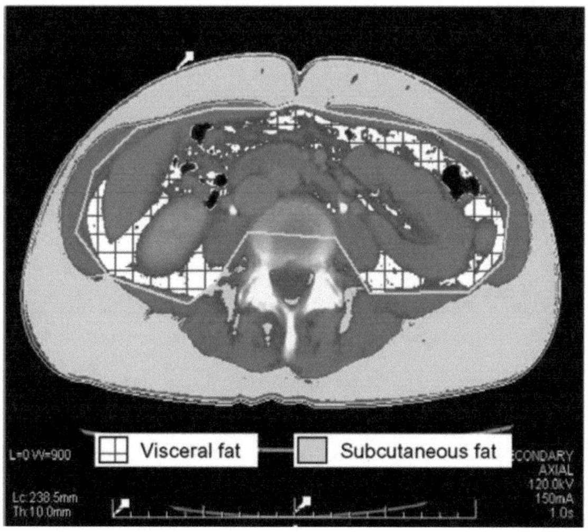

Fig. 1b.

tissue was strongly and significantly correlated with operation time (P = 0.002, R^2 = 0.285, Fig. 2A), but the area of SF tissue was not correlated with operation time (P = 0.229, R^2 = 0.052, Fig. 2B). The correlation between fat accumulation and operative blood loss was also analyzed. The area of VF tissue was strongly and significantly correlated with operative blood loss (P = 0.0003, R^2 = 0.365, Fig. 2C), but the area of SF tissue was not significantly correlated with operative blood loss (P = 0.060, R^2 = 0.120, Fig. 2D). These findings suggest that VF accumulation rather than SF accumulation may be a risk factor in LADG. Because BMI has commonly been used as a marker of obesity, the correlation between BMI and operation time or operative blood loss was also analyzed. BMI was significantly correlated with both operation time and operative blood loss (P = 0.044, R^2 = 0.138, and P = 0.042, R^2 = 0.139, respectively) (Fig. 2E and 2F). VF accumulation was, however, much more strongly correlated with both operation time and operative blood loss than BMI. These data suggest that VF accumulation may be strongly associated with operative difficulty in LADG.

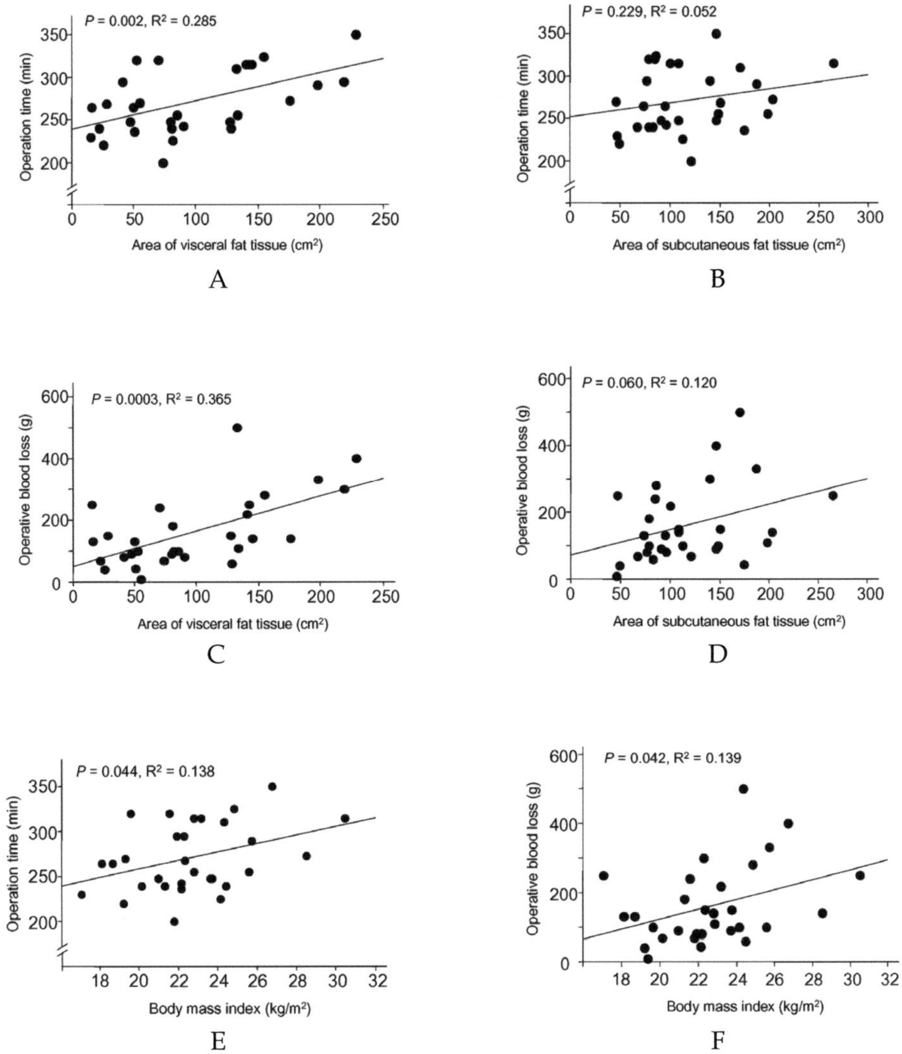

Fig. 2.

3.2 The impact of VF accumulation on operative difficulty and outcome of LADG

To confirm the impact of VF accumulation on LADG, patients were divided into high VF accumulation (160.4 ± 35.9 cm^2) and low VF accumulation (53.9 ± 24.9 cm^2) groups. Operative difficulties, operation time, operative blood loss, number of dissected lymph nodes, time to first flatus, time to food intake, duration of fever (> 37.5℃), white blood cell count on day 1 and 7, serum CRP level on day 1 and 7, postoperative complications, and conversion to laparotomy were compared between the two groups. Age, concurrent illnesses, tumor location, tumor size, tumor type, depth of tumor infiltration, and lymph node metastases were similar between the groups. The male to female ratio was significantly higher in the high VF accumulation group than the low VF accumulation group (Table 1).

The operative outcomes are given in Table 2. Operation time was significantly longer in the high VF accumulation group than the low VF accumulation group (294 ± 34 minutes versus 255 ± 32 minutes, P = 0.003). Operative blood loss was also significantly higher in the high VF accumulation group than the low VF accumulation group (240 ± 129 g versus 109 ± 64 g, P = 0.001). There was no significant difference in the number of dissected lymph nodes, time to first flatus, time to food intake and duration fever between the groups. White blood cell count on day 7 and serum CRP level on day 1 and 7 were significantly higher in the high VF accumulation group than the low VF accumulation group. The frequency of postoperative complications and conversion to laparotomy was not significantly different between the groups, but major complications (anastomotic leakage) and conversion to laparotomy occurred only in the high VF accumulation group. There were no recurrences or deaths due to cancer during the follow-up period (range: 8 - 75 months, mean: 32 months).

4. Discussion

The present study showed a significantly longer operation time and significantly more operative blood loss in patients with high VF accumulation than with low VF accumulation. However, time to first flatus, time to food intake, duration of fever elevation and postoperative complications were similar in the two groups. There were no operative deaths or requirements for blood transfusion in either group. These results suggest that LADG is as safe and beneficial for patients with high VF accumulation as for patients with low VF accumulation.

In Japan, dietary changes favoring Western eating habits may have resulted in an increased rate of obesity in the population. BMI has been increasing in Japanese patients with gastric cancer (Kubo et al., 2005). Obesity is characterized by an excess of fat accumulation, and VF accumulation has been reported to be associated with obesity-related diseases such as cardiovascular disease, diabetes and hypertension (Fujioka et al., 1987; Kanai et al., 1990; Despres & Lemieux, 2006). VF accumulation may also be of great interest to surgeons, who consider excess fat accumulation to be a risk factor because of the limited visualization of surgical fields and increased difficulty of dissecting vessels. In this study, both operation time and operative blood loss were strongly correlated with VF accumulation, even though VF accumulation did not affect the operative death rate or postoperative complication rate. Our data suggests that VF accumulation may be a risk factor for operative difficulty in LADG. Two procedures were converted to open laparotomy, one because of difficulty isolating the root of the right gastroepiploic vessels in abundant fatty tissue, and the other because of difficulty in performing appropriate lymphadenectomy around the common hepatic vessels due to abundant fatty tissue. It is also recently reported that visceral fat accumulation increase operation time in laparoscopic resection of a rectosigmoid carcinoma (Seki et al., 2007). These data strongly supports the surgical opinion that VF accumulation is a risk factor in laparoscopic surgery.

Although the obese population is increasing, severely obese patients are still uncommon in Japan compared to Europe and the United States. None of the patients in our study were severely obese, with the maximum BMI being 31 kg/m^2 and the maximum VF being 230 cm^2. VF accumulation in severely obese patients may affect postoperative complications.

The effect of VF accumulation in severely obese patients undergoing LADG should be further investigated.

Interestingly, the postoperative CRP and white blood cell count were significantly higher in the high VF accumulation group than the low VF accumulation group. VF accumulation is considered to contribute to systemic inflammation (Lyon et al., 2003). It has been shown recently that adipose tissue secretes inflammatory cytokines such as tumor necrosis factor-alpha (TNF-α) and interleukin 6 (IL-6), and that IL-6 production by human adipose tissue increases with obesity (Ronti et al., 2006). Gletsu et al. demonstrated recently that IL-6 content in adipose tissue increased dramatically after laparoscopic surgery, especially in VF tissue, and that plasma IL-6 concentration is strongly correlated with IL-6 content in adipose tissue (Gletsu et al., 2006). Our data suggests that VF accumulation may play an important role in postoperative inflammation after LADG.

5. Conclusions

In conclusion, LADG for the treatment of early gastric cancer is as safe and beneficial for patients with high VF accumulation as for patients with low VF accumulation. VF accumulation may, however, be a risk factor in LADG because VF accumulation had a strong correlation with both operation time and operative blood loss. VF accumulation should be considered as a possible risk factor when making the decision to perform LADG.

6. References

Adachi Y. et al. (2000). Laparoscopy-assisted Billroth I gastrectomy compared with conventional open gastrectomy. *Arch Surg* 135(7):806-10.

Despres JP & Lemieux I. (2006) Abdominal obesity and metabolic syndrome. *Nature* 444(7121):881-7.

Dhar DK. et al. (2000). Body mass index determines the success of lymph node dissection and predicts the outcome of gastric carcinoma patients. *Oncology* 2000; 59(1): 18-23.

Fujioka S. et al. (1987). Contribution of intra-abdominal fat accumulation to the impairment of glucose and lipid metabolism in human obesity. *Metabolism* 36(1): 54-9.

Gletsu N. et al. (2006). Increased plasma interleukin 6 concentrations and exaggerated adipose tissue interleukin 6 content in severely obese patients after operative trauma. *Surgery* 140(1):50-7

Inagawa S. et al. (2000). Effect of fat volume on postoperative complications and survival rate after D2 dissection for gastric cancer. *Gastric Cancer* 3(3):141-144.

Kadowaki T. et al. (2006). Japanese men have larger areas of visceral adipose tissue than Caucasian men in the same levels of waist circumference in a population-based study. *Int J Obes* 30(7):1163-5.

Kanai H. et al. (1990). Close correlation of intra-abdominal fat accumulation to hypertension in obese women. *Hypertension* 16(5):484-90.

Kanazawa M. et al. (2005). Criteria and classification of obesity in Japan and Asia-Oceania. *World Rev Nutr Diet* 94:1-12.

Kim KH. et al. (2006). The impact of obesity on LADG for early gastric cancer. Gastric *Cancer* 9(4):303-7.

Kitano S. et al. (2002) A randomized controlled trial comparing open vs laparoscopy-assisted distal gastrectomy for the treatment of early gastric cancer: an interim report. *Surgery* 131(1 Suppl):S306-11.

Kitano S.et al. (2007) A multicenter study on oncologic outcome of laparoscopic gastrectomy for early cancer in Japan. *Ann Surg* 245(1):68-72.

Kubo M. et al. (2005) Increasing body mass index in Japanese patients with gastric cancer. *Gastric Cancer* 8(1):39-41.

Leroy J. et al. (2005) The impact of obesity on technical feasibility and postoperative outcomes of laparoscopic left colectomy. *Ann Surg* 241(1):69-76.

Lyon CJ. et al. (2003) Minireview: adiposity, inflammation, and atherogenesis. *Endocrinology* 144(6):2195-200.

Noshiro H. et al. (2003) Laparoscopy-assisted distal gastrectomy for early gastric cancer: is it beneficial for patients of heavier weight? *Ann Surg* 238(5):680-5.

Noshiro H. et al. (2005) Laparoscopically assisted distal gastrectomy with standard radical lymph node dissection for gastric cancer. *Surg Endosc* 19(12):1592-6.

Ogden CL. et al. (2006) Prevalence of overweight and obesity in the United States, 1999-2004. Jama 295(13):1549-55.

Ronti T. et al. (2006) The endocrine function of adipose tissue: an update. Clin Endocrinol 64(4):355-65.

Shimizu S. et al. (2000) Laparoscopically assisted distal gastrectomy for early gastric cancer: is it superior to open surgery? *Surg Endosc* 14(1):27-31.

Shimizu S. et al. (2003) Laparoscopic gastric surgery in a Japanese institution: analysis of the initial 100 procedures. *J Am Coll Surg* 197(3):372-8.

Senagore AJ. et al. (2003) Laparoscopic colectomy in obese and nonobese patients. *J Gastrointest Surg* 7(4):558-61.

Seki Y. et al. (2007) Evaluation of the technical difficulty performing laparoscopic resection of a rectosigmoid carcinoma: visceral fat reflects technical difficulty more accurately than body mass index. *Surg Endosc* 21(6):929-34.

Tanaka S. et al. (2003) Ethnic differences in abdominal visceral fat accumulation between Japanese, African-Americans, and Caucasians: a meta-analysis. *Acta Diabetol* 40 Suppl 1:S302-4.

Tsukada K. et al. (2004) Body fat accumulation and postoperative complications after abdominal surgery. *Am Surg* 70(4):347-51.

Ueda J. et al. (2009) The impact of visceral fat accumulation on laparoscopy-assisted distal gastrectomy for early gastric cancer. *J Laparoendosc Adv Surg Tech* 19(2): 157-62.

Yasuda K. et al. (2004) Laparoscopy-assisted distal gastrectomy for early gastric cancer in obese and nonobese patients. *Surg Endosc* 18(8):1253-6.

Yoshiike N. et al. (2002) Epidemiology of obesity and public health strategies for its control in Japan. *Asia Pac J Clin Nutr* 11 Suppl 8:S727-31.

Yoshizumi T. et al. (1999) Abdominal fat: standardized technique for measurement at CT. *Radiology* 211(1):283-6.

14

Small Bowel Obstruction After Laparoscopic Roux – En - Y Gastric Bypass

Hugo Sánchez and Miguel F Herrera
The Obesity clinic. ABC Medical Center
México

1. Introduction

Obesity is an important health problem that has almost reached epidemic proportions. Morbid obesity, defined as body mass index (BMI) ≥ 40kg/m^2 leads to a number of chronic-degenerative diseases with high morbidity, mortality, and costs of health care services. Conservative treatment has an elevated average of failure, being Bariatic surgery the best treatment. Surgical treatment results in sustained weight loss and control of co morbidities. (Sjöström, 2004; Buchwald, 2004). The Laparoscopic Roux-en-Y Gastric Bypass (LRYGB) is one of the most commonly performed bariatric procedures. Although the risk-benefit balance is highly favorable, it is important for the people in the field to be aware, understand and prevent potential complications. The aim of this chapter focuses on one of the potential complications of the LRYGB which is small bowel obstruction (SBO).

2. General characteristics of the LRYGB

This procedure was originally described by Masson and cols. in the 60's, based on the observation that patients who underwent gastrectomy presented weight loss. From the beginning it was found that factors such as size of the gastric pouch, diameter of the gastrojejunostomy, and length of the alimentary limb had an impact on the amount of weight loss.
Surgical steps include:

1. Construction of a divided small gastric pouch along the lesser curvature, and
2. A small Roux-en Y gastrojejunostomy and a standard side to side jejunojejunostomy.

Although there are several technical variations, volume of the gastric pouch is intended to be close to 30cc, length of the alimentary limb approximately 1m and length of the biliopancreatic limb ≤ 50cm.
Physiologic changes involved in the RYGB include:

- Early satiety due to the small size of the gastric pouch and elevation of the PYY in the lower part of the bowel.
- Delay in the gastric empting as a result of the small diameter of the gastrojejunostomy, resulting in persistent satiety.
- Decrease of appetite as a consequence of reduction of the levels of Grhelin in the excluded stomach.

- Reduction of the intestinal absorption as a result of the shortening of the small bowel by 1,5m or more.
- Intolerance to meals with high content of carbohydrates and fat.

Among the many advantages of laparoscopic surgery in general, one is the reduction in adhesions which is a known factor for the development of SBO. LRYGB has demonstrated to improve patient recovery, to reduce postoperative pain, to diminish abdominal wall related problems but to increase the number of SBO from internal hernias. (Nguyen ,2004; Champion, 2007). When performing a LRYGB, the alimentary limb can be brought up in an antecolic or retrocolic fashion. In both techniques it is important to realize that there are some potential defects where the small bowel may be introduced producing an internal hernia. As it is shown in Figures 2 and 3, the mesenteric defect at the jejuno-jejunostomy takes place in both techniques, there is also a space between the alimentary limb and the mesocolon in both, and in the retrocolic fashion, the opening at the mesocolon is added as a potential defect.

3. Small bowel obstruction from internal hernias

In Figures 4 and 5, the way how a loop of small bowel can herniate through both the mesenteric defect at the jejunojejunostomy and the Petersen's space are shown. As we can presume, the major risk for an internal hernia is to leave the spaces open. However, it has been demonstrated that in some patients after significant weight loss, the intraabdominal fat

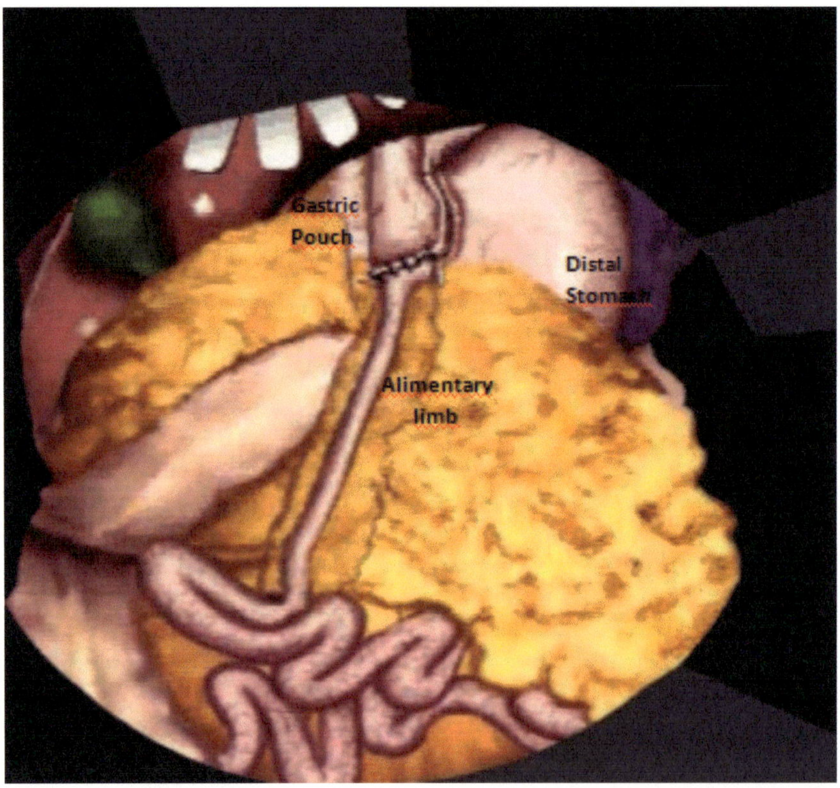

Fig. 1. Antecolic and antegastric LRYGB.

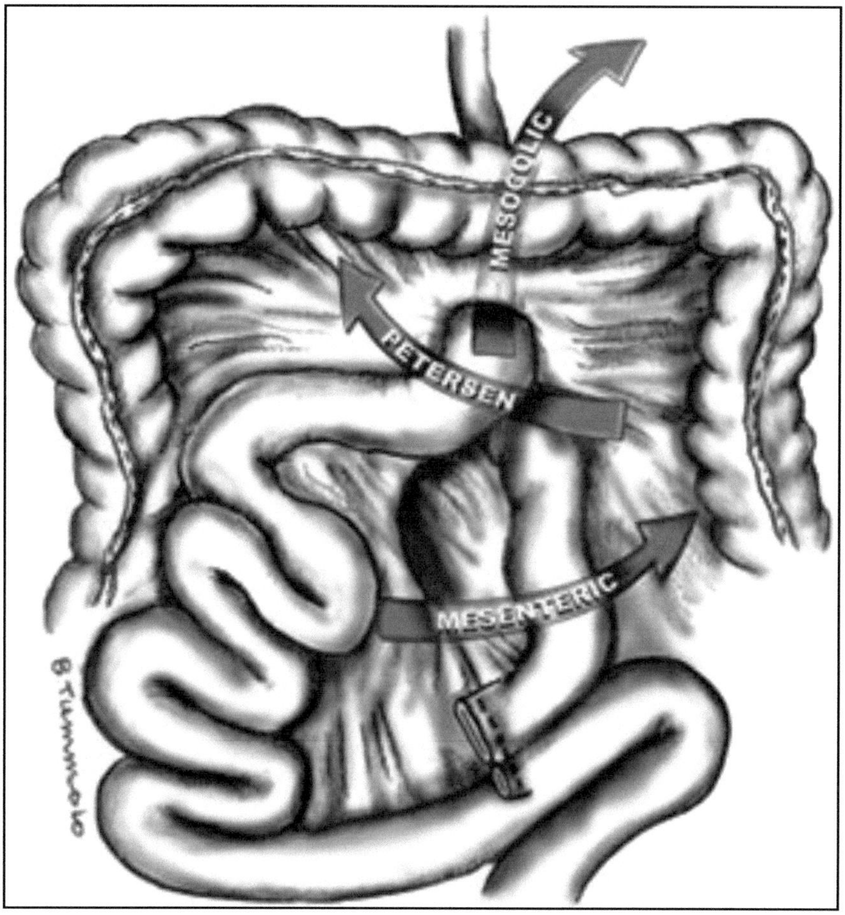

Fig. 2. Mesenteric potential defects. Retrocolic RYGBP (from Capella RF,Lannace VA, Capella JF. Bowel Obstruction after Open and Laparoscopic Gastric Bypass Surgery for Morbid Obesity. J Am Coll Surg 2006; 203:328-335.)

tissue is also significantly reduced and the defects may be reopened. Small bowel obstruction in these patients has some peculiarities. Significant amount of small bowel can be introduced in the defect before symptoms appear. In many cases, the clinical feature becomes evident until the jejunojejunostomy passes through the defect. This has as a consequence that patients may experience nonspecific symptoms for long time or that symptomatic periods can be intermittent.

4. Clinical presentation

The most important symptom in patients experiencing small bowel obstruction after a RYGB is severe abdominal pain induced by food intake. Pain is associated to nausea but vomit is very rare. Some patients refer a history of repetitive episodes of abdominal discomfort that are resolved without medical management or with minimum dose of analgesics/antispasmodics. Opposite to the clinical feature of intestinal occlusion in non bariatric patients, bloating is rarely present.

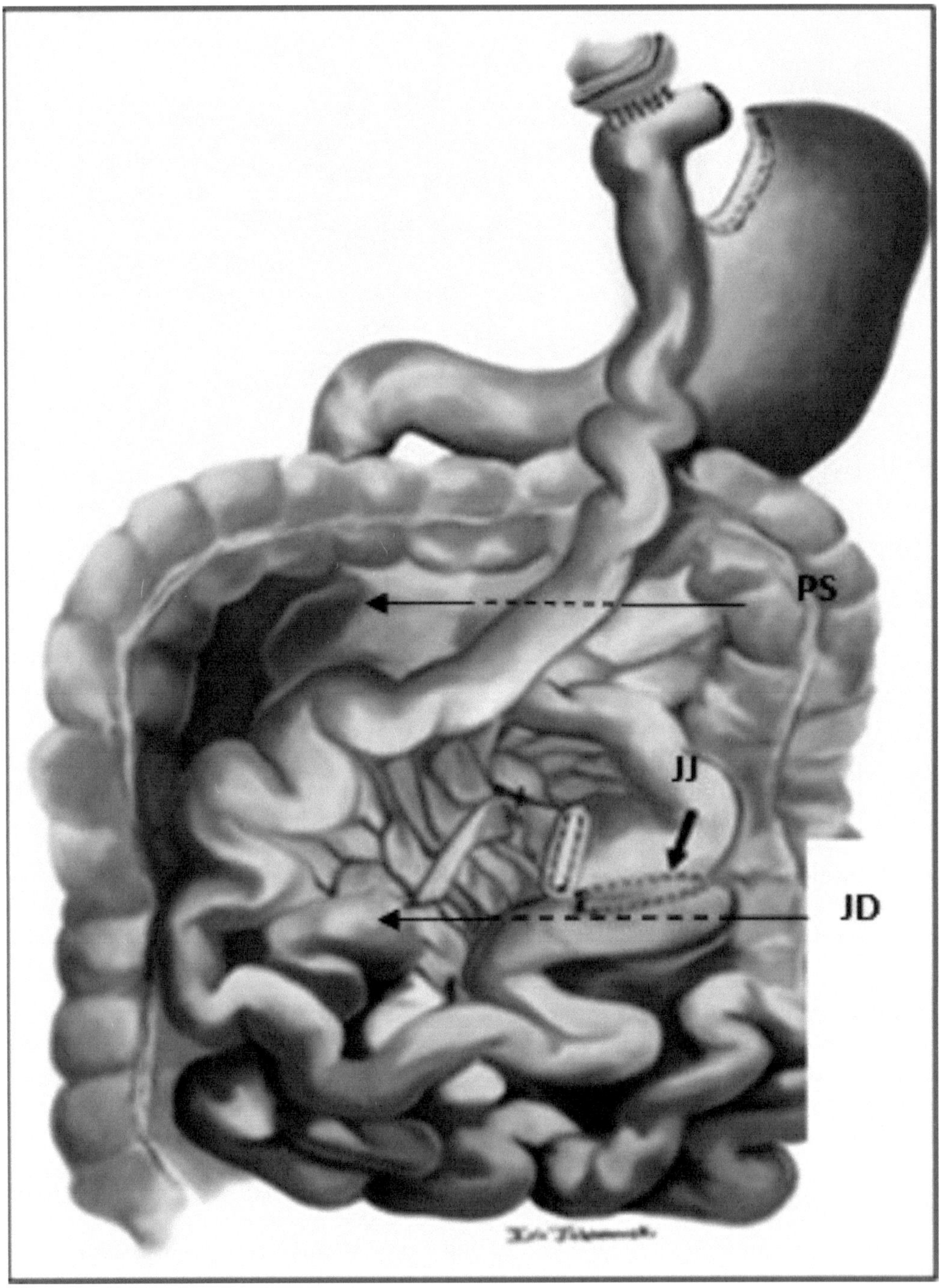

Fig. 3. Mesenteric potential defects. Antecolic RYGBP. PS Petersen´s defect. JJ jejuno-jejunostomy. JD Jejunal mesenteric defect (From Blachar A. Gastrointestinal complications of laparoscopic Roux-en-Y gastric bypass surgery: clinical and imaging findings. Radiology 2002; 223: 625-632)

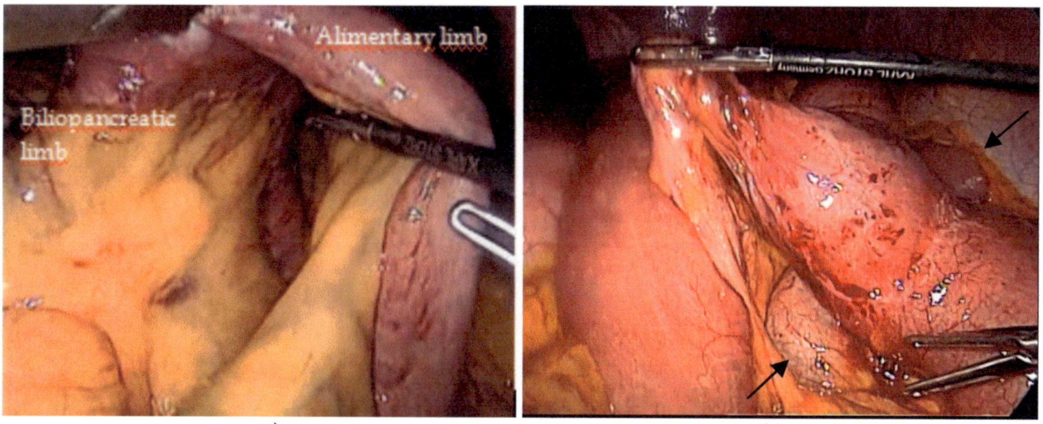

a) b)

Fig. 4. a. Surgical view of the mesenteric defect at the jejunojejunostomy. b. A loop of the common limb (arrows) is herniated into the mesenterium of the jejunojejunostomy

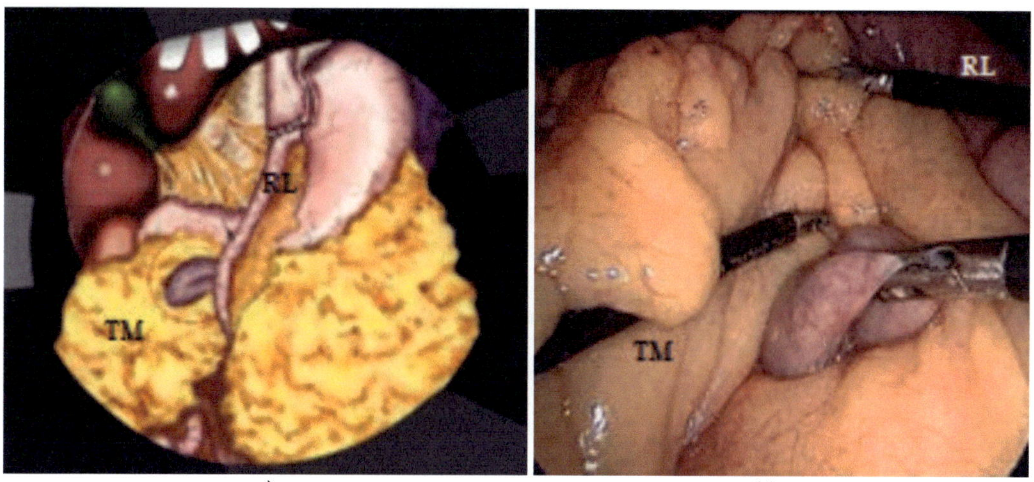

a) b)

Fig. 5. a and b. A loop of small bowel is herniated through the Petersen´s space. (TM Transverse mesocolon, RL Roux limb)

According to the limb that gets obstructed, the clinical characteristics may be different. Cho and colleagues for example have divided SBO into 3 types (Figure 6). In Type I, the intestinal segment blocked is the alimentary limb, and because it is not connected to the bilio-pancreatic fluids, patients vomit only gastric juice and food remnants without bile content. In the Type II, the biliopancreatic limb is obstructed. Clinically there is no abdominal distention and radiological findings rarely show air-fluid levels; a contrast gastrointestinal series shows progression of radiological contrast along the entire small bowel up to the colon. The diagnosis is made on the basis of a high medical suspicion, a big air bubble in the left upper quadrant or by CT scan. Fortunately this type of hernia is very rare. The most common small bowel obstruction is Type III. Obstruction on any segment along the common channel occurs and the clinical picture is very similar to the classic bowel obstruction due to adhesions. The clinical features include abdominal pain, bloating, nausea and vomiting. Multiple air-fluid levels are seen on X-rays and there is also enlargement of the gastric remnant. The diagnosis is established through the clinical feature and radiological studies including abdominal x-ray, contrasted upper gastrointestinal series and CT scan.

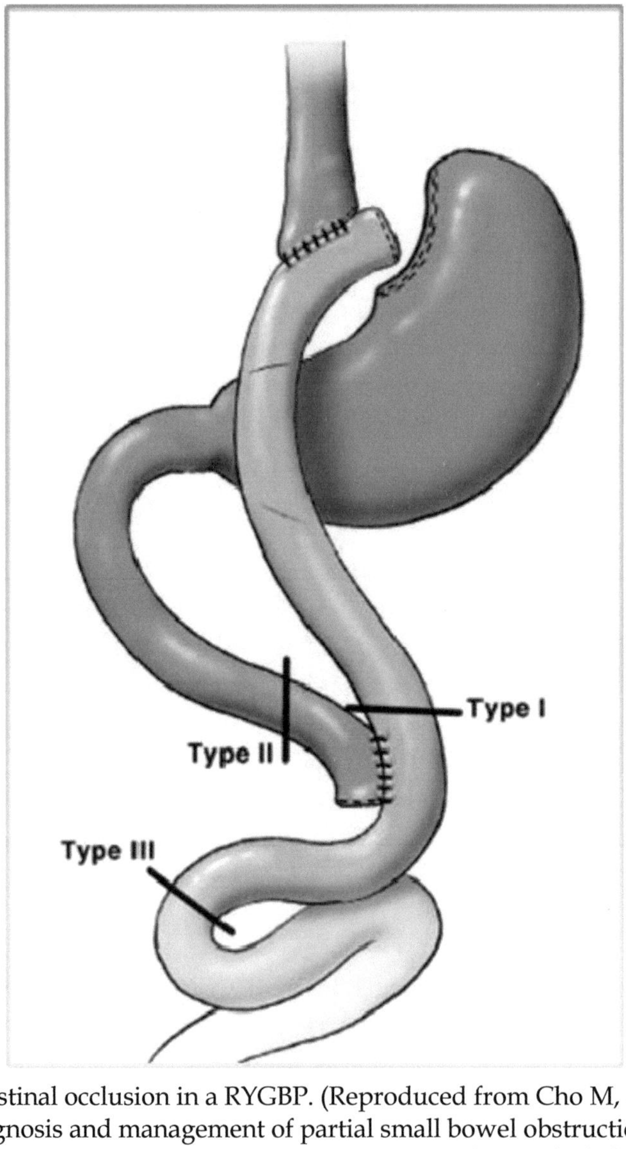

Fig. 6. Sites of intestinal occlusion in a RYGBP. (Reproduced from Cho M, Carrodeguas L, Pinto D, et al. Diagnosis and management of partial small bowel obstruction after laparoscopic antecolic antegastric Roux-en-Y gastric bypass for morbid obesity. J Am Coll Surg. 2006; 202:262 - 268).

For the diagnosis of SBO it is very important a complete clinical history and physical exam. Patients undergoing a RYGBP may present other medical conditions causing abdominal pain such as gastric ulcer, marginal ulcer, gallstones, irritable bowel syndrome, etc. Once other causes of abdominal pain are ruled out, a plain abdominal X-ray may help with the diagnosis. In Fig 7, radiological characteristics of SBO are shown. Multiple air-fluid levels and dilation of bowel loops proximal to obstruction are highly suggestive of intestinal obstruction. The most sensitive and specific radiologic test to confirm the diagnosis is an abdominal CT (Iannuccilli, 2009). A gastrographin upper gastrointestinal series may be used as an alternative (Fig 8). It is important to highlight however, that in up to 20% of the patients the diagnosis cannot be established before surgery (Hwang, 2004; Higa, 2003).

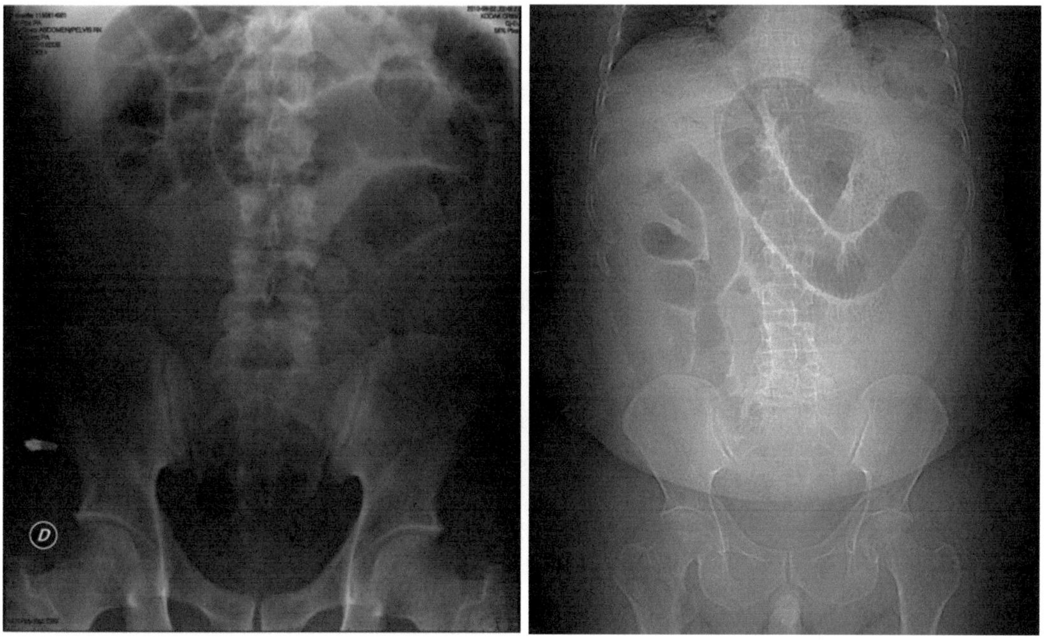

Fig. 7. Plain abdominal X-ray films showing a proximal small bowel obstruction after a LRYGB. An internal hernia at the mesenteric defect of the jejunojejunostomy was confirmed at surgery

Radiological signs of small bowel obstruction on CT are:

- Dilatation of the small bowel proximal to the obstruction with multiple air-fluid levels.
- Normal or collapsed bowel distal to the obstruction.
- The "mushroom sign" which is the result of the herniated mesenteric root through the jejunojejunostomy defect, bordered by the superior mesenteric artery and distal mesenteric branches. (Fig 9a)
- The mesenteric swirl sign. Due to twisting of mesenteric vessels and fat around the mesenteric artery.
- A jujunojeunostomy displaced to the right side of the midline which suggests torsion of the mesenteric root. (In the normal situation the jejunojejunostomy is located on the left side of the abdomen. (Fig 9b)
- Loops of small bowel clustered at the left lower quadrant.
- The hurricane eye sign created by mesenteric fat surrounded by tightly packed bowel loops.(Fig 10 a)
- Multiple enlarged lymph nodes clustered together within the mesentery around a central vascular axis. (Fig 10 b)

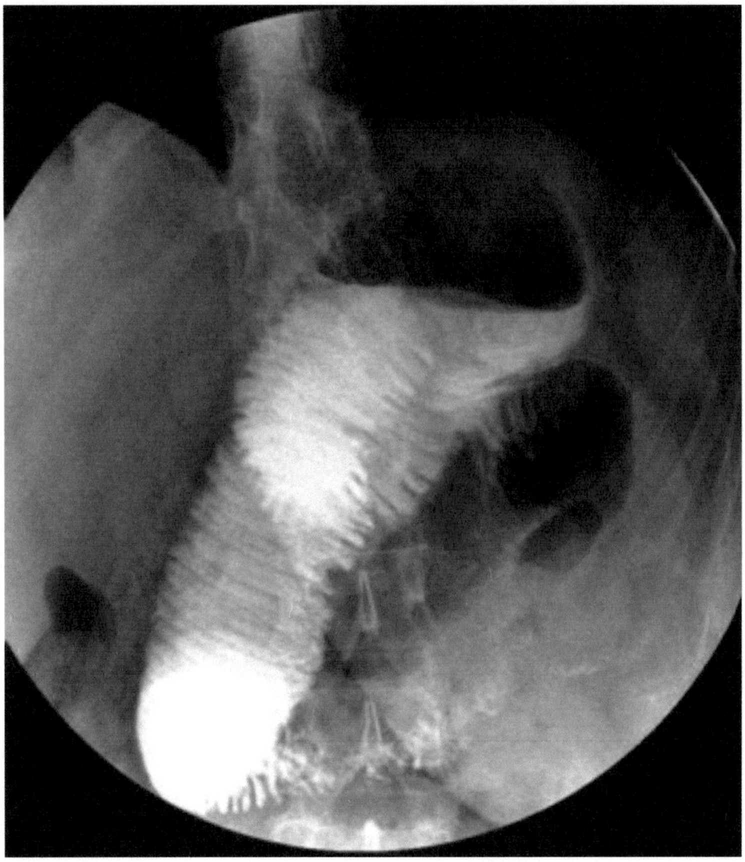

Fig. 8. Gastrographin upper gastroinestinal study showing small bowel obstruction in a patient with internal hernia at the jejunojejunostomy

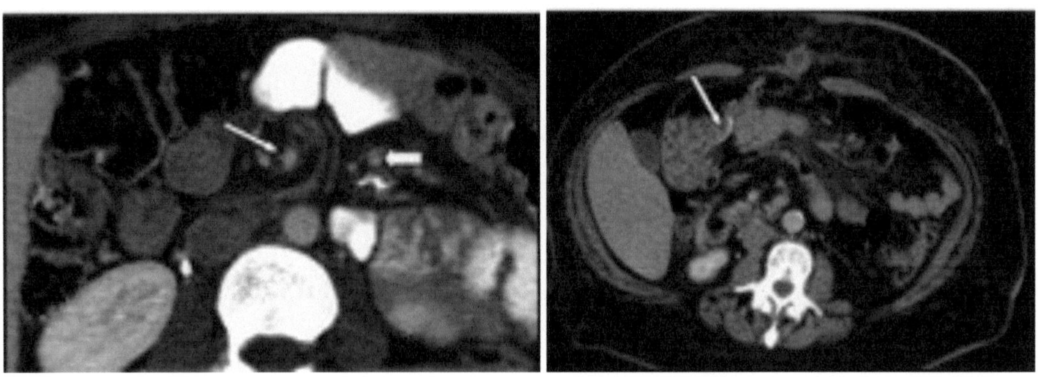

a) b)

Fig. 9. Signs of SBO on CT. a) The mushroom sign. Note the mesenteric root passing through the jejuno-jejunostomy defect, bordered by the superior mesenteric artery (thin arrow) and the distal mesenteric branches (thick arrow). b) The jejunojejunostomy is displaced to the right side of the abdomen. (arrow)

(Reproduced from Iannuccilli J, Grand D, Murphy B et al. Sensitivity and specificity of eight CT signs in the preoperative diagnosis of internal mesenteric hernia following Roux-en-Y gastric bypass surgery. Clinical Radiology 2009; 64: 373-380.)

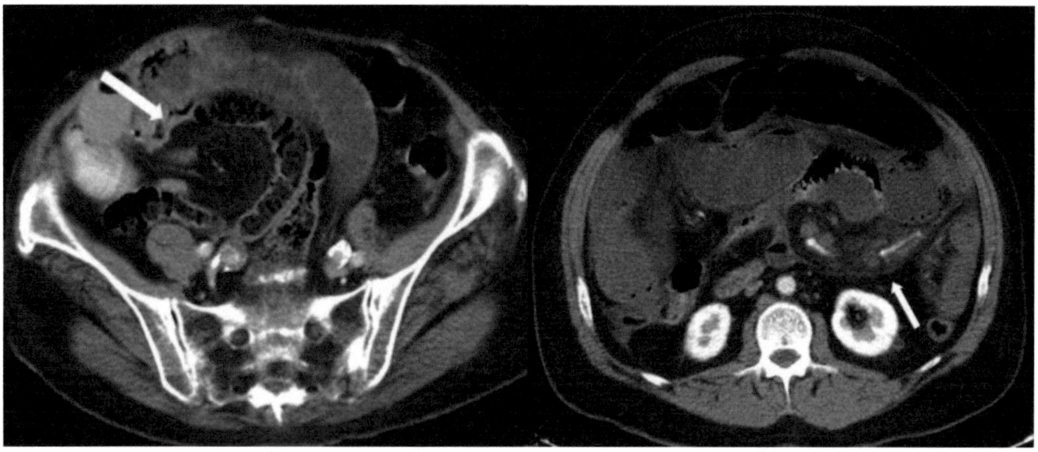

a) b)

Fig. 10. CT scans showing a) the Hurricane sign (arrow) and b) enlargement of lymph nodes (arrow)

In a patient with history of a RYGBP who present with abdominal pain associated to abdominal bloating, nausea, vomiting and radiological findings suggestive of small bowel obstruction, the diagnosis is very easy. However, patients with episodic abdominal pain and no radiological findings may represent a real challenge. Because untreated internal hernias have a potentially high risk of complications, diagnostic by laparoscopy is recommended in those patients. (Pitt, 2008)

5. Management

Initial management of patients with SBO includes proper assessment and reposition of fluids and electrolytes. A nasojejuneal tube may be needed for decompression in order to ameliorate the pain and to reduce the risk of bronchial aspiration at the time for surgery. Prophylactic antibiotics are highly recommended to prevent infections from bacterial translocation.

Once the diagnosis is established, surgical management is the only therapeutic option. The time between the diagnosis and surgery must be just the necessary to stabilize the patient, to get pain control and take care of additional problems that may be present such as severe hyperglycemia in diabetics.

Most patients may be treated by laparoscopy. Rapid sequence intubation is preferred in most patients. In the authors experience (Rodriguez & Herrera, 2010) the first step during the systematic surgical exploration is to explore Petersen's space by lifting the mesocolon on the right side of the alimentary limb. A loop of bowel protruding behind the alimentary limb makes the diagnosis of a Petersen's hernia. To assess the jejunojejunostomy, identification of the distal ileum is recommended. Once the ileocecal valve is identified, the small bowel is run between forceps all the way up. A cluster of dilated small bowel loops above the mesocolon in a patients in whom the RYGP was performed retrocolic, makes the diagnosis of hernia through the mesocolic defect. Any bowel herniation must be reduced by gentle traction using atraumatic forceps and the defects should be closed using non-absorbable sutures. All potential sites for obstruction should be explored and all open defects must be closed even in the absence of an overt hernia. Figure 10 shows a hernia through the Petersen's space and proper closure of the defect after the hernia was reduced. In figure 11, a hernia through the mesenterium at the jejunojejunostomy is shown as well as the space after closure

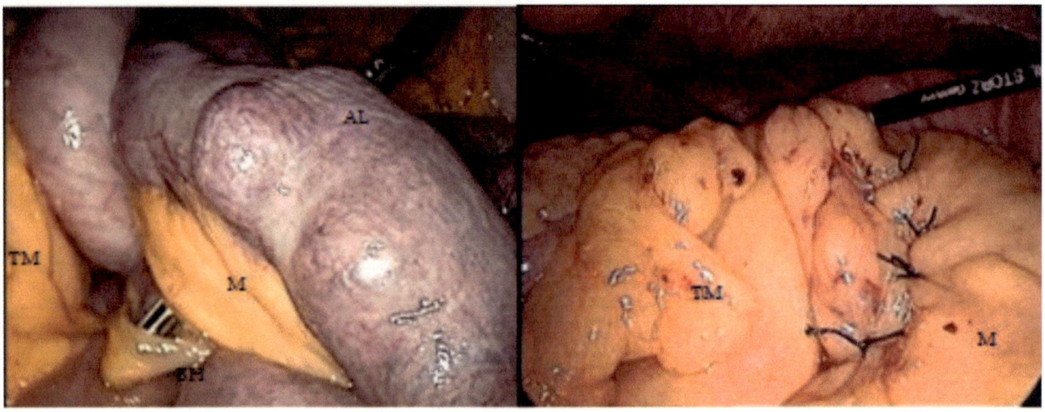

a) b)

Fig. 10. a) Hernia through the Petersen's space and b) Petersen's space properly closed. TM transverse mesocolon, M mesenterium, AL alimentary limb, BH bowel herniated.

Intestinal function usually recovers soon after surgery and patients are able to take liquid diet on the 1st postoperative day. Prokinetics may help in the process. Many patients can be discharged from the hospital within 24 hrs.

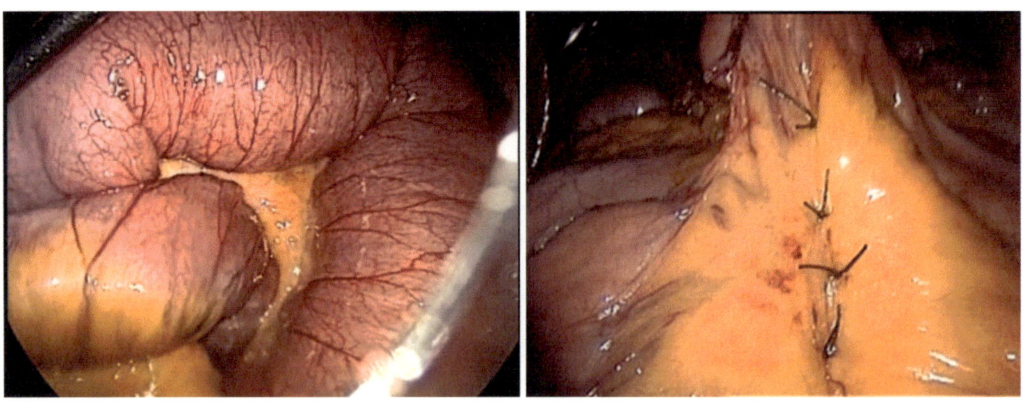

a) b)

Fig. 11. a) Internal hernia through the Jejunal mesenteric defect and b) The mesenteric defect has been closed

The reported incidence of SBO from of internal hernias has important variations in the surgical literature. In our experience, proper closure of all potential defects with non

absorbable sutures significantly reduces the incidence of internal hernias. (Rodriguez, 2010). In a recent study two different techniques in patients undergoing an antecolic and antegastric RYGB were comparatively analyzed. In the first group, the surgical technique included a wide opening of the mesentery at the level of the jejunojejunostomy and the Petersen´s space was left open. In the second group, only a small mesenteric window at the jejunojejunostomy was opened and both, the Petersen´s space and the mesenteric folds at the jejunojejunostomy were meticulously closed. The incidence of internal hernia was excessively high in the first group and it significantly dropped in the second group.
Just as in an abdominal wall defect, mesenteric defects are potential sites of SBO. Because of the peristaltic and random movement of the intestine, it is feasible that at some point a loop of small bowel may get into the defect and become obstructed. Table 1 shows the comparative analysis of SBO in different series

1st Author, year	Total No. Patients	SBO No (%)	Roux limb fashion	Internal Hernia No (%)	Jejunal defect	Petersen´s space	Trans mesocoli c defect
Higa 2003	2000	-	Retrocolic	63 (3.1)	14	5	44
Champion 2003	711	13 (1.8)	Both	6 (0.8)	1	1	4
Hwang 2004	1715	55 (3.2)	Both	17 (0.9)	8	-	9
Nguyen 2004	225	9 (4)	Retrocolic	4 (1.7)	2	-	2
Cho 2006	1400	21 (1.5)	Antecolic	3 (0.21)	-	-	-
Authors 2010	187¶	-	Antecolic	27 (14.4)	17	10	-
	172§	-	Antrecolic	2 (1.1)	2	0	-

* Transverse mesocolic hernia
¶Wide opening of jejunal mesentery and without closure of the Petersen´s defect.
§ Without wide opening of jejunal mesentery and closure of the Petersen´s defect.

Table 1. Comparative results of revision from SBO after laparoscopic gastric bypass

It is important to mention that there are other sources of SBO after LRYGB such as kinking or narrowing of the intestinal anastomosis, intussuception and adhesions. Since internal hernias are more prevalent in these patients we decided to focus on the pathogenesis, diagnosis and treatment of internal hernias. Most surgeons agree that jejunojejunostomy should be performed using at least a 45 mm stappler. In order to reduce the risk of stenosis we recommend a 60mm anastomosis with manual closure of the common enterotomy or even a larger anastomosis (90mm using double firing of a 45mm stapler) when the common opening is also stapled.
In the experience of the authors the most common site of an internal hernia when all defects were closed at the initial operation is the jejunojejunostomy.

6. Conclusions

SBO is a common complication after antecolic and antegastric LRYGB if mesenteric defects are not closed. Clinical presentation may be nonspecific, and the diagnosis frequently requires contrast imaging studies. Internal hernias can be successfully treated by laparoscopy in most patients. The occurrence of internal hernias can be significantly reduced by careful closure of the mesenteric defects.

7. References

Buchwald H, Avidor Y , Braunwald E, et al. (2004). Bariatric Surgery. A systematic review and meta-analisys. *JAMA*, vol 292, No.14, (October 2004), pp. 1724-37.

Sjöström L, Lindroos A, Peltonen M, et al. (2004). Lifestyle, Diabetes and Cardiovascular Risk Factors After Bariatric Surgery. *N Engl J Med*, vol 351, No. 26 (December 2004), pp. 2683-93.

Scopinaro N, Papadia F, Camerini G, et al.(2008) A comparison of a personal series of biliopancreatic diversion and literature data on gastric bypass help to explain the mechanisms of resolution of type 2 diabetes by the two operations. *Obes surg*, Vol 18, No.8, (August 2008), pp. 1035-8.

Buchwald H, Estok R, Fahrbach K, et al. (2009). Weight and Type 2 Diabetes after Bariatric Surgery: Systematic Review and Meta-analysis. *Am J Med* vol 122, No. 3, (March 2009), pp. 248-56.

Wittgrove AC, Clark GW. (1994) Laparoscopic gastric bypass, Roux-en-Y: preliminary report of five cases. Obes Surg ;vol 4 No.4 (april 1994) pp 353–7.

Nguyen N, Huerta S, Gelfand D, et al. (2004). Bowel obstruction after laparoscopic Roux-en-Y gastric bypass. *Obes Surg*, Vol 14, No. 2, (February 2004), pp. 190–6.

Champion JK, Williams M. (2003) Small bowel obstruction and internal hernias after laparoscopic Roux-en-Y gastric bypass. *Obes Surg*, vol 13 No4 (april 2003) pp 596–600.

Hwang RF, Swartz DE, Felix EL. (2004) Causes of small bowel obstruction after laparascopic gastric bypass. Surg Endosc. vol.18 No 11 (November 2004) pp1631-1635.

Higa KD, Tienchin H, Boone KB. (2003) Internal hernias after laparoscopic Roux-en-Y gastric bypass: incidence, treatment and prevention. Obes Surg vol 13 No. 3 (march 2003) pp350–4.

Cho M, Carrodeguas L, Pinto D, et al. (2006) Diagnosis and management of partial small bowel obstruction after laparoscopic antecolic antegastric Roux-en-Y gastric bypass for morbid obesity. J Am Coll Surg. vol. 202 No. 2 (February 2006) pp 262 - 268.

Rogers A, ionescu A, Pauli E et al. (2008) When is a Petersen´s hernia not a Petersen´s hernia. J am coll surg. Vol 207 No 1 (January 2008) pp 121-4.

Iannuccilli J, Grand D, Murphy B et al. (2009) Sensitivity and specificity of eight CT signs in the preoperative diagnosis of internal mesenteric hernia following Roux-en-Y gastric bypass surgery. Clinical Radiology vol. 64, no. 4 (april 2009) pp373-380.

Gunabushanam G, Shankar S, Donald R et al. 2009 Small-Bowel Obstruction After Laparoscopic Roux-en-Y Gastric Bypass Surgery. J Comput Assist Tomogr vol 33 No.3 (march 2009) pp 369 - 375.

Pitt T, Brethauer S, Sherman V et al. (2008) Diagnostic laparoscopy for chronic abdominal pain after gastric bypass. Surg Obes Related Dis 2008 vol, 4 No 3 pp 394-398.

Rodriguez A, Mosti M, Herrera MF et al. (2010) Small Bowel Obstruction After Antecolic and Antegastric Laparoscopic Roux-en-Y Gastric Bypass: Could the Incidence be Reduced? Obes Surg vol 20, no. 1 (November 2010) pp 1380-1384.

15

Laparoscopy and Well-Differentiated Papillary Mesothelioma of the Peritoneum

María Eugenia Aponte-Rueda, Ramón Saade-Cárdenas and Salvador Navarrete-Aulestia
Endoscopic Surgery Unit, Service of Surgery 2, Caracas University Hospital, Central University of Venezuela
Venezuela

1. Introduction

Mesothelioma, is a rare and poorly understood disease that arises from mesothelial cells lining serous cavities. From a histopathologic point of view there are epithelial, connective tissue and mixed varieties. Although commonly found in the pleura, the peritoneum is involved in 20-40% of cases.[1-5]
Well-Differentiated Papillary Mesothelioma of the Peritoneum (WDPMP) is a type of epithelial mesothelioma which typically shows benign biological behavior,[6-12] although several cases with a more aggressive form have been reported.[13-18] Being uncommon, it lacks of specific clinical and radiological manifestations,[19-21] and it is difficult to obtain precise information regarding its natural history and optimal management. The diagnosis is challenging and the delay is a component of the clinical picture of these patients. This chapter evaluates the applicability of laparoscopy when this entity is suspected.

2. Diagnosis

There is nonspecific presentation for peritoneal mesothelioma and the clinical diagnosis is difficult. Symptomatology is insidious, undefined and unspecific, but it can appear as a surgical emergency,[22-23] although usually the disease is diagnosed incidentally during a laparoscopy, done for another other reason. Generally, the patient with peritoneal mesothelioma shows up with one or two types of symptoms and signs: those with abdominal pain, usually localized and related to an abdominal mass with little or no ascites and those, without abdominal pain, but with ascites and distension.[24] A history of asbestos exposure is common in patients with pleural mesothelioma, but this association has not been firmly established in the case of the peritoneal mesothelioma.[25]
One of the clinical poorly understood aspects of this disease is the low diagnostic yield of the cytologic analysis of ascites. In a study of 51 patients with peritoneal mesothelioma, Sugarbaker et al[26] found that only two patients had a definitive diagnosis established by paracentesis of the intrabdominal fluid and the cytology. The analysis of the ascitic fluid usually reveals an exudative process, varying from clearly, mucinosous or serohematic. The cytology can be diagnostic in approximately 80% of cases with an adequate sample, but it has to be related to an abdominal mass.[27] In some cases it has been reported to be useful for

the diagnosis of Well-Differentiated Papillary Mesothelioma.[28-29] No tumor marker is reliable for diagnosis.

Peritoneal Mesothelioma does not have specific radiological characteristics. Therefore, a precise diagnosis based on imaging findings alone is not possible; in addition, distinguishing between benign and malignant processes, as well as primary and metastatic processes is also difficult (Figure 1). Lovell et al[19] found that the Computed Tomography Scan is clearly superior to the ultrasound, specifically detecting small tumoral nodules and mesenteric or peritoneal thickening. The Tomography can reveal a peritoneal enhancing soft-tissue mass within the mesentery, omentum or peritoneum thickening, multiple small nodules surrounding the peritoneum, mesentery and omentum. Other findings include ascites, infiltrating mass involving the serous of the bowels, direct invasion within the liver, spleen and abdominal wall, retroperitoneal adenopathies and metastasis at distance.[30] The pelvic involvement can suitably be evaluated by ultrasound as well as a small amount of liquid at cul-de-sac.[19] Few data has been published about the magnetic resonance imaging and PET-CT imaging manifestations. Due to no specificity in clinical characteristics and the low trust of the conventional techniques in the diagnosis of mesothelioma, the laparoscopic surgery will allow assuring the definitive diagnosis and nowadays it is preferable to laparotomy, due to lower invasiveness. Application of diagnostic laparoscopy allows direct visualization of the abdominal-pelvic peritoneum and organs, and may disclose laparoscopic characteristics, which beside the direct vision biopsy allows the diagnostic accuracy of this uncommon medical entity.

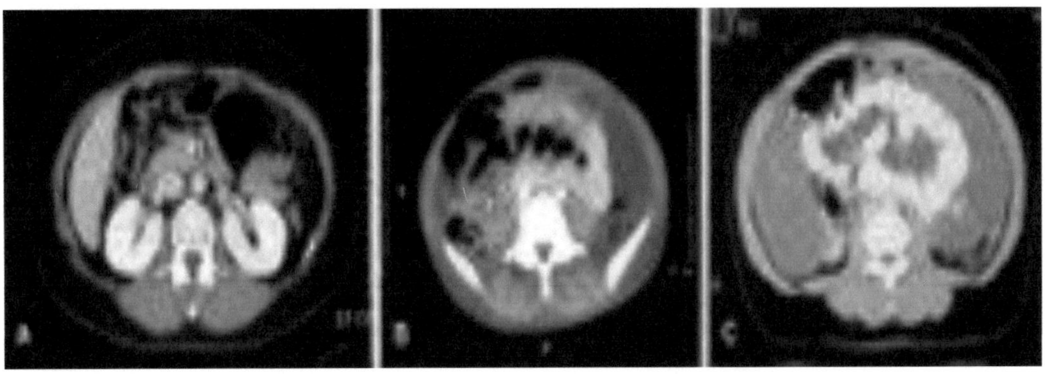

Fig. 1. Axial Contrast Abdominal-Pelvic Computer Tomography shows multiple round nodules and mesenteric and peritoneal thickening and ascites. A. WDPM (courtesy of Dr. Hyuong Sun Jang and Ki Young Ru) ,B. Peritoneal Carcinomatosis, C. Peritoneal Tuberculosis (courtesy of Dr Suárez-Grau and Dr Morales-Conde).

3. Laparoscopic surgery

The first case of peritoneal mesothelioma, involving the laparoscopic surgery and the peritoneal biopsy, was published in 1974.[31] Nowadays the diagnostic laparoscopic surgery offers a fast, safe and less invasive form to confirm the diagnosis of peritoneal mesothelioma. We must consider the laparoscopic approach as the main technique for correct visualization of the peritoneal cavity, peritoneal fluid and multiple peritoneal biopsies obtained from intra-abdominal locations, to diagnose a multitude of gastrointestinal diseases showing abdominal pain and ascites of unknown etiology. Yoon et al[39] reported a diagnostic yield of 87.2% for diagnostic laparoscopy in patients with ascites of unknown origin. Piccigallo et al[40] reported the correct diagnosis using the laparoscopic surgery and the histological examination of biopsy specimens, reaching a percentage of diagnostic security near 90%, in patients diagnosed with Malignant Peritoneal Mesothelioma. In patients with Well Differentiated Papillary Mesothelioma of the Peritoneum the laparoscopic surgery reduces the period of observation and for that reason, the repetition of examinations and other explorations, as well as avoiding the inherent complications related to laparotomy, with a more comfortable post-operative evolution by the smaller surgical trauma. Accurate diagnosis allows a precise therapy to be promptly started. The majority of authors recommend multiple biopsies with or without adjuvant therapy, instead of an extensive surgery due to its low malignant potential. We reported a case of WDPMP showing its resolution after adjuvant chemotherapy.[41]

Diagnostic laparoscopic surgery is useful for staging pleural mesothelioma[42] (although only two cases of Well Differentiated Papillary Mesothelioma, involving the peritoneal and pleural cavities, have been published).[16-43] In cases of isolated pelvic nodules it can provide anatomic information, allows definitive management and pathologic diagnosis, therefore, to diagnose and treat WDPMP the laparoscopic approach can be used effectively and safely.[21,44]

3.1 Surgical technique

The diagnostic laparoscopic surgery can be done under general anesthesia or under local anesthesia and sedation. The table essentially will be moved into: steep anti-Trendelenburg + left tild, anti-Trendelenburg + right tild, steep Trendelenburg + left tild, steep Trendelenburg + right tild during the examination to mobilize the ascitic fluid and the intestine. The surgeon and assistants are positioned on the patient's left side. The monitor is placed right to the patient´s head. The normally used instrument is a rigid endoscope with the optic connected to a cold light source, of 5 mm with a forward viewing angle of view of 0° and oblique viewing of 30°. For the exploration of the peritoneal cavity, it is necessary to create a suitable pneumoperitoneum that is induced by CO_2 insufflation, an intraabdominal pressure of 10 to 12 mm is the adopted to secure a good vision. At the same time there it is introduced a supra or transumbical trocar and the laparoscope is passed through it, inspecting the peritoneal cavity. A second and third trocar (10 mm and 5 mm, respectively) can be positioned under visual control for biopsy and introduction of accessory instruments, according to the particular requirements in each case. In order to avoid complications, it is recommended to follow carefully a entry procedure technique due to adhesions between the small bowel loops and the abdominal wall. We use a blunt tip trocar described by Hasson,[45] to enter the abdominal cavity, a small incision must be done under direct vision and the aponeurotic hole has to be adjusted by stitches to the Hasson trocar to avoid neumoperitoneum leaks.

3.2 Abdominal cavity exploration

Begin the exploration with the table in horizontal position. The presence of ascites in abdominal cavity is evaluated and its characteristics. Cytology and bacteriology samples should be taken under direct vision and finally the ascites should be completely emptied. The situation and degree of alterations must be defined.

Then, the laparoscopic exploration must follow a defined systematic plan, covering the different quadrants of the cavity (Figure 2).

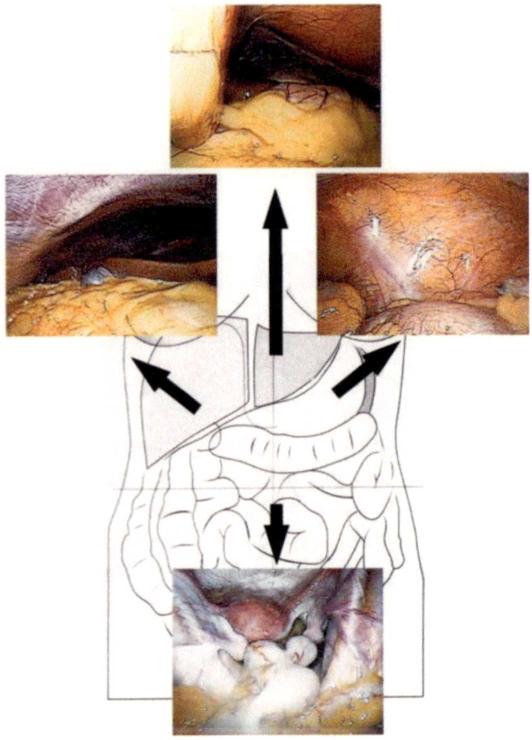

Fig. 2. Laparoscopic Exploration

Henning and Look[46] described four positions that allow a good vision of the entire peritoneal cavity; such positions can be modified according to the particular requirements of each case. In position I, it turns the table slightly (15-20^0) towards the left and raise to the head other 15-20^0. Being the explorer to the left of the patient, the laparoscope is introduced towards the right hypochondrium, which allows to observe the gallbladder, the hepatic edge, the surface of the right lobe and right side of the falciform ligament. The rotation of the optics, the variation of the intensity of the position or the cephalic elevation of the table provides a vision of the entire region.

Position II is the same as I, but laparoscope moves under the round ligament, until reaching the left hypochondrium. If the light goes towards the right, the left hepatic lobe could be observed, the left side of the falciform ligament and the diafragm. If it goes towards the left side, it could see the anterior face of the stomach and the epiploic fat.

Position III is achieved changing the position towards the right side (45^0) and lifting the head on the exploration table (40^0), with the surgeon at the right side. In this case, the spleen, the frenic and colonic ligament, good part of the anterior face of the stomach, including fornix and possibly, also the esofagic hiatus can be seen, if the gastrohepatic ligament allows it.

Position IV is to inspect the inferior quadrants (pelvic region) and the rest of intraabdominal organs. This position requires the Trendelenburg´s position, turning the table towards the side that we wish to explore. The changes from one position to another require a lateral displacement of the optic, which always must be done in the sense of the iluminated field, to avoid tears of adhesions. In this case, the monitor should be placed down and to the right side of the patient.

3.3 Laparoscopic findings

WDPMP, due to its rarity the surgeons are usually not sensitive with the disease. Laparoscopic findings of mesothelioma are indistinguishable of peritoneal tuberculosis, metastatic adenocarcinoma or primary tumour of the mesentery, from the gross standpoint, the common presentation sign of peritoneal nodules in WDPMP may lead to confusion during the diagnostic laparoscopic surgery, therefore a diagnosis is frequently difficult. However, the increased use of laparoscopic surgery to identify pathologic causes of ascitis of unknown origin, as well as pelvic pain, particularly in young women, which implies that the surgeons must be conscious of the laparoscopic characteristics of this tumor and distinguished from other common neoplasms involving the peritoneum to be enabled to properly recognize and treat the tumor.

The laparoscopic features of the Peritoneal Mesothelioma, are:[40]

a. The presence of homogeneous spreading of nodules, plaques or masses on both parietal and visceral peritoneum (Figure 3). The nodules become more confluent plaque like masses and eventually omental span is observed with the progression of the disease [41](Figure 4).

The nodules usually are:

- Heterogenous size: The size of nodules is variable. Most of them appeared to be in the range of 0.5 cm to 2.0 cm, located in the abdomen and pelvis.[18] If they appear under the form of a fine dissemination to miliar, therefore they can simulate the typical aspect of the tuberculous elements.[47] They can one or multiple be distributed by the totality of the peritoneal cavity, omentum and mesentery. Occasionally, small foci of tumor are present in the surface of the ovary[18](Figure 5).
- White color.
- Firm consistency.

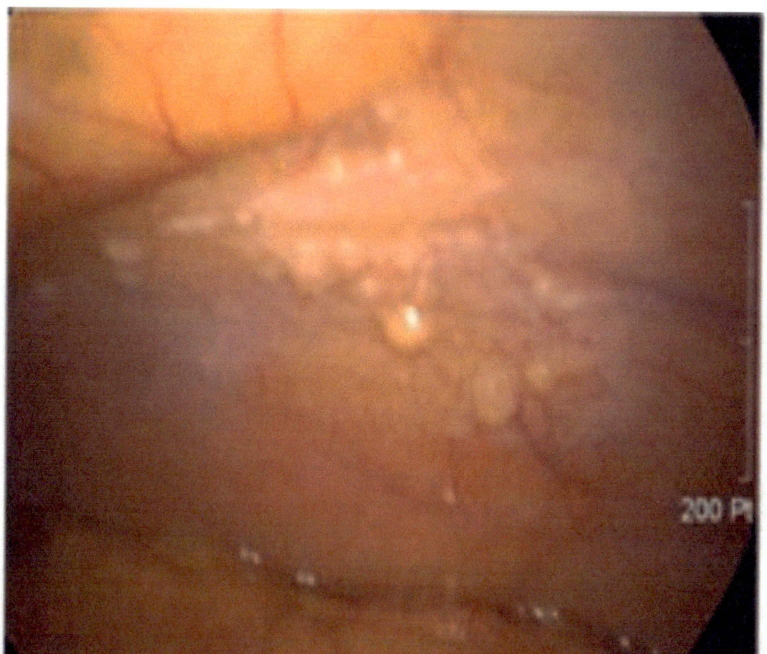

Fig. 3. Laparoscopic view of tumor whitish nodules on parietal peritoneum (courtesy of Dr. Hyuong Sun Jang and Ki Young Ru)

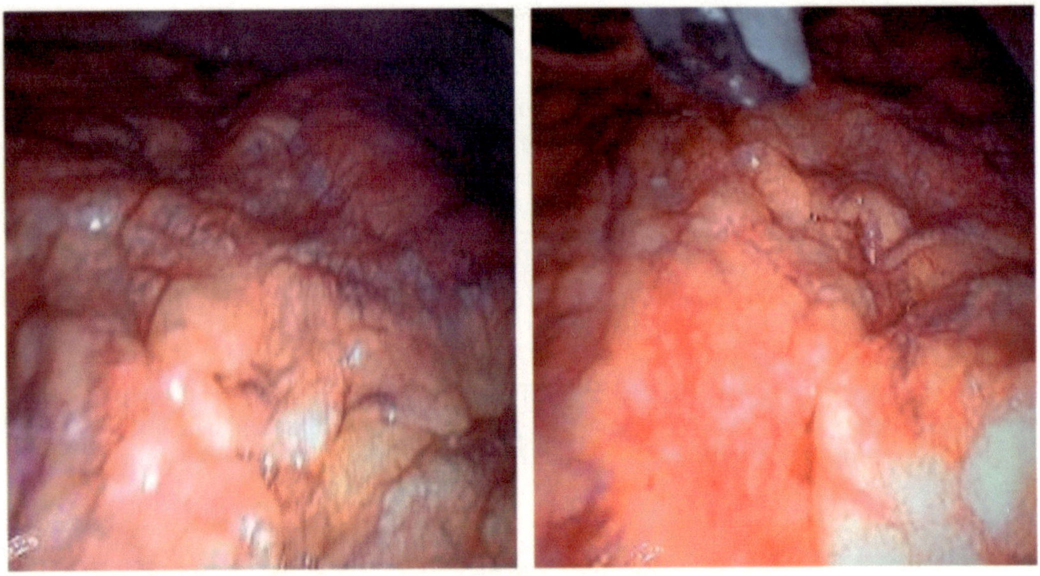

Fig. 4. Laparoscopic view of omental ¨caking¨ due to confluent nodules.

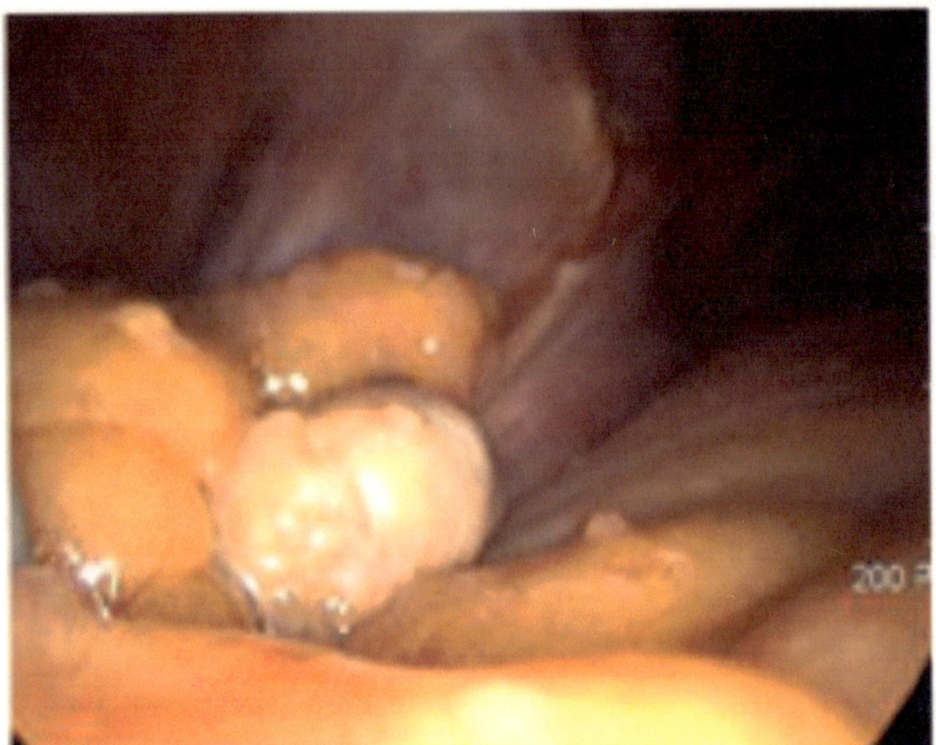

Fig. 5. Laparoscopic view of multiple nodules in the ovarian surface (courtesy of Dr. Hyuong Sun Jang and Ki Young Ru).

b. The absence of direct or indirect signs of other abdominal neoplasms.
c. The absence of hepatic metastases or the possible presence of nodules or plaques on Glisson´s capsule without parenchyma envolvement. Just in the advanced states of the disease, the tumor infiltrates the capsule of the liver with later extension within the parenchyma and retroperitoneal structures.
d. Ascites is practically constant and is variable in color from yellowish to cloudy to bloodstained. The ascitic fluid is usually serosanguinous or grossly blood-stained, but does not constitute a definitive diagnosis of peritoneal tumor.
e. Little hyperemia that extends to all the peritoneum. It serves to the gross differentiation criterion of the inflammatory form, where the parietal peritoneum is erythematous.
f. The presence of adhesions between the intestinal loops and the abdominal wall, that is typical of active tuberculosis, can in addition be seen in mesothelioma. In the case of Tuberculosis, when entering the cavity a multitude of adhesions between the different abdominal organs are present, emphasizing the hepatic adhesions[47] (Figure 6).

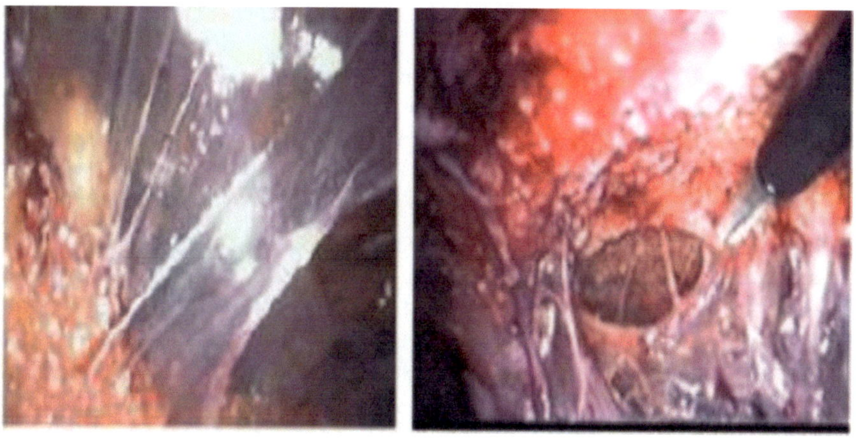

Fig. 6. Laparoscopic view of Peritoneal Tuberculosis: numerous small yellow-white nodules on the parietal peritoneum and adhesions (courtesy of Dr Suárez-Grau and Dr Morales Conde)

3.4 Biopsy

The laparoscopic surgery, in comparison with its diagnostic effectiveness, goes naturally considered as a whole and therefore not only with the inspection of the abdominal cavity, but with the biopsy for the histological diagnosis it is of extraordinary effectiveness[48] adding diagnostic accuracy, due to the following reasons:

- It can be done on several organs: Multiple biopsies of the parietal peritoneum, diaphragm, omentum and lesion of the pelvic cavity.
- It comes often on the guide from the laparoscopic, reason why it is of particular importance when the injuries are unique. The biopsy must be taken near the edges close to the nodule and the peritoneum in order to avoid the central necrosis.
- The site of the biopsy is not forced as by the transcutaneous biopsy; it can be taken with direct vision.
- The histological fragment has the sufficient quality to assure the most precise examination (Figure 7).

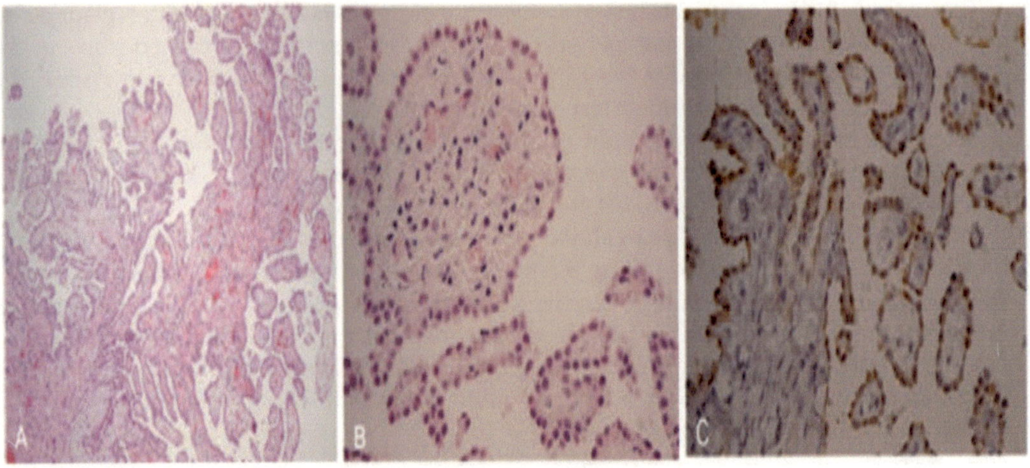

Fig. 7. Well-differentiated Papillary Mesothelioma of Peritoneum Microscopic Findings. A. Well-developed papillae lined by uniform mesothelial cells with minimal cytologic atypia. B. Neoplastic mesothelial cell shows strong positive staining for Cytokeratins. C. Inmunohistochemical staining for Calretin.

3.5 Complications

3.5.1 Tear of Adhesions

In some cases the adhesions are present, the small intestine loops tightly adherent to abdominal wall, with a careful open technique using a Hasson trocar to enter the abdominal cavity, these complications are rare. Beside, the substitution of the view field by a red veil indicates that the window of the optics has been applied on the small intestine or the adhesion; in these cases avoid to continue the movement, because it could originate a tear of the adhesions.

3.5.2 Hemorrhage

The observation of the biopsy site is a fundamental requirement to avoid any type of haemorrhagic complication. The laparoscopic biopsy is practically risk free, due to the use of coagulation to form a clot or by positioning fibrin dressings.

3.5.3 Port-site metastases

Recurrences at the insertion site of the laparoscope or other instruments for malignant mesothelioma as well as WDPMP have been reported, this source of disease usually progresses fast compared to the intraabdominal component and requires extensive surgery for the local control.[13,22,38,49] The aggressive nature of such recurrences is evident. According to Sugarbaker,[27] any invasive procedure used to establish the diagnosis of mesothelioma, including the paracentesis, should be carried out with great precaution and they recommend that paracentesis or laparoscopic surgery should be carried out along the midline of the abdominal wall, allowing the port site and the needle tract to be excised as part of the cytoreductive surgery.

4. Conclusion

Well-Differentiated Papillary Mesothelioma is an entity rarely observed and difficult to diagnose. Laparoscopy with biopsy under direct vision is an accurate and safe technique to confirm the diagnostic.

5. Acknowledgment

We acknowledge Fritz Dorries for his expert assistance in the preparation of the manuscript.

6. References

[1] Legha SS, Muggia FM.(1977). Pleural mesothelioma: clinical features and therapeutic implications. *Annals of Internal Medicine,* Vol.87, No.5, (November 1977), pp.613-21, ISSN 0003-4819.

[2] Asensio JA, Goldblatt P, Thomford NR.(1990). Primary malignant peritoneal mesothelioma. A report of seven cases and a review of the literature. *Archives of Surgery,* Vol.125, No.11, (November 1990),pp. 1477-81. ISSN 0004-0010.

[3] Reuter K, Raptopoulos V, Reale F, Krolikowski FJ, D'Orsi CJ, Graham S, Smith EH. (1983). Diagnosis of peritoneal mesothelioma: computed tomography, sonography, and fine-needle aspiration biopsy. *American Journal of Roentgenology,* Vol.140, No.6, (June 1983),pp.1189-94. ISSN 1546-3141.

[4] Bridda A, Padoan I, Mencarelli R, Frego M. (2007). Peritoneal Mesothelioma: A Review. *Medscape General Medicine,* Vol.9, No.2, (May 2007),pp.32. ISSN 1531-0132.

[5] Kass EM.(1996). Pathology of Peritoneal Mesothelioma. Pathology of Peritoneal Mesothelioma. *Cancer Treatment and Research,* Vol.81, pp.213-225. ISSN 0927-3042.

[6] Butnor K, Sporn TA, Hammar SP, Roggli VL.(2001). Well-Differentiated Papillary Mesothelioma. *The American Journal of Surgical Pathology,* Vol.25, No.10, (October 2001), pp.1304-1309. ISSN 1532-0979.

[7] Daya D, McCaughey WT. (1991). Pathology of the peritoneum: A review of select topics. *Seminars in Diagnostic Pathology,* Vol. 8, No.4, (November 1991), pp.277-89. ISSN 0740-2570.

[8] Daya D, McCaughey WT. (1990). Well-differentiated papillary mesothelioma of the peritoneum: a clinicopathologic study of 22 cases. *Cancer,* Vol.65, No.2, (January 1990), pp.292-296. ISSN 1097-0142.

[9] Goldblum J, Hart WR. (1995). Localized and Diffuse Mesothelioma of the genital tract and peritoneum in women: a clinicopathologic study of nineteen true mesothelial neoplasm other than adenomatoid tumors, multicystic mesothelioma and localized fibrous tumors. *The American Journal of Surgical,* Vol.19, No.10, (October 1995), pp. 1124-37. ISSN 1532-0979

[10] Hoekman K, Tognon G, Risse EKJ. (1996). Well-differentiated papillary mesothelioma of the peritoneum a separate entity. *European Journal of Cancer,* Vol.32A, No.2, (February 1996), pp.355-8. ISSN 1879-0852

[11] McCoughey WTE. (1985). Papillary Peritoneal Neoplasm in Females. *Pathology Annual,* Vol.20, (1985), pp.387-404. ISSN 0079-0184

[12] Roggli VL, Kolbeck J, SanFilippo F. (1987). Pathology of Human Mesothelioma: etiologic and diagnostic considerations. *Pathology Annual*, Vol.22, (1987), pp.91-131. ISSN 0079-0184

[13] Min-Jung KI, Moon EJ, Park YJ, Roh JW, Park YS, Park SY, Kim HS, Sim JS, Park SY. (2001). A Case of well-differentiated Papillary Mesothelioma developing malignant mesothelioma with seeding mass on the trocar insertion site of diagnostic laparoscopy and malignant change. *Cancer Research and Treatment*, Vol 33, No.4, (January 2001), pp. 357-361. ISSN 2005-9256.

[14] Foyle A, Al-Jabi M, McCaughey WT. (1985). Papillary Peritoneal Tumors in Women. *The American Journal of Surgical Pathology*, Vol.5, No.3, (April 1985), pp.241-9. ISSN 1532-0979

[15] Goepel JR. Benign Papillary Mesothelioma of Peritoneum: A Histological, Histochemical and Ultrastructural Study of Six Cases. *Histopathology*, Vol.5, No.1, (January 1981), pp.21-30. ISSN 1365-2559

[16] Hollinger P, Gaeng D. (1997). Simultaneous bilateral spontaneous pneumothorax in a patients with peritoneal and pleural papillary mesothelioma. *Respiration; International Review of Thoracic Diseases*, Vol.64, No.3, (1997), pp.233-5. ISSN 1423-0356

[17] Hejmadi R, Ganesan R, Kamal NG. (2003). Malignant transformation of a well-differentiated peritoneal papillary mesothelioma. *Acta Cytologica*, Vol.47,No.3,(May-June 2003).pp.517-8. ISSN 1938-2650

[18] Burrig KF, Pfitzer P, Hort W.(1990). Well-differentiated papillary mesothelioma. Report of two cases and review of literature. *Virchows Archiv. A, Pathological anatomy and histopathology*. Vol. 417, No.5, (1990), pp. 443-7, ISSN 0174-7398

[19] Lovell FA, Cranston PE. (1990). Well-Differentiated Papillary Mesothelioma of the Peritoneum. *American Journal of Roentgenology*, Vol.155, No.6, (December 1990), pp.1245-1246. ISSN 1546-3141

[20] Meister T, Birkfellner T, Poremba C, Becker JC, Menzel J, Domschke W, Lerch MM. (2003). Papillary Mesothelioma of the Peritoneum in the absence of asbestos exposure. *Zeitschrift für Gastroenterologie*, Vol.41, No.4, (April 2003), pp.329-32. ISSN 1439-7803

[21] Porpora MG, Bracato V, D´Elia C, Natilli M, Alo PL, Cosmi EV. (2002). Laparoscopic Diagnosis and Treatment of Well Differentiated Papillary mesothelioma of the Peritoneum. *The Journal of the American Association of Gynecologic Laparoscopists*, Vol.9, No. 3, (August 2002), pp.384-8. ISSN 1074-3804

[22] Averbach AM, Sugarbaker PM. (1996). Peritoneal Mesothelioma Treatment approach based on natural history. *Cancer Treatment and Research*, Vol.81, (1996), pp.193-211. ISSN 0927-3042

[23] Jang HS, Kim SR, Ryu KYU, Kim JW, Cho SH. (2009). A Laparoscopy Diagnosis of Well-Differentiated Papillary Mesothelioma of the Peritoneum in a women with ascitis: A case report. *Journal Of Women`s Medicine*, Vol.2, No.2, (2009), pp.81-84. ISSN 2233-6222

[24] Sugarbaker PH, Acherman YIZ, González-Moreno S, Ortega-Pérez G, Stuart OA, Marchettini P, You Di. (2002). Diagnosis and Treatment of Peritoneal Mesothelioma: The Washington Cancer Institute Experience. *Seminars in Oncology*, Vol 29, No.1, (February 2002), pp.51-61. ISSN 1532-8708

[25] Welch LS, Acherman YIZ, Haile E, Sokas Rk, Sugarbaker PH. (2005). Asbestos and Peritoenal Mesothelioma among college-educated men. *International Journal of Occupational and Environmental Health*, Vol.11, No.3, (July-September 2005) pp.254-258. ISSN 1077-3525
[26] Acherman YIZ, Welch LS, Branley CM, Sugarbaker PH. (2003). Clinical presentation of peritoneal mesothelioma. *Tumori*, Vol.89, No.3, (May-Jun 2003), pp.269-273, ISSN 2038-2529
[27] Tanimu S, Centeno B, Klapman J. (2009). Diagnosis of Malignant Peritoneal Mesothelioma by Rectal Endoscopic Ultrasound with Fine-needle Aspiration. *Gastroenterology & Hepatology*, Vol.5, No.2, (February 2009), pp.142-145. ISSN 1440-1746.
[28] Gong Y, Ren R, Ordóñez NG, Sun X, Sneige N. (2005). Fine needle aspirations cytology of Well-Differentiated Papillary Mesothelioma: A case Report. *Acta Cytologica*, Vol.49, No.5, (September-October 2005), pp.537-42. ISSN 1938-2650
[29] Aramburu JA, Nájera L, Rodríguez JM.(2005) Hallazgos citomorfológicos del mesotelioma papilar bien diferenciado. A propósito de un caso y revisión de la Literatura. *Revista Española de Patología*, Vol. 38, No.3, (2005), pp.172-175. ISSN 1988-561X
[30] Hassan R, Alexander R, Antman K, Boffetta P, Churg A, Coit D, Hausner P, Kennedy R, Kindler H, Metintas M, Mutti L, Onda M, Pass H, Premkumar A, Roggli V, Sterman D, Sugarbaker P, Taub R, Verschraegen C. (2006). Current treatment options and biology of peritoneal mesothelioma: meeting summary of the first NIH peritoneal mesothelioma conference. *Annals of Oncology*, Vol.17, (April 2006),pp. 1615-1619. ISSN 1569-8041
[31] Eslami B, Lutcher CL. (1974). Ante Morten Diagnosis in Two Cases of Malignant Peritoneal mesothelioma. *The American Journal of the Medical Sciences*, Vol.267, No.2, (February 1974), pp. 117-121. ISSN 1538-2990
[32] McCallum RW, Maceri DR, Jensen D, Berci J. (1979). Laparoscopic Diagnosis of peritoneal Mesothelioma. Report of a Case and Review of the Diagnostic Approach. *Digestive Disease and Sciences*, Vol. 24, No.2, (February 1979), pp. 170-174. ISSN 1573-2568
[33] Milingos S, Protopapas A, Papadimitriou C, Rodolakis A, Kallipolitis G, Skartados N, Markaki S, Dimopoulous MA, Antsaklis A. (2007). Laparoscopy in the evaluation of women with unexplained ascites: an invaluable diagnostic tool. *Journal of Minimally Invasive Gynecology*, Vol. 14, No.1, (Jan-Feb 2007), pp. 43-48. ISSN 1553-4669
[34] Van de Walle P, Blomne Y, Van Outryve L. (2004). Laparoscopy and primary diffuse malignant peritoneal mesothelioma: a diagnostics challenge. *Acta Chirurgica Belgica*, Vol. 104, No.1, (Feb 2004), pp. 114-7. ISSN 0001-5458
[35] Stamat JC, Chekan EG, Ali A, Ko A, Sporn TA, Eubanks WS. (1999). *Laparoscopy and mesothelioma. Journal of laparoendoscopic & advanced surgical techniques. Part A*, Vol. 9, No.5, (October 1999),pp. 443-7. ISSN 1557-9034
[36] Estrada-Saiz RV, Loscos JM, García-Paredes J, Del Pozo A, Estrada V. (1995). The role of laparoscopy in the diagnosis of primary peritonealmesothelioma. *Revista Española de Enfermedades Digestivas*, Vol.87, No.5, (May 1995), pp.403-6. ISSN 1130-0108

[37] Chu CM, Lin SM, Peng SM, Wu CS, Liaw YF. (1994). The role of laparoscopy in the evaluation of ascites of unknown origin. *Gastrointestinal Endoscopy*, Vol. 40, No.3, (May 1994), pp.285-9. ISSN 1097-6779

[38] Muensterer OJ, Averbach AM, Jacquet P, Otero SE, Sugarbaker PH. (1997). Malignant peritoneal mesothelioma. Case-report demonstrating pitfalls of diagnostic laparoscopy. *International Surgery*,Vol.82, No.3, (Jul-Sep 1997), pp.240-3. ISSN 0020-8868

[39] Yoon YJ, Ahn SH, Park JY, Chon CY, Kim Do Y, Park YN, Han KH. (2007). What is the role of diagnostic laparoscopy in a gastroenterology Unit? *Journal of Gastroenterology*, Vol.33, No.5, (November 2007), pp.633-638, ISSN 1435-5922

[40] Piccigallo E, Jeffers LJ, Reddy Kr, Caldironi MW, Parenti A, Schiff ER. (1988). Malignant Peritoneal Mesothelioma. A clinical and Laparoscopic Study of ten cases. *Digestive Diseases And Sciences*, Vol. 33, No.5, (May 1988), pp. 633-638, ISSN 1573-2568

[41] Aponte-Rueda ME, Nieves M. (2009). Mesotelioma Papilar Bien Diferenciado. *Revista Venezolana de Oncología*, Vol.21, No.4, (2009), pp.229-236, ISSN 0798-0582

[42] Conlon K, Rusch V, Gillern S.(1996). Laparoscopy: An Important Tool in the Staging of Malignant Pleural Mesothelioma. *Annals of Surgical Oncology*, Vol.3, No.5, (September 1996), pp.489-494, ISSN 1534-4681

[43] Shukunami K, Hirabuki S, Kaneshima M, Kamitani N, Kotsuji F.(2000). Well-Differentiated Papillary Mesothelioma involving the peritoneal and pleural cavities: successful treatment by local and systemic administration of carboplatin. *Tumori*, Vol.86, No.5, (September-Octuber 2000) pp.419-2. ISSN 2038-2529

[44] Nezhat FR, DeNoble Shaghayegh M, Brown DN, Shamshirsaz Amir, Hoehn D. (2010). Laparoscopic Management of Peritoneal Mesohelioma associated with pelvic endometriosis. *The Journal of Minimally Invasive Gynecology*, Vol 17. No.5, (September-October 2010), pp.646-650, ISSN 1553-4669

[45] Hasson HM. (1971). A modified instrument and method for laparoscopy. *American Journal of Obstetrics and Gynecology*, Vol.110, No.6, (July 1971), pp.886-7. ISSN 1097-6868

[46] Henning H, Lightdale CJ, Look D. (1994). Color Atlas of Diagnostic Laparoscopy, G. Thieme Verlag, ISBN 9780865772892, Stuttgart, Germany.

[47] Suárez-Grau JM, Rubio C, García JL, Martín JA, Socas M, Álamo JM, López F, Cadet H, Bustos M, Tutosaus JD, Morales S. (2007). Presentación atípica de tuberculosis peritoneal. Caso clínico diagnosticado por laparoscopia. *Revista Española de Enfermedades Digestivas*, Vol. 99, No.12, (2007), pp.725-728, ISSN 1130-0108.

[48] Roskos M, Popp MB. (1999). Laparoscopic Diagnosis and Management of Malignant Ascites. *Surgical Laparoscopy, Endoscopy & Percutaneous Techniques*, Vol. 9, No.5, (October 1999), pp.365-368, ISSN 1534-4908

[49] Carmignani CP, Sugarbaker PH. (2004). Regional lymph node metastases from port site implants after laparoscopic surgery. *Surgical Endoscopy*, Vol. 18, No.12, (December 2004), pp.1818, ISSN 1432-2218